DATE DUE

OCT - 1 1997	
OCT 17 1997	
FEB 2 5 1998	
OCT - 5 1998	
JAN 1 8 1999	
APR 1 7 1999	
OCT 1 5 1999	
OCT - 6 2000	
JUL 2 3 2001	

The Making of a Social Disease

Tuberculosis in Nineteenth-Century France

David S. Barnes

UNIVERSITY OF CALIFORNIA PRESS
Berkeley · Los Angeles · London

University of California Press
Berkeley and Los Angeles, California

University of California Press
London, England

Copyright © 1995 by The Regents of the University of California

Library of Congress Cataloging-in-Publication Data

Barnes, David S.
    The making of a social disease : tuberculosis in nineteenth-
century France / David S. Barnes
        p.   cm.
        ®
    Includes bibliographical references and index.
    ISBN 0-520-08772-0 (cloth : alk. paper)
    1. Tuberculosis—France—History—19th century.   I. Title
    [DNLM: 1. Tuberculosis—history—France.   2. History of Medicine,
19th Cent.—France.   3. Disease Outbreaks—history—France.
4. Socioeconomic Factors.   WF 11 GF7 B2m 1995]
RC316.F8B37   1995
614.5'42'094409034—dc20
DNLM/DLC
for Library of Congress   94-15230
                                                                                CIP

Printed in the United States of America

1 2 3 4 5 6 7 8 9

The paper used in this publication meets the minimum requirements of American National Standard for Information Sciences—Permanence of Paper for Printed Library Materials. ANSI Z39.48-1984 ♾

To my parents,
Richard and Helena Barnes,
and to the memory of my grandmother,
Helena Borcic,
and my great-grandmother,
Rose Stepanek

Contents

Acknowledgments

The research for this project was funded in part by the French government's Chateaubriand fellowship program and the Lurcy Charitable Trust. Dissertation writing support was provided by the Mellon Fellowships in the Humanities. In France, many people went out of their way to help me in my efforts to track down and make sense of my sources. Jean Legoy, Philippe Manneville, and Didier Nourrisson in Le Havre helped me understand what makes that city so fascinating for historical study and guided me in situating tuberculosis within a local social and political context. Colette Chambelland and Françoise Blum of the Musée social in Paris helped me find many elusive and invaluable materials. Jérôme Renaud of the Service des Archives, Assistance publique de Paris, graciously facilitated access to hospital records and other holdings. My research benefited from many helpful strategic discussions with, among others, Patrick Fridenson, Alain Corbin, Olivier Faure, Pierre Guillaume, Bernard-Pierre Lécuyer, Alain Cottereau, Lion Murard, and Patrick Zylberman. Allan Mitchell was generous with source material and drafts of his own work and cordially agreed to disagree with me on certain matters of interpretation. Annie Lenhart provided moral support and vital French newspaper clippings.

Back in the Bay Area, a number of discussion groups and the cooperative atmosphere fostered by the History Department of the University of California, Berkeley, provided a friendly and comfortable academic environment in which to write and discuss the dissertation from which this book developed. From the very earliest stages of this project, Catherine Kudlick has been an acute reader and supportive critic of countless drafts. She has also been my mentor in the history of disease and a trusted friend, and I owe her more than the devoted thanks I can express here. Denise Herd of the School of Public Health contributed her expertise to this project as a member of my dissertation committee, as did Thomas Laqueur, who cheerfully challenged me with his eclectic and imaginative sense of the history of the human body. Reggie Zelnik offered sage advice and gave freely of his time from the beginning.

Tim Lennon and Lisa Schiff generously gave me thorough readings and helpful comments on the dissertation version of this study. I owe many thanks to Neil Leonard for his editorial and strategic advice over the years. Deirdre O'Reilly and Elizabeth Aife Murray gave immeasurable assistance during the preparation of the manuscript, and Stuart Kogod of RayKo Photo Center in San Francisco did yeoman's service on the illustrations. I am grateful to my sisters, Elizabeth Barnes and Ann Deschamps, and the Batistas, Roy, Kathy, Peggy, Matthew, and Marc, for their support. I would also like to thank Mary Jo Savage and the Rev. James Kolp for their insights concerning Saint Thérèse of Lisieux.

Guenter Risse and Jack Pressman, my colleagues in the History of Health Sciences Department at the University of California, San Francisco, have greatly enlarged my view of the history of medicine and have never failed to engage me in fruitful discussion and debate. Jack also volunteered extensive advice on graphing and computing. The members of the Berkeley–San Francisco History, Medicine, and Culture group (affectionately and irreverently known as the "Med-Heads") were repeatedly exposed to tuberculosis; Lisa Cody, Caroline Acker, and Robert Martensen were particularly helpful. The meetings of the Northern California French History group also brought kindred spirits together for serious yet convivial historiographical discussion. In this latter group, I am especially grateful to Lou Roberts, Gabrielle Hecht, and Tyler Stovall for their insightful critiques and suggestions.

For the participants in the illustrious French History dissertation group at Berkeley, the long and arduous process of dissertation writing is truly a collective enterprise. Countless evenings of fine food, drink, and scholarly exchange at the Barrows household—always enlivened by the wise and stylish Alexandra Barrows—punctuated our hard work with critical analysis, solidarity, and even occasional joy. I am grateful to Marjorie Beale; Joshua Cole, Sarah Farmer, Megan Koreman, Doug

Mackaman, Jeff Ravel, Vanessa Schwartz, Matt Truesdell, Jeffrey Verhey, and Tami Whited. I owe special thanks to Ian Burney, Nicoletta Gullace, Regina Sweeney, and Sylvia Schafer, who helped me survive graduate school with their intellectual companionship and friendship.

I first glimpsed the joys of studying history through the teaching of John Merriman. Bon vivant, raconteur, and archive connoisseur of world renown, he breathes life into the subject matter of French history as few other historians can. William Cronon's analytical rigor, mastery of style, and devotion to teaching taught me a great deal about the craft of history. The opportunity to work with these two historians as an undergraduate first instilled in me the desire to become one myself.

In a profound way, my work bears the imprint of Susanna Barrows. I could not dream of a more inspiring and dedicated mentor. Her love of history and her ability to evoke its human dimension, both comic and tragic, serve as a model for all of her students. When she first suggested tuberculosis to me as a research topic, I recall thinking that with background in neither medicine nor opera, I was ill equipped for (and little interested in) the task. She knew better. Over the years, her advice has been demanding, surprising, constructive, counterintuitive, and unfailingly on target.

My parents have encouraged me at every step of my academic career. Their love of France is more contagious than any disease, and I caught it at an early age; for that alone I am eternally grateful. They have lived the historian's life vicariously through me, housed me under their roof at various times on both sides of the Atlantic during my research, and provided critical readings of my chapter drafts along the way; they have been instrumental in seeing this project through to fruition. This book is dedicated to them and to the memory of my grandmother and my great-grandmother, who between them taught me to read and taught me to love learning. Finally, I owe a constant and profound debt of gratitude to Joan Batista, teacher, confidante, partner. She has put up with endless talk of germ theory and syndicalism, accompanied me—if not to the ends of the earth—as far as Lisieux and Le Havre, and made setbacks tolerable and good times better. It is both true and inadequate to say that my work and my life are richer because of her.

Chronology

Tuberculosis in France, 1819–1919

1819	First edition of René-Théophile-Hyacinthe Laënnec's *Traité de l'auscultation médiate* published
1829	*Annales d'hygiène publique et de médecine légale,* France's first journal of public health, founded
1830	Louis-René Villermé's study of differential mortality in Parisian neighborhoods published in *Annales d'hygiène publique*
1865	Jean-Antoine Villemin demonstrates transmissibility of tuberculosis in laboratory
1867–1868	Academy of Medicine debates contagiousness of tuberculosis
1870–1871	Franco-Prussian War, Prussian siege of Paris, Paris Commune
1879	Inauguration of municipal health department and casier sanitaire des maisons in Le Havre
1882	Robert Koch isolates and identifies tubercle bacillus, causal agent of tuberculosis
1894	Casier sanitaire des maisons begins operation in Paris
1894–1897	First major revolutionary syndicalist writings on tuberculosis published by Fernand Pelloutier and by the

	Groupe des étudiants socialistes révolutionnaires internationalistes
1898	Academy of Medicine report "On the Prophylaxis of Tuberculosis," first major manifesto of mainstream War on Tuberculosis, delivered by Joseph Grancher
1899	First government-appointed commission on tuberculosis convened
1901	Lionel Amodru reports to parliament on necessary measures to halt spread of tuberculosis
	"Permanent" commission on tuberculosis established under Ministry of Interior
	First antituberculosis dispensary opened in Lille under direction of Albert Calmette
1902	Public health law passed, mandating creation of municipal health departments in large cities
1904	Revolutionary syndicalist Marc Pierrot's lengthy series, "The War on Tuberculosis," published in *Les Temps nouveaux*
1905	International Tuberculosis Congress meets in Paris
1906	Revolutionary syndicalist campaign for eight-hour day culminates in strikes and protests beginning May 1
1914–1918	World War I
1916	Léon Bourgeois law passed, providing for widespread establishment of antituberculosis dispensaries
1919	André Honnorat law passed, providing for widespread establishment of sanatoriums

Introduction

Tuberculosis is back. In most developed nations, a steady decline throughout most of the twentieth century reversed itself beginning in the mid-1980s, and cases of the disease have increased ever since. New bacterial strains resistant to various antituberculosis drugs have caused considerable alarm in major cities, where tuberculosis is often associated with AIDS, drug abuse, homelessness, and poverty. Meanwhile, in less developed countries, where tuberculosis never left the scene, it continues apace. Experts offer dire warnings of "the greatest health disaster since the bubonic plague"[1]; World Health Organization officials estimate that three million people worldwide die of tuberculosis every year and that fully one-third of the world's population is infected with the tubercle bacillus.[2] The increased incidence has been paralleled by increased public attention, as each week brings new press reports of epidemiological studies and antituberculosis strategies.

France is no exception; recently, legislation has been introduced to revive that country's antituberculosis dispensaries. Recourse to such an old-fashioned institution, thought by most to be "outmoded,"[3] suggests that the latest biomedical techniques can neither explain nor solve the problem of chronic illness in society. Indeed, the story of tuberculosis in France provides a revealing glimpse into the history of this problem. Or perhaps *stories* of tuberculosis would be more accurate. Cauldron of wealth and poverty, reform and revolution, social anxiety and scientific hubris, nineteenth-century France was the stage for several parallel dramas in which tuberculosis played key roles. French medicine, struggling to maintain its international preeminence, contributed crucial discoveries regarding the nature of the disease and oversaw the birth of germ theory. Intensifying worry over France's low birthrate and stagnating population contributed to increased concern over the nation's leading cause of death. Industrialization and urbanization radically altered the rhythms and material conditions of life. An ambitious, nationalistic bourgeoisie largely committed to economic liberalism finally assumed political power and debated how best to hold onto it. Meanwhile, a disastrous war with Prussia and the threat of class warfare made all of these issues more pressing during the early decades of the Third Republic. These and other stories will serve as the backdrop for this examination of tuberculosis as a social problem.

The comeback of tuberculosis confounds the familiar history of medicine's incremental advances and triumphs. More than a century after the bacterial agent of tuberculosis was discovered and nearly half a century after the advent of effective antibiotic treatments, some very old questions are being asked about the disease, including, what is it about society that facilitates the spread of tuberculosis, and what can be done about it? These same questions were being asked with great urgency a century ago, and despite the vast technological and scientific changes of the intervening years, the answers most commonly proposed today bear a striking resemblance to the answers of the past. They range from a reliance on greater governmental intervention in public health matters (such as heightened surveillance by local authorities of those infected or "at risk") to forced isolation of active cases.[4] A few scattered voices target poverty as the chief cause of tuberculosis and call for improvements in standards of living as the only means of effectively combating the disease.[5] The questions and the answers seem to be preserved intact from the first time tuberculosis emerged as a major social problem in many countries in the nineteenth century.

Meanwhile, since the mid-1980s, the AIDS crisis has forced increasingly technocratic, medicalized, welfare-state societies to confront the basic question of how and why a culture assigns particular meanings—especially moral meanings—to disease. Scientific knowledge, it has become clear, does not provide a single and exclusive "truth" about health and disease, and the clash of conflicting truths can be as traumatic (in a cultural sense) as any epidemic.[6] Although they certainly do not impose a definitive reading on the past, present-day struggles to address the social meaning of AIDS and tuberculosis add relevance and urgency to an examination of the history of such efforts. Before considering the factors that came to bear on the understanding of tuberculosis in the unique circumstances of nineteenth-century France, it is worth briefly discussing the basic characteristics of that elusive pathological entity—characteristics that, if not timeless or absolute, at least correspond to the current consensus in medical science.

Tuberculosis is a contagious disease. That simple fact is both indisputable and misleading. The causal agent of tuberculosis—variously known as the Koch bacillus (after Robert Koch, the German bacteriologist who first identified it in 1882), the tubercle bacillus, and *Mycobacterium tuberculosis*—is a bacterium transmitted from person to person most often through inhalation of "aerosolized" sputum droplets expelled through coughing. In the majority of cases, the infection is localized as a lesion in the respiratory tract and contained by immune reactions, never producing symptoms of illness (although it does, for example, cause a positive reaction to a skin test). When resistance is compromised for any reason, at the time of infection or at any subsequent time, the bacilli can spread and attack the body's tissue. This "active" or "open" tuberculosis occurs most often in the lungs but can also affect the lymphatic glands (scrofula), bones, intestines, brain, liver, kidneys, and other organs. Nonpulmonary forms of tuberculosis can also be acquired by ingesting milk or meat from infected cows. This form of transmission was the object of a certain amount of concern in the nineteenth century, before widespread pasteurization of milk and regulation of meat supplies, but it was always perceived as a minor danger compared to inhalation.[7] (Pulmonary tuberculosis is by far the most common form of the disease. Both in the nineteenth-century sources and in these pages, the word "tuberculosis" indicates primarily the pulmonary localization, although in prophylaxis, as opposed to diagnosis or treatment, there was often little practical distinction to be made among the various forms.)

The recent resurgence of tuberculosis in the United States and other industrialized countries has taken place among certain clearly identifiable communities and "risk groups": homeless people, drug addicts, prison inmates, poor immigrants, migrant farm workers, the elderly, and people with HIV infection and AIDS.[8] All of these groups share one common trait: immunodeficiency, the central element in the acronyms "HIV" and "AIDS." Most of them share another closely related trait: poverty, with all of its concomitant physical effects. This present-day epidemiology, so divergent at first glance from the observed and reported incidence of tuberculosis in nineteenth-century societies, may at least provide some questions (if not answers) with which to address the historical dimension of tuberculosis.

In both present and past societies in which tuberculosis is prevalent, far more people are infected with (that is, exposed to) the bacillus than ever experience symptoms. A still smaller subset of the population dies of the disease. Even at the historical peaks of the disease's incidence, the seemingly vast numbers of deaths from tuberculosis each year represented just a fraction of those infected. Indeed, it is possible that a near-totality of the population of many large European cities in the nineteenth century technically "had" tuberculosis—that is, would have tested positive for exposure to the tubercle bacillus.[9] It is widely believed today that in the United States, only 10 percent of those infected with the disease ever develop active or "symptomatic" tuberculosis; in other words, even those who test positive for exposure (and therefore have *Mycobacterium tuberculosis* in their bodies) have only a one-in-ten chance of ever "getting" tuberculosis (becoming ill). This ratio is a widely quoted rule of thumb,[10] although there is evidence that this "risk of disease" (as opposed to "risk of infection") varies considerably and is often much lower than 10 percent. Detailed long-term studies of certain populations have shown (1) that the risk of disease among those infected with tuberculosis drops off considerably after the first one to two years, and (2) that even as long as ten years following infection, the risk of developing active disease is often considerably less than one in ten, with rates varying between 0.6 and 3.7 percent in U.S. studies and reaching as high as 9.4 percent in others.[11]

It is impossible to know whether these proportions hold true for other geographic and historical contexts; yet even if the precise figures differ, there is reason to suppose that in many industrial cities a century ago, nearly the entire population was infected with tuberculosis.[12] In late-nineteenth-century Le Havre and Paris, when the disease was at its deadliest and accounted for one-fifth to one-fourth of all deaths, it killed only a fraction of those infected. It follows, therefore, that all or nearly all of those cities' residents were infected with the tubercle bacillus by the time they reached adulthood. Most people lived their entire lives without any inkling of their infection. Exposure does not equal illness. However, any circumstance that compromises the body's resistance by depressing immune reaction can cause latent tuberculosis infections to reactivate, no matter how long ago the original exposure took place. Today, such circumstances range from malnutrition, drug abuse, and alcoholism to cancer (especially following chemotherapy) and AIDS.[13]

It is certain that similar immunosuppressive factors were at work in nineteenth-century France. Particularly among the working classes, where tuberculosis claimed most of its victims, the obstacles to maintaining a decent standard of living were formidable. The influence of any individual factor on the incidence of tuberculosis at the time is impossible to determine. It is not the aim of this book to develop a retrospective epidemiology of tuberculosis in nineteenth-century France, even if such a project were feasible. The primary sources for such an endeavor—even statistical reports and surveys—are so thoroughly imbued with the categories, preconceptions, and concerns of the time that to wrench them from this context would rob them of all meaning. Even to condemn them as "biased" would be to suggest misleadingly that they could have been otherwise. Juxtaposing the medical and public health texts of the nineteenth century with present-day judgments regarding the true causes or incidence of disease borders on reproaching the doctors and authorities of the time for not knowing then what is known now, an enterprise of little historiographical value. It is quite another matter, however, to examine orthodox or mainstream knowledge in light of conflicting views that were being expressed on the same issues at the same time. This book undertakes to trace what was known about tuberculosis in the nineteenth century, the conditions under which that knowledge was produced, and how it was used.

A recent historiographical controversy has resuscitated the question of the "true" causes of tuberculosis in the nineteenth century. This debate illustrates the difficulties and uncertainties inherent in historical epidemiology as well as the implications of such scholarly questions for present-day tuberculosis control efforts. The exhaustive and pioneering work of Thomas McKeown in Britain had over several decades—in the view of most historians—established that the decline of tuberculosis and other infectious diseases in the industrial world was largely a result of rising standards of living rather than medical advances or state intervention in matters of public health.[14] This revisionist thesis opened up new horizons of scholarly inquiry, but it also stepped on some toes. In the past few years, a strong backlash against McKeown has emerged. A series of articles has attacked the standard-of-living thesis and argued that the real reasons for the decline of tuberculosis in France, Britain, and the United States can be found in government sanitary reforms and in the isolation of those suffering from the disease.[15]

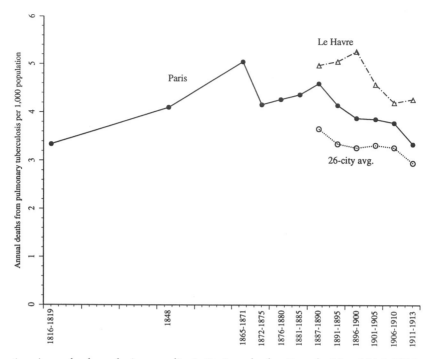

1.   Annual tuberculosis mortality in Paris and other French cities, 1816–1913.

Allan Mitchell, an expert in the history of France's relations with and attitudes toward Germany, has contended that the public powers' inaction in the face of tuberculosis explains France's relatively high death rate from the disease around the turn of the century. France lagged behind, the argument goes, while its neighbors in Britain and Germany pursued concerted campaigns to improve public health. Therefore, tuberculosis rates declined in both of the latter countries—but not in France—during the decades leading up to World War I.[16] Actually, the experience of the three major western European powers at the close of the nineteenth century can be read quite differently. The available evidence, in fact, clearly indicates (1) that tuberculosis mortality was declining in France, albeit more slowly than in Britain and Germany, and (2) that France's higher death rate and slower decline in tuberculosis corresponded to a standard of living that was lower and improving more slowly than that of the other two countries.[17]

It is difficult to establish with any certainty the curve of tuberculosis mortality over the course of the nineteenth century in France. Nation-wide statistics were not kept on such matters until after the First World

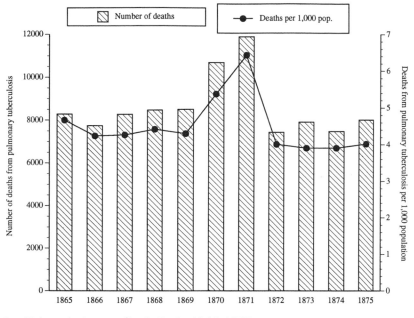

2. Tuberculosis mortality in Paris, 1865–1875.

War; even for large cities, the figures date back only as far as 1887. However, Paris was under a microscope for most of the century, and the occasional publication of tuberculosis death rates for the capital begins in 1816. Calculating per capita and combining the early Paris numbers with the later figures for all of urban France, it is possible to approximate the direction, if not the overall magnitude, of the disease's incidence.

According to this method, tuberculosis increased gradually in France until its peak in the late 1880s and early 1890s, whereupon it decreased, also gradually, through most of the twentieth century. Figure 1 depicts tuberculosis mortality for Paris over the entire nineteenth century, alongside Le Havre (France's tuberculosis leader) and an aggregate of the twenty-six largest French cities for the Belle Epoque, averaged out over census periods to give a more reliable long-term picture.[18] Figures 2 and 3 focus on periods of particular interest. One apparent anomaly is a dramatic increase in Paris in 1870 and 1871, during the Franco-Prussian War and the subsequent siege of Paris; figure 2, with annual figures not averaged out over census intervals, shows its magnitude and suddenness. Figure 3, also showing year-by-year changes, suggests that although statistics for cities other than Paris were kept only beginning

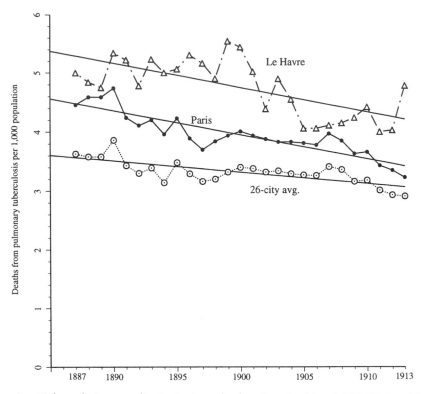

3. Tuberculosis mortality in Paris and other French cities, 1887–1913, with lines showing closest-fitting equations for long-term trends.

in 1887, the overall peak of tuberculosis mortality in urban France may have come around 1890, give or take five years; outside of 1870–1871, the long-term experience of Paris bears this out. The decline of tuberculosis was long and gradual; by the time vaccination and effective medication were made widely available in the 1950s, most of the historical decline in the industrialized nations had already occurred.[19]

A closer look at the sudden surge of tuberculosis mortality during the Franco-Prussian War and siege may also shed some light on the McKeown debate. After averaging 8,250 deaths per year from pulmonary tuberculosis between 1865 and 1869, Paris suddenly saw this figure balloon to 10,691 in 1870 and 11,900 in 1871 before falling back to a mere 7,436 in 1872. The per capita tuberculosis mortality rose from a prewar average of 4.38 per thousand per year to 5.38 and 6.44 before settling back to 4.01 in 1872—a nearly 50 percent rise within two years, followed by a decline just as precipitous in a single year.[20]

Such drastic yearly fluctuations in tuberculosis death rates were unknown in France both before and after this episode; there is only one
plausible explanation for this sudden rise and fall. The overriding facts
of material life in Paris during the siege of 1870–1871 were the Prussian
blockade and the ensuing food shortage. Only the severe hunger and
impoverishment that resulted can conceivably explain the sudden rise
(and equally sudden fall) in tuberculosis mortality in these years. Likewise, on a less dramatic scale, the early Third Republic as a whole appears to have been a time of slowly but noticeably improving standards
of living in France. For example, the best estimate of real wage growth
(synthesizing the work of four respected economic historians) shows a
33 percent increase between 1882 and 1909—from wages in 1882 that
had only recently rebounded from levels far below that of 1824.[21]
Slowly but appreciably declining death rates from tuberculosis beginning in the early 1890s may be related to this trend.

Much more difficult to explain is the puzzling shift in sexual inequality where tuberculosis was concerned. In Paris, until around 1860, more
women than men died of the disease; thereafter, the differential was
reversed. Moreover, the proportions were significant: in the 1830s, for
example, nearly two-thirds more women than men succumbed to tuberculosis, whereas by 1890, it claimed almost two-thirds more men than
women.[22] For the later period, other French cities showed a sex differential similar to that of Paris. On the rare occasions when early-
nineteenth-century doctors and "hygienists"[23] referred to the overrepre-
sentation of women among victims of tuberculosis, they attributed it
variously to women's inherent weakness, to the constricting effect of
corsets on the chest, or to workplace conditions specific to certain predominantly female occupations.[24] Later, around the turn of the century,
authorities failed to point out that the sex differential had reversed itself,
but they did use the higher mortality among men to bolster the contention that alcoholism (thought to be a predominantly male affliction)
contributed to tuberculosis. (See chap. 5, below.)

Alain Cottereau, one of the few historians to point out this shift,
attributes it to two trends. Without citing any evidence, he claims that
improving conditions of childbirth lessened the susceptibility of women
to tuberculosis. Meanwhile, he argues, accelerating industrial capitalism, with its debilitating physical labor affecting a mostly male workforce, weakened the resistance of men to infection.[25] There may be validity in Cottereau's argument, as well as in the alcoholism thesis.
However, far more detailed research is needed before this significant

historical change can be satisfactorily explained by these or any other factors. Whatever the case, the sizable and changing sex differentials in tuberculosis mortality cannot be explained by the late-nineteenth-century emphasis on unsanitary housing and on exposure to the bacillus among the causes of the disease, since the sexes could not have been subject to these factors to an appreciably different extent.

Every attempt to single out *the* determinant factor or factors in the incidence of tuberculosis in the nineteenth century must inevitably run up against the only indisputable fact that emerges from all the available evidence: the lives of many tuberculosis victims were lived inside a constellation of social conditions that affected their overall well-being. These conditions included debilitating, draining labor; little or no job security; meager wages; poor diets; slum housing; filthy bodies and surroundings; and heavy drinking. It seems obvious in retrospect that these conditions were interrelated, even inseparable. Any attempt to extract from this constellation a single social cause of tuberculosis is doomed to failure, or at best to irrelevance, because it presupposes that one or more of these conditions could have operated independently of the others.

Most historians have chosen to avoid speculating on the "true" causes of tuberculosis, with Mitchell and Cottereau among the exceptions. By and large, however, even when they have averted such pitfalls, histories of tuberculosis—in France and elsewhere—have operated within an unfortunately narrow and limiting conceptual framework. The historiography has tended to downplay politics, ideology, and contestation, orienting itself instead toward medical triumphalism and consensus, with the romantic allure of "consumption" occasionally given attention as well. While these have become somewhat shopworn complaints among historians of medicine, and they no longer apply to much of the field, they unfortunately characterize much of the work on the history of tuberculosis in the past twenty years.[26] Especially for the period after the rise of germ theory, conflict and opposition within the medical profession regarding the causes and prevention of disease recede from the historiographical picture. This is regrettable and misleading; in fact, one can find a great deal of tumult, strife, and uncertainty in the archival and published sources relating to tuberculosis.

A recent spate of works has drawn increased scholarly attention to the history of tuberculosis. Since 1988, two books on Great Britain, three on the United States, one on France, and one covering both Europe and the United States have appeared, in addition to two others on France published in the mid-1980s—all specifically dealing with tuberculosis.[27] These works send mixed signals about the fate of the old triumph-and-consensus model. Pierre Guillaume's *Du désespoir au salut: Les tuberculeux aux 19e et 20e siècles* is a useful survey with some valuable insights. However, its title, *From Despair to Salvation,* sends a naively positivist message that simply does not correspond to the history of tuberculosis. Guillaume pays homage to the "intrepid practitioners" and "obstinate men of science" and "men and women of good will" who "led a . . . victorious combat" against the disease.[28] As noted above, to attribute the decline of tuberculosis to "men of science" is a dubious enterprise at best. Guillaume's book dwells at length on the existential suffering of the sanatorium patient in the twentieth century (and gives considerable attention to the romantic literary sensibility), while passing over the social dimension of the disease relatively quickly. One is left with the impression of an emotional and spiritual affliction, devoid of social or political significance.

Two students of Roland Barthes, Isabelle Grellet and Caroline Kruse, are also fascinated with the twentieth-century world of the sanatorium, but they reject medical triumphalism. Their *Histoires de la tuberculose: Les fièvres de l'âme* contains brilliant insights, particularly concerning the surveillance impulse in medical thought and the invisible power of multiple, intertwined stigmas woven around a disease. Grellet and Kruse proudly proclaim their method of mixing up genres within their source material, reading literary, medical, and autobiographical "discourses" "pell-mell."[29] Indeed, the range of material from which the authors coax information and interpretation is their strong suit. However, in their eagerness to transcend artificial intellectual barriers, they ignore the importance of the genres themselves. In the words of the historian Joan Scott, interdisciplinary analysis should "take seriously the boundaries of disciplines and the different genres they represent but make these a matter for investigation, rather than a set of preconditions for scholarly work."[30]

Alongside the continuing interest in the spiritual and literary significance of tuberculosis and the attempts to discover a true historical epidemiology, there seems to be a sustained effort to tell the empirical story of various societies' responses to the disease. For example, Linda Bryder's *Below the Magic Mountain* revives the debates and the politics behind medical treatment and state antituberculosis intervention in early-twentieth-century Britain. Similarly, several of the essays in *Peurs et terreurs face à la contagion,* a 1988 collection organized by the

French Society for Historical Demography, exemplify a critical and historically sensitive attitude toward the ostensibly neutral domain of medical knowledge. The essay by Dominique Dessertine and Olivier Faure
on sanatorium policy in the interwar years shows the degree to which
the "sanatorial network," instead of being a set of strictly therapeutic
institutions, involved elements of a repressive, carceral strategy. Didier
Nourrisson's contribution to the volume retraces the vagaries of the
official French dogma concerning alcoholism's role in tuberculosis during the years surrounding the First World War. His identification of the
interests at stake in national alcohol policy and the social imperatives
behind official orthodoxy testifies to both a critical temperament and a
careful attention to primary texts and subtexts.[31]

Perhaps the most exciting and promising trend in the historiography
of health and disease over the last fifteen years—a trend that has informed my approach to the history of tuberculosis—is best exemplified
by the work of William Coleman and Richard Evans. Both of these
historians have highlighted the myriad interrelationships—some obvious, some quite subtle—between political economy and public health
practices. Coleman's *Death Is a Social Disease* inserts the early-nineteenth-century hygienic investigations of Louis-René Villermé and his
colleagues into the context of liberalism and nascent socialism outside
of which they are incomprehensible. Coleman acutely depicts the dilemma in which Villermé, one of the pioneers in the study of public
health in France, found himself: compelled to point out appalling social
inequality but incapable of recommending remedial public action.
Evans's *Death in Hamburg* examines the 1892 cholera epidemic—and
indeed the material life of an entire city—against the backdrop of a
society dominated by a merchant elite dedicated to the principles of
laissez-faire.[32]

Many of the variables that governed society's understanding of and
response to tuberculosis were material ones. Yet there were also less
concrete forces at work, forces that operated through language and systems of thought and that deserve equal attention. Many scholars, inspired by the work of Michel Foucault and other theorists, have tried
to pry apart "discourses" and expose the politics behind "objective"
scientific knowledge. At its best, this effort remains attuned to empirical
and material modes of explanation as well. One exemplar of this approach, David Armstrong, has looked for the "political anatomy of the
body" in twentieth-century British public health policies. Among his
findings of particular relevance to this study is the "dispensary gaze," a

strategy of controlling space within the city by mapping the movement of pathology within it.[33] Ways of seeing combine with other material and ideological imperatives to constitute responses to disease. As Allan Brandt has put it, "Medicine is not just affected by social, economic, and political variables—it is embedded in them."[34] In a sense, this is both the premise and conclusion of all social history of medicine, including this book.

The "truth" about tuberculosis changed drastically in France over the course of the nineteenth century. Around 1820, during the Bourbon Restoration, consumption, or *phthisis,* was an individual, inscrutable, and all but random killer, probably hereditary and somehow related to passion. In the 1830s, under the July Monarchy, the disease was for the first time seen as socially discriminating, choosing its victims from certain professions and from poor neighborhoods. Beginning in the 1840s, being a consumptive woman signified in certain circles heightened sensibility and emotion as well as the redemptive power of suffering. From the late 1860s through the early 1880s, as the Third Republic established itself, the disease was possibly contagious. Around 1900, tuberculosis was a national scourge, highly contagious, lurking around every corner and symptomatic of moral decay. These successive truths, or stages of knowledge, about tuberculosis do not just show the developing *content* of medical science. They also reveal the changing social *context* within which that knowledge was embedded. It is the fit of content into context—and the changes that each wrought in the other—that will be examined here.

For a disease that throughout the nineteenth century was the leading cause of death in France, the chronology of official concern and mobilization is surprisingly limited. While the pace of medical work on the social aspects of tuberculosis accelerated after Jean-Antoine Villemin's 1865 experiments on transmissibility and again after Koch's 1882 identification of the tubercle bacillus, it was not until the late 1890s—after death rates from the disease had begun to *fall* in French cities—that governmental and philanthropic organizations began to mount what they called *la lutte contre la tuberculose.* (I have translated this as "the War on Tuberculosis," a proper noun, to suggest the extent to which it was referred to as a formal institution or event, regardless of its actual impact. In this respect, its twentieth-century counterparts in the United States might be the War on Poverty and the War on Drugs.) Ten years later, much of the public and private energy behind the campaign had waned, and it was only after World War I that the battle was reengaged,

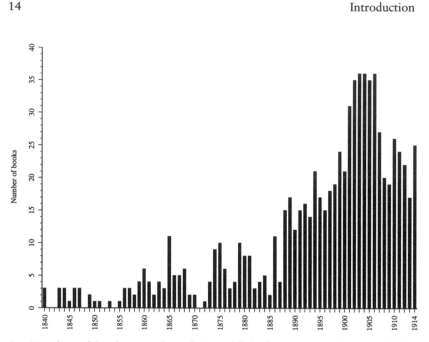

4. Number of books on tuberculosis published per year in France, 1840–1914.

this time in a very different form. The timing of the campaign is significant, in that it coincided neither with significant medical discoveries nor
with any upturn in the incidence of tuberculosis. The magnitude of attention as measured by the printed word follows roughly the same curve.
More than thirty-five books on tuberculosis were published per year between 1902 and 1906 in France, as compared to just four in 1887 and
around fifteen per year in the early 1890s. The figure dropped off to just
over twenty books per year on the eve of World War I.[35] (See fig. 4.) Despite its brief duration, the turn-of-the-century War on Tuberculosis represents a revealing episode in French social and cultural history, whose
roots and legacy extend far beyond its short life span.

Several milestones can be looked to for indications of France's developing public concern about tuberculosis. Each of them generated considerable paperwork, discussion, and headlines—in the lay press as well
as in medical journals. The first major salvo in the War on Tuberculosis
was fired in the Academy of Medicine in 1898. The eminent physician
Joseph Grancher delivered a lengthy report on behalf of an academy
committee charged with proposing preventive measures against the disease. Grancher lamented the fact that tuberculosis had previously been
discussed without any thought at self-defense on the part of a society

armed only with "passivity and indifference." He singled out one target for the thrust of his attack: contagious spittle. "The danger of contagion," he wrote, "is underestimated every day, even by doctors. Far from the terror that it should inspire, tuberculosis is . . . accepted with resignation in families that take no precautions whatsoever." It was not medical knowledge that was lacking, according to Grancher; it was the will to turn that knowledge into action.

> We know . . . that the *tuberculeux* who spits or secretes his bacilli is dangerous and that we must be protected from him.. . . Bacillus-laden spittle . . . is the usual vehicle of the germ of tuberculosis! *Therefore,* that [spittle] is what we must destroy—right away—before it dries . . . .[36]

Here is one of the central logical operations guiding the War on Tuberculosis: the tubercle bacillus is transmitted most often through spitting; therefore, our strategy must focus on discouraging spitting and on disinfecting spittle. Grancher, like nearly all his colleagues, saw exposure and bacilli as the vital point of attack. An important corollary was that people with tuberculosis were "dangerous."

The following year, in 1899, Prime Minister René Waldeck-Rousseau appointed a blue-ribbon panel to investigate preventive policies against tuberculosis. The group, chaired by France's leading hygienist, Paul Brouardel, returned in 1900 with a detailed study of mortality from tuberculosis and a set of recommendations that focused on population density and alcoholism, in addition to spitting, in the social etiology of the disease.[37] (Although it is a scientific term not in common usage, the word *etiology* will figure prominently in these pages, for lack of a convenient alternative. It denotes the body of knowledge and opinion concerning the causes of a given disease; its usage here generally refers to social causes.) In 1901, the government named a "permanent" tuberculosis commission that would meet periodically for the next decade, issuing reports on nearly every imaginable aspect of the disease's place in public policy and making occasional practical recommendations to the bureaucracy. The commission's members included well-known doctors, government functionaries, and politicians—including Léon Bourgeois and Jules Siegfried, two of the Third Republic's most influential figures in the area of social welfare reform.[38]

In that same year, 1901, another landmark report also sounded a call to arms. This time, the audience was the French parliament, whose committee on public health took the legislature's first public stand on the tuberculosis problem. Written by Deputy Lionel Amodru, the par-

liamentary report contained a full statement of what was by then the
dominant etiology of tuberculosis—the official consensus of the medical
community and public officials regarding the principal social causes of
the disease. The dominant etiology isolated three key factors in the
spread of tuberculosis: widespread exposure to the bacillus (in which
spitting was the main culprit), slum housing, and immoderation (especially in drink).

Amodru's report noted that tuberculosis claimed most of its victims
among those between the ages of twenty and forty-five, adults "in the
period of full activity," that is, in the most productive sector of the
workforce. "In these conditions," he wrote, "tuberculosis can no longer
be regarded simply as an accidental by-product of contemporary society."

> It is a fearsome, advancing scourge that is gaining ground every day with no
> obstacles in its contagious path; one is justified in saying that in France,
> where the population is not growing, [tuberculosis] is more than a threat to
> individuals—it is truly a national peril. [39]

Amodru rehearsed what was becoming a familiar litany of enemies.
Contagion meant that in modern city life one was never safe from tuberculosis. At work, at home, or at play, "if he is well, his companions are
a danger to him; if he is sick, he is dangerous to them." Like Grancher,
Amodru contended that because spittle, le crachat, could contain the
bacillus, "it is therefore the enemy" (c'est donc lui qui est l'ennemi).
Even healthy citizens should aid in the effort to eliminate spitting by
setting an example and refraining from a practice "as contrary to hygiene as it is to decorum." [40]

In the aggressive rhetoric of antituberculosis education, if spitting
was the "single greatest cause" of the disease's spread, it appears to
have shared that distinction with alcoholism and housing. Amodru's
report to parliament claimed that "of all the intervening causes of the
illness, none is more formidable nor more frequently observed at the
present time than alcoholism.. . . But it is above all unsanitary housing,
lacking air and sunlight, that is the great auxiliary of tuberculosis."
Hyperbole aside, these were the two other social factors (along with
contagion) consistently denounced by the official antituberculosis campaign. Amodru quoted Professor Louis Landouzy of the Paris Faculty
of Medicine, noted authority on tuberculosis and source of numerous
such aphorisms, to the effect that "alcoholism makes the bed for tuber-

culosis." Brouardel, also from the Paris medical faculty, was Amodru's
source for material on housing:

> "If somebody," writes Professor Brouardel, "predisposed by birth or by hab-
> its to tuberculosis, lives in . . . housing where air and sunlight penetrate
> abundantly, he can escape from contagion. Conversely, if a vigorous man,
> with no hereditary or acquired taint, lives in unsanitary housing, he will not
> escape contagion.. . ." One has to have seen in Paris certain poor workers'
> housing to understand the extent to which hygiene can be misunderstood.[41]

This transition, too, from "slum housing is bad for one's health" to
"slum residents' ignorance of hygiene is dangerous," typified the dominant etiology and the War on Tuberculosis. At the same time, parliament was considering a bill—eventually passed into law in 1902—that
mandated municipal health departments and generally increased both
the capacity and the obligation of local authorities to keep the health of
their populations under close surveillance.

After these developments, tuberculosis had become inscribed as one
of the burning issues of the day in the French polity and in public awareness. The last major milestone in this progression was the 1905 International Tuberculosis Congress at the Grand Palais in Paris. During the
week in October that the congress was in session and for several months
before and after, tuberculosis was front-page news in Paris and the
provinces, and controversies that otherwise would never have left the
medical world were the subject of nationwide debate. For example,
when a German doctor announced that he had discovered a substance
that might be effective as either a vaccine or a cure for tuberculosis, the
intense press coverage that ensued bore all the marks of a political scandal or a true-crime detective story. During the congress itself, crowds
thronged the public lectures and exhibits concerning tuberculosis and
its prevention. Several police brigades and a cordon of Republican
Guards were needed to control the crowd of "curious" onlookers at
the official opening of the congress. More than three thousand official
participants, not including invited guests, vied for places in the two-
thousand-seat auditorium of the Grand Palais.[42] For a short time, the
eyes of the international medical community were on Paris, and the eyes
of France were on tuberculosis.

After 1906, the intensity of public attention to tuberculosis subsided
somewhat, reviving periodically when new legislative or philanthropic
initiatives were launched. With the outbreak of World War I, the entire

political, social, and administrative climate changed radically. Laws sponsored by Bourgeois in 1916 and André Honnorat in 1919 began the process of covering the nation with networks of antituberculosis dispensaries and sanatoriums, respectively. This process, along with the leading role taken by American philanthropy (through the Rockefeller Foundation) in postwar campaigns against tuberculosis, signaled a new phase in French society's response to the disease.[43]

The zenith of the nineteenth-century War on Tuberculosis, then, lasted only from the late 1890s to around 1906. Why these years? There was no sudden upsurge in the incidence of tuberculosis at this time, nor were there any major medical discoveries about the disease. The timing of official worry points to reasons beyond epidemiology and medicine. The middle of the so-called Belle Epoque was a time that Susanna Barrows has artfully termed "the apogee of anxiety and anomie" in France.[44] The republic, its legitimacy consolidated since the late 1870s, was coming under increasing attack from both Left and Right. Gen. Georges Boulanger nearly engineered a coup d'état in 1889, and in the late 1890s, the Dreyfus Affair split the nation, pitting church, army, and tradition against secularism, modernity, and individual rights. Meanwhile, the amnesty of exiled Communards in 1880 and the legalization of labor unions in 1884 laid the groundwork for a revived workers' movement. Strike-related protests and violence at Anzin, Decazeville, Fourmies, and Carmaux between 1884 and 1892 crystallized in many bourgeois minds the threat posed by a savage working class to private property and public order; a series of anarchist bombings culminating with the assassination of President Sadi Carnot in 1894 reinforced the immediacy of this perceived threat. A new wave of strikes beginning in 1904 and the formation of a unified Socialist party in 1905 intensified mutual class resentment and fear.

Other equally acute anxieties were also at work in France at the turn of the century. The economic, military, and biological vitality of the nation itself appeared to be threatened by dangerous trends to which its neighbors seemed immune. The German and British populations (and therefore their pools of potential workers and soldiers) were increasing rapidly. Meanwhile, France's birthrate was low and falling fast, and the other side of the demographic equation was no more encouraging. Europe's leading cause of death, tuberculosis, claimed far more lives per capita in French cities than in German or British ones, where it was also declining more rapidly. When French scientists took a close look at the French population during this period, they saw these trends as well as, in Robert Nye's words, "a host of social pathologies that appeared to call into question both the quantity and the quality of the French population."

> Under the spur of the internal and external events of the era, a medical model of cultural crisis developed that exercised a linguistic and conceptual imperialism over all other ways of viewing the nation's plight. If this model of crisis was *medical* in nature, it served the thoroughly *cultural* aim of explaining to the French the origins of national decadence and the weaknesses of their population.[45]

According to Nye, such anxieties crystallized in "the literary generation of 1890" and gained strength through 1900. They most often involved an implicit or explicit comparison with Germany, the upstart power that had humiliated France in 1870.[46]

It is true, of course, that much of French history has been marked by anxiety and contentiousness; the entire nineteenth century in particular, with cataclysmic industrialization, urbanization, and revolutions, fits this description quite well. Yet the fin de siècle period was unique in several respects. The domestic and international political context of the period gave added intensity to concerns about France's fragile status among nations. Both the perception and the reality of demographic decline added a new dimension to social fears that had been expressed in biological terms since the early nineteenth century.[47] Later, after 1906, the relative waning of public attention to tuberculosis coincided with rising international tensions and concerns over the imminent threat of war.[48]

French responses to tuberculosis cannot be understood outside of this political and cultural context. Birthrates, mortality, moral decay, political subversion, the filth and danger represented by the working classes in bourgeois eyes—tuberculosis allowed all these diverse and threatening themes to be assembled into a single coherent package. To be sure, the illness was not just a metaphor, not just a sign through which social relations or anxieties expressed themselves. Real people got sick and died from tuberculosis, just as they are getting sick and dying today. That seemingly self-evident proposition must not be forgotten. However, neither should that truth mislead historians into a fruitless search for the single true explanation of those real deaths. Even if much more historical evidence were available regarding the incidence and causes of tuberculosis, it would still represent the inescapable biases, preoccupations, and blind spots of the society in which it was produced.

All scientific knowledge is—and has always been—conditioned by social factors. Industrialization, urbanization, class conflict, religious piety and charity, bourgeois sexual morality, demographic stagnation, military defeat, and international rivalry all contributed to the peculiar shape of the French understanding of tuberculosis. In turn, worry over the nineteenth century's leading cause of death inevitably colored perceptions of these and other aspects of French politics, culture, and society, lending an air of vital, bodily urgency and scientific certainty to discussions of problems outside the immediate realm of medicine. Ultimately, to write the history of tuberculosis in nineteenth-century France, one must write a history of nineteenth-century French society.

This particular social history, like all others, has biases and blind spots of its own. Recently, many social historians of medicine have trained their sights on the history of health care "from the bottom up." They have resurrected the patient as a salient actor in the series of negotiations and complex interactions that constitute the history of healers and hospitals.[49] A great deal of information has come to light regarding the impressively varied sorts of medical care (both "traditional" and "scientific," with a great deal in between) to which different segments of society had recourse in various epochs of history.[50] This has not been my approach here. Epidemiology and public health figure more prominently in this study than medical practice per se. In medical terms, this is a history of etiology and prophylaxis rather than of therapeutics. Conceptions of the causes and prevention of tuberculosis are my chief concern here, insofar as they provide keys to the vital question, how does a society make sense of a widespread and deadly disease? As a result of this preoccupation, the saga of medications and treatment regimens in the nineteenth century is given short shrift, as is that of the sanatorium (largely the province of the elite, particularly during the period covered by this study), and the voice of the individual patient is rarely heard. While stories of the doctor-patient interaction and of hospitals and other medical institutions do reveal important aspects of social change, they are peripheral to this account of how the healthy (in medicine, government, and elsewhere) explained tuberculosis to each other and to the not-yet-sick in the rest of society. Similarly, much of this study concerns the writings, teachings, and actions of influential men or committed propagandists; how the general population received their ideas must necessarily remain an open question. No simple method exists for determining the nature and extent of popular attitudes toward tuberculosis in nineteenth-century France. There are, however, scattered bits of evidence suggesting varying degrees of public receptivity to the agendas of medicine, government, philanthropy, and labor where tuberculosis was concerned. This evidence is considered carefully here, but the resulting picture of popular perceptions is, unfortunately, a partial one at best.

The first two chapters of this book cover the first two-thirds of the nineteenth century, when "essentialist" explanations of tuberculosis predominated. Chapter 1 examines the early social and epidemiological investigations of Villermé and other hygienists during the July Monarchy in the context of bourgeois concern over the rapid growth of cities (especially Paris) and the resulting poverty and social dislocation. It also discusses the controversy surrounding Villemin's 1865 experiments purporting to show the transmissibility of tuberculosis and takes seriously the arguments of the since-discredited anticontagionists. Chapter 2 suggests that during these same pre-germ theory years, outside the realm of medicine, a certain age-old ideal of womanhood took a distinctive nineteenth-century form, appropriating tuberculosis as a vehicle of redemptive suffering. This ideal survived both the decline of romanticism and the Pasteurians' demystification of disease and manifested itself at the end of the century in the strange and fascinating career of Saint Thérèse of Lisieux.

Chapters 3 through 5, the heart of the book, detail the development of the dominant etiology in the late nineteenth century and its implementation in the War on Tuberculosis. Chapter 3 explains how fear of microbes led doctors and public officials to mount a concerted campaign against spitting (except in approved, disinfectant spittoons) and fostered a certain "tuberculophobia" among the population, as infected people were discriminated against or even shunned. Disgust at the deplorable state of working-class slum lodgings prompted an unprecedented surveillance effort (notably in Paris and Le Havre), the *casier sanitaire des maisons,* which kept track of all buildings and apartment units whose occupants died of tuberculosis, so as to track down hotbeds of infection. Chapter 4 analyzes this administrative strategy as well as the role of women as vectors in what was diagnosed as the dangerous domestic spread of tuberculosis. Chapter 5 traces the way in which, by medically associating alcoholism and syphilis with tuberculosis, doctors and hygienists were able to link deviant behavior and marginal classes with the perceived moral and demographic decline of the French nation.

Chapter 6 focuses on the experience of Le Havre, which experienced tremendous urban growth as well as France's highest tuberculosis mortality during the nineteenth century. What makes this Norman seaport a particularly salient case study is the convergence of these dramatically changing material conditions with the maturation of an activist group of city fathers led by the mayor (and occasional cabinet minister), Jules Siegfried. The city's paternalistic bourgeoisie attempted to translate its fervent positivism into action, mobilizing on the local level to fight the scourges of slum housing, alcoholism, and tuberculosis—all perceived as serious threats to Le Havre's prosperity. Among other examples, the story of France's first municipal health department (established in 1879) testifies to the energetic (if unsuccessful) efforts directed against tuberculosis by an emerging cadre of hygienists, bureaucrats, and politicians.

Chapter 7 describes at length the origins and elaboration of a defiantly oppositional body of medical knowledge, which arose on the far left of French politics around the turn of the century. While some socialists sought to represent a working-class point of view within the terms of debate of mainstream medicine, doctors and other militants associated with revolutionary syndicalism rejected those terms of debate. They put forward a theory of tuberculosis based on diminished bodily resistance rather than on exposure to the bacillus (which they considered to be all but universal) and blamed overwork and low wages as the chief reasons for workers' susceptibility to the disease. In the workers' movement as in nearly every sector of French society, the turn of the century was a critical period of change, instability, and anxiety. Questions of power, identity, and survival increasingly focused on the leading killer of the time, at once familiar and mysterious. Throughout France, whether in medicine, politics, literature, or theology, knowledge of tuberculosis became valuable—and contested—terrain.

Social Anxiety, Social Disease, and the Question of Contagion

During the first half of the nineteenth century, France watched in fascination and horror as its capital showed every sign of imminent implosion. A city whose physical facilities had changed little in centuries saw its population double in less than thirty years. "In these years Paris looked around and was unable to recognize itself," the historian Louis Chevalier wrote.

> Another, larger city had overflowed into the unaltered framework of streets, mansions, houses and passageways . . . filling every nook and corner, making over the older dwellings of the nobility and gentry into workshops and lodging houses, erecting factories and stockpiles in gardens and courts where carriages had been moldering quietly away, packing the suddenly shrunken streets, . . . overloading the forgotten sewers, spreading litter and stench even into the adjacent countryside and besmirching the lovely sky of the Ile-de-France with [its] vast and universal exhalation.[1]

Already a cauldron of volatile social and political forces, Paris suddenly had to accommodate hundreds of thousands of mostly poor migrants from the countryside and provincial cities who had come to the capital seeking a better life. Even before this massive influx, discontent and unruliness among the city's population had been known to trigger political crises, including the events leading up to the great revolution of 1789. Occasional uprisings in the densely populated central quarters of Paris and two more full-scale revolutions—in 1830 and 1848—accompanied the city's growth in this period. An emergent bourgeoisie assumed greater economic and political power under the July Monarchy (1830–1848) and began to perceive the swelling ranks of the urban poor as filthy, criminal, and politically dangerous. In an atmosphere of such political instability and class antagonism, the cataclysmic growth of Paris was regarded with extreme apprehension. When Asiatic cholera devastated the capital in 1832 and again in 1849—in both cases coinciding with civil unrest in the aftermath of revolutions—the worst fears of many seemed confirmed.[2] Paris was headed for material and social catastrophe.

This dread expressed itself in a sizable literature of concern over the transformation Paris was undergoing. In the picturesque literature of crime and poverty as well as in public health investigations, a tone of fascinated disgust infused all descriptions of the pathological city. Honoré de Balzac, for one, was well known for his "filthy descriptions" of the capital's poor neighborhoods. "Nothing escapes him," wrote Jules Janin of Balzac, "not a wrinkle, not a sticky scab of this foul tetter."[3] In his own novel, *Un Hiver à Paris*, published in 1845, Janin also refused to shrink from the unpleasant details of life in Paris. Here is his description of the city at night.

> Bespattered carts draw up to the door of the sleeping houses to carry off every kind of filth. . . . In the hideous lairs which Paris hides away behind its palaces and museums . . . there lurks a swarming and oozing population that beggars comparison. . . . A vile bohemian world, a frightful world, a purulent wart on the face of this great city.[4]

Others lamented the disappearance of the great and proud city of recent memory, drowned in a sea of overcrowded buildings and people.

> If you contemplate from the summit of Montmartre the congestion of houses piled up at every point of a vast horizon, what do you observe? . . . One is tempted to wonder whether this is Paris; and, seized with a sudden fear, one is reluctant to venture into this vast maze, in which a million beings jostle one another, where the air, vitiated by unhealthy effluvia, rising in a poisonous cloud, almost obscures the sun.[5]

Common to nearly all of the literature—fictional, political, and hygienic—on the growth of Paris in the early nineteenth century was a profound and fearful disgust at the city's filth, smells, and overcrowding. Vivid descriptions of "purulent warts," "sticky scabs," "unhealthy effluvia," and "a million beings jostl[ing] one another" fill many such accounts, in which few aspects of Parisian life could be depicted in any tone other than that of sheer physical revulsion.

In the historiography of medicine, the rise of germ theory is the great divide of the nineteenth century, in light of which all preceding and subsequent developments are interpreted. Where tuberculosis in France is concerned, the decisive dates have been 1865 and 1882, when Villemin demonstrated the inoculability of the disease and when Koch identified the tubercle bacillus, respectively. However, several significant elements of the pre-germ theory etiology of tuberculosis survived intact through the late nineteenth century. Among these elements are filth, stench, and overcrowding, all symptomatic of the underlying pathology of the city. Furthermore, the history of early-nineteenth-century medicine and public health includes some pivotal debates and revealing preoccupations underlying the search for the incidence and causes of tuberculosis.

The first half of the nineteenth century was not a time of great innovation in the realm of etiology. "Among the intervening causes of pulmonary consumption, I know of none more certain than sorrowful passions [*passions tristes*]," wrote René-Théophile-Hyacinthe Laënnec in 1826. Forty years later, the opinion of Laënnec, the inventor of the stethoscope and one of the most revered figures in the history of French medicine, continued to enjoy the status of virtually unquestioned dogma among physicians concerned with tuberculosis. When Professor Michel Peter of the Paris Faculty of Medicine reviewed the latest medical thinking in his 1866 book on tuberculosis, he reproduced Laënnec's analysis almost unchanged. Tuberculosis, Peter wrote, arose within the body itself, determined by inherited predisposition and often also by "intervening causes" (*causes occasionnelles*) such as "sorrowful passions."[6]

It would be rash, however, to conclude that those four decades had been a time of stasis or inertia in the development of French society's understanding of tuberculosis. In fact, they had seen not only the beginnings of a systematically "social" perspective on health and disease but also the modification of some key tenets of Laënnec's "morbid spontaneity" and even the first nineteenth-century expressions of germ theory and contagionism relating to tuberculosis.

Historians have long regarded the Bourbon Restoration and the July Monarchy (1815–1848) as a crucial era in the development of French medicine and public health. Erwin Ackerknecht called Paris "the center of world medicine" and its medical school "the first faculty of the universe" during this time. He identified "a quite specific and unique type of medicine" characteristic of the time and place—he called it "hospital medicine"—based on firsthand physical examination, pathological anatomy, and statistics.[7] Other historians have emphasized developments outside medicine itself; one recently claimed that this period saw the French "creat[e] . . . the modern notion of public health and . . . the scientific discipline of public hygiene."[8] William Coleman and Bernard-Pierre Lécuyer in particular have reevaluated the social investigations of Villermé and the other early hygienists—those who for the first time attempted to prove that "it was society rather than nature that produced inequality before death."[9] On the heels of these changes, during the Second Empire, Pasteurian bacteriology boldly asserted the contagiousness of tuberculosis.

The two most salient developments in early-nineteenth-century French knowledge about tuberculosis were (1) the shift from hereditary essentialism to contagionism in the *etiology* of tuberculosis and (2) the rise of various social *epidemiologies* of the disease in the emergent field of public health. It should be emphasized that these two trends were not necessarily related to each other. Coleman's history of yellow fever in early- and mid-nineteenth-century Europe has shown the mutual independence of epidemiology and etiology—that is, that the development of epidemiology as a method of social investigation bore no necessary relation to the status of knowledge regarding disease causation.[10] In fact, the increasing awareness of social factors in tuberculosis—if it was related at all to the competing etiologies—was associated with the older "miasmatic," anticontagionist point of view. This chapter reviews the shift from essentialism to contagionism and the rise of the "social" perspective in light of the intensifying fear and anxiety with which many French social critics viewed the urban environment and the urban poor during the middle third of the nineteenth century.

LAËNNEC AND ESSENTIALIST MEDICINE

One cannot help but think of the label "romantic medicine" when contemplating Laënnec's remarks concerning *les passions tristes* and seeing their echo in subsequent decades. Such comments seem to replicate in medicine a common theme in romantic literature and art: the tragic, fatalistic determination of illness and death by "psychogenic" factors. Some have called the early nineteenth century the heyday of romantic medicine for other reasons, referring to the search for transcendent explanations and the tendency to speculative, idealistic, universal system building (in opposition to rationalist empiricism).[11]

In France, as far as the etiology of disease is concerned, a better term might be "essentialist medicine": the belief that disease in general (and tuberculosis in particular) was part of a person's *essence*. Illness, in this view, arose spontaneously from internal causes and constitutional predisposition rather than from external causes, although external factors could influence the outcome of internal tendencies and predispositions. (This last corollary would become quite significant when essentialist medicine confronted the unequal incidence of tuberculosis in French society.) Some doctors even attributed epidemic disease to an "epidemic constitution." According to Ackerknecht, a strong political and philosophical aversion to contagion brought about this "regression to older, classic causal explanations." After all, in his words, "things had to be explained somehow." Heredity served as an especially popular explanation of many diseases, including tuberculosis. Through heredity, it was assumed, a constitutional predisposition to the disease—or "diathesis"—transmitted itself from generation to generation.[12]

Laënnec, whose opinions on tuberculosis influenced medical teaching and practice throughout the first two-thirds of the nineteenth century, rejected contagion in favor of heredity in his landmark *Traité de l'auscultation médiate*.

> If the question of contagion may be regarded as highly dubious relative to tubercles, the same cannot be said of hereditary predisposition. Experience proves to all physicians that the children of consumptives are more frequently attacked by this disease than are other subjects.[13]

In Laënnec's treatise, however, the entire question of etiology was tinged with uncertainty and equivocation. Even his denial of contagion was less than rock solid.

> Tuberculous phthisis has long been thought contagious, and it is still thought to be so by the common people, by magistrates, and by some doctors in certain countries, especially in the southern parts of Europe. In France, at least, it does not seem to be [contagious].[14]

He based this curiously qualified opinion on his experience with many patients whose spouses remained healthy despite sharing a bed even in the late stages of the illness and with poor families who slept crowded together in a small room, where the tuberculosis of one family member did not endanger the health of the others. Yet Laënnec admitted that, "fortunately," many countervailing examples existed for heredity as well, cases in which only one of several children in a family contracted

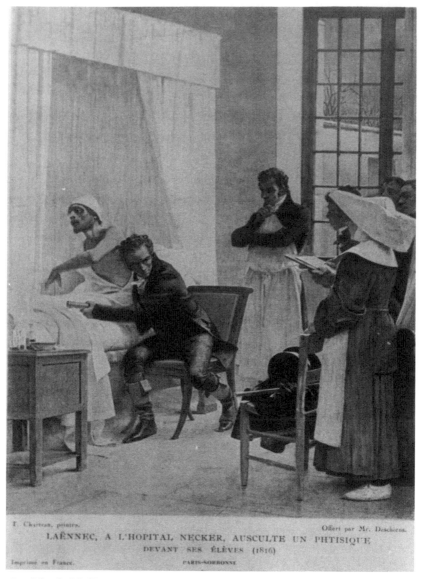

T. Chartran, peintre.   Offert par Mr. Deschiens.

LAËNNEC, A L'HOPITAL NECKER, AUSCULTE UN PHTISIQUE
DEVANT SES ÉLÈVES (1816)

Imprimé en France.   PARIS-SORBONNE

5. Théobald Chartran's painting of Laënnec auscultating a consumptive patient, 1816. Photo courtesy of the National Library of Medicine.

the disease; conversely, he added, tuberculosis occasionally wiped out entire families who showed no signs of it in previous generations.[15]

It is possible that this uncertainty, which was by no means unique to Laënnec, can be traced to the relative neglect of etiology itself in early-nineteenth-century medicine. The star of pathological anatomy was ascendant in French medicine, and most of its innovations concerned semiology and nosology: the symptoms and diagnosis of various disorders. The history of Laënnec's landmark book on diseases of the chest is itself instructive on this point. The first edition, published in 1819, contained none of this material on the causes of tuberculosis in its thousand-plus pages. He added the section "Intervening Causes of Pulmonary Consumption" to the book's second edition, which came out in 1826, just before his own death from tuberculosis. In the ensuing years (as will be seen below), epidemiological investigations associated with the early public health movement brought etiology and the social determinants of health under closer scrutiny. Still, forty years later, Michel Peter stated confidently, "If there is a universally accepted proposition, it is that of the heredity of [tuberculosis]." He called it "the most considerable cause" of the disease's development.[16] Heredity reigned supreme among causal explanations until it was displaced by contagion through the work of Villemin in the 1860s and, finally, Koch in 1882.

Meanwhile, equivocation, uncertainty, and emphasis on heredity did not prevent Laënnec and others from pointing out the contribution of various *causes occasionnelles* to the onset of tuberculosis. Significantly, the two chief factors invoked by the hereditarians were sorrowful passions and unhealthy sexual activity (including masturbation and "venereal excesses"). Both of these factors reinforced the impression that disorders such as tuberculosis were part of an individual's essence. Neither factor was innate, certainly, but both were widely portrayed (in romantic and postromantic literature, among other genres) as aspects of fate, intimately related to identity and individuality.

As noted above, Laënnec found sorrowful passions to be one of the few *certain* causes of tuberculosis. Among other things, it explained why the disease was so common in cities and so rare in the countryside.

> It is perhaps to this reason alone that the frequency of pulmonary consumption in large cities must be attributed: there, men have more relations with each other, and so have cause for more frequent and profound sorrows; bad morals and poor conduct of all sorts are more common there and are often the cause of bitter regrets that cannot be consoled and that even time cannot soften.[17]

Here the connection between sorrow and "bad morals" was made explicit. Implicit was the conclusion that medicine was therapeutically impotent in the matter (no consolation, not even time itself, could heal these emotional wounds). The passage also came closer than most such texts to explaining the epidemiology of tuberculosis, or at least its concentration in large cities.

"Chagrin," "regrets," and "poor conduct" were exceedingly vague, but there was a consensus that more specific moral weaknesses also contributed to tuberculosis; namely, masturbation and venereal excesses. Laënnec glossed over the matter, calling "very probable" the chance that "excesses [and] . . . syphilitic conditions" were "sometimes the intervening cause" in the onset of tuberculosis, although he cautioned that these factors would be unlikely in and of themselves to cause the disease "in subjects who were not naturally predisposed to it." However, many others, writing both before and after Laënnec, stressed the twin dangers in both "onanism" and "the abuse of coitus." Both involved what Peter called "a double loss": the loss of vital bodily fluids, which was "costly to the organism," and the loss of "nerve impulses" through the convulsions of the *spasme cynique* at climax. It was also suggested that the "shock" of orgasm could cause harmful congestion in the heart and lungs.[18]

It would be a mistake to confuse references in medical texts, however frequent, with a concerted social and political campaign aimed at stigmatizing certain groups and practices (such as the one that arose later in the century through the association of alcoholism and syphilis with tuberculosis). Nevertheless, these references show that there was in the early nineteenth century a significant and established current of thought connecting perceived moral failings with physical illness. They also prefigure later etiological debates in another respect. Essentialist medicine implicated venereal excesses as a cause of tuberculosis because they represented uncompensated "organic losses." Peter especially decried such losses; they were part of "physiological poverty" (*la misère physiologique*), a combination of "excessive [bodily] expenditure and insufficient restoration." Rest and nourishment did not match physical exertion. The same phrases recurred in the later leftist critique of capitalism and official medicine, in which overwork and low wages were seen as the principal causes of tuberculosis. Peter cited such factors explicitly, though few of his contemporaries followed suit.[19] For the most part, medicine left social investigation to the emerging science of public health.

THE EARLY HYGIENISTS' SOCIAL PERSPECTIVE

Death is a social disease, according to the title of Coleman's study of Villermé and the early public health movement in France. But "social disease" can mean many different things, even when applied to a specific illness such as tuberculosis. Later polemics would revolve around whether the term meant a disease inherent in the lifestyle of the working classes or a disease determined by the dictates of industrial capitalism and wage labor. Moreover, the very notion of contagion added an inherently social dimension to the antituberculosis campaigns of the late nineteenth century. The singular achievement of Villermé and his fellow hygienists in the 1830s and 1840s was to establish that mortality in general and tuberculosis in particular were socially determined in that they were not randomly distributed throughout society. Simply put, social status conferred relative susceptibility to or immunity from disease. The particulars of the poverty–mortality relationship or the specific social factors that contributed to tuberculosis were not fully explored in this period. Nonetheless, the breakthrough was significant and had lasting repercussions for French society's response to tuberculosis.

As Coleman and other historians have shown, Villermé was the leading figure of the "party of hygiene" during the July Monarchy. Two of his projects in particular broke new ground for public health research: a series of articles around 1830 on mortality in Paris (based on the *Recherches statistiques* published periodically beginning in 1821 by the prefecture of the Seine), and the two-volume monograph published in 1840 on conditions among textile workers.[20] The exhaustively documented and statistically measured conclusion of Villermé's work was inescapable: the poor were sicker and died earlier than the rich. Although the simplicity of the proposition may seem almost self-evident, it was neither proven nor widely accepted—in fact, it was not given much consideration one way or the other—before Villermé's time. Little of the subsequent work of the nineteenth-century hygienists would have been possible or plausible if this basic social connection had not been established.

However, Coleman overstated his case when he wrote that the early hygienists "created a *thoroughly social* view of the process of industrialization," going out of their way to expose themselves to "the harsh reality of the daily life of the laboring population."[21] Villermé and the other pioneers in the field of public health could hardly have been expected to transcend their intellectual environment, class, and culture.

Their work inevitably reflected the preoccupations and prejudices of their milieu, and, viewed in retrospect, it contained numerous gaps and silences. Although it is risky to criticize any work on the basis of what it does not say, such blind spots are noteworthy in several respects. The early hygienists held themselves to a high standard by their explicit claim to have enlarged the study of health and disease to encompass all of society. Furthermore, they self-consciously sought to address the "social question" at a time when socialism was in its crucial early stages of development in France and to provide alternative, nonsocialist answers through their work. As Lécuyer has pointed out, many hygienists considered it their duty to absolve industry of responsibility for death and disease.[22] This attitude obviously colored, for example, their investigations of occupational health and even in other matters closed off certain areas of inquiry and excluded certain conclusions. Instead of a "thoroughly social" perspective, theirs was an *innovatively* social one, which opened the door for later ways of understanding disease but did not point them in a single clear direction.

From this perspective, the crucial point at which the social epidemiology of tuberculosis was set in motion seems to have been Villermé's studies of differential mortality in the arrondissements of Paris. Taken together, the works (published between 1826 and 1830) represent a manual in statistical interpretation as well as a methodical review of possible causes of insalubrity in the capital. (Coleman and Lécuyer have each separately established Villermé's—and these articles'—pivotal place in the history of sociological and statistical inquiry.)[23] One by one, Villermé considered and rejected factors that had been proposed by various observers to explain mortality differences: climate, soil drainage, water supply, miasmatic filth, altitude, wind patterns. None correlated with the city's death rates by arrondissement. Population density received the most detailed attention, as it was widely believed to be a contributing cause of ill health. Still, on close inspection, no clear correlation emerged. In Villermé's mind, only one possibility remained: poverty. Using a considerable array of tables and charts, he presented the data in various different ways. Estimating or excluding deaths in hospitals, calculating average rental costs or percentage of untaxed rental housing units by arrondissement, the results were the same: the rank of arrondissements by mortality matched the inverse rank by wealth nearly exactly. "So, wealth, affluence, and poverty are . . . for the residents of the various arrondissements of Paris—by the conditions in which they place them—the principal causes (I do not say the only causes) to which one must attribute the great differences . . . in mortality."[24]

Given Villermé's aims and approach, this was a final conclusion rather than an intermediate one or a starting point, notwithstanding the suggestive reference to the unnamed "conditions" in which wealth and poverty place Parisians. This was as far as he wanted to go, and he readily admitted as much. "It is enough for me here to have established this truth; I do not want to follow all of its medical consequences, nor by any means address it in a moral or economic light."[25] Later in his career, Villermé did touch on the specific conditions of poverty, and he certainly did not shy away from adopting an economic or moral point of view on these issues. But he never took the next step—the basis for so much of the later campaigns concerning tuberculosis—of relating the constituent elements of poverty to specific causes of death. Nor could he bring himself, committed as he was to the principles of liberal political economy, to recommend remedial public action on the scale of the problems he described.[26] Several of his contemporaries, however, did go so far as to investigate the role of certain social and environmental factors in the specific disease of tuberculosis, without Villermé's focus on wealth and poverty as variables. The questions these hygienists asked—and did not ask—and their tentative answers shed some light on the attitudes of public health experts toward the rapidly changing social fabric in the early nineteenth century.

WORK AND ENVIRONMENT: THE DIAGNOSIS OF OCCUPATIONAL PREDISPOSITION

Several studies focused on the occupational incidence of tuberculosis, most often seeking to determine if particular toxins or environmental influences could be shown to have deleterious health effects. Lécuyer has analyzed this preoccupation with occupational exposure in terms of two related tendencies unique to this period: first, the fact that this class of hygienic investigation originated as inquiries into specific industries reputed to be harmful (for example, mines and tobacco factories); and second, the philosophical and political background of the hygienists themselves, which led them to place as much emphasis on absolving industry of responsibility as on identifying harmful conditions. "As a result," according to Lécuyer, "anything that has to do with physical strenuousness, or even with a lack of air or with cramped working quarters, seems negligible to them."[27]

Two reports in particular, which appeared in the *Annales d'hygiène publique* in the early 1830s, merit closer attention because they illustrate the loose connection between epidemiology and etiology in these years: even the most exhaustive epidemiological studies bore no necessary relation to any established theory of disease causation.[28] Henri Lombard's 1834 article, "The Influence of Professions on Pulmonary Consumption," attempted to draw a direct correspondence between the professions of tuberculosis victims (as gleaned from municipal death registers) and occupational conditions. By reviewing many different types of occupations, this relentless hymn to the statistical method gives the impression of comprehensiveness while actually considering only the immediate impact of certain types of work on the chest and lungs.[29]

Lombard began by assembling data from five sources covering four cities: Paris, Geneva, Hamburg, and Vienna. All the sources indicated to some extent the professions and causes of death for all patients who died in certain of the cities' hospitals over certain periods of time. For each city, Lombard compiled a list of all professions specified for tuberculosis victims and ranked the professions by the number of tuberculosis victims belonging to each of them. He then did the same for all causes of death combined, and he compared the two rankings of professions.

If a profession ranked higher on the tuberculosis list than it did on the overall list in a majority of cities, it was classified as "positive" for correlation with tuberculosis, no matter how high or low the actual ranks were. Those that ranked lower on the tuberculosis list than on the overall list for most cities were considered to have negative correlations with the disease. For example, day laborers ranked very high on both the tuberculosis list and the general list for all cities, but because they ranked higher on the general list, they were classified as negative. In effect, the classification said nothing about the actual mortality of day laborers from tuberculosis (the ratio of tuberculosis deaths to the total number of those workers in the population) but suggested that they were more likely than workers in the positive category to die of causes other than tuberculosis. Lombard considered this evidence that the occupation did not contribute to the disease.

Lombard's unstated assumption that there was something inherent in the nature of the work for the "positive" occupations that was conducive to tuberculosis (and conversely, that the negatively correlating professions were inherently salutary) led him to venture explanations for the correlations of nearly every profession on his lists. Differences in workers' physical well-being derived from three factors, according to Lombard: degree of wealth or poverty, forced exercise or inaction of certain parts of the body, and "purity or impurity of the surrounding atmosphere." Tuberculosis was no exception, and by analyzing the various professions according to these three categories, he felt he could determine which aspects of work predisposed workers to contract the disease.[30]

The first category, wealth and poverty, was quickly disposed of. Because one-fourth of the professions (not workers) in the below-average group were *professions aisées* and only one-eighth of the above-average occupations were of that class, Lombard deduced confidently that the poor were twice as likely as the rich to die of tuberculosis.[31] The method was somewhat more clear for the bodily exercise category. Grouping the professions according to whether they were "inactive" or "active," Lombard found more *inactive* jobs correlating positively than negatively with tuberculosis and more *active* occupations negative than positive. Therefore, he concluded, muscular activity warded off tuberculosis and inactivity invited it. Lombard rejected the long-held belief that constant arm movement, vocal activity, and bent-over body position caused tuberculosis. Professions corresponding to these characteristics did not correlate uniformly in the positive category, so he deemed the effects of such activity negligible.[32]

The most significant feature of all in professional life, though, was neither economic status nor muscular activity but *air*. "Of all the circumstances to which workers in the various professions are submitted, none is as important as the surrounding atmosphere, because it acts directly on the lungs, the seat [*siège*] of consumption." [33] Lombard was most concerned about the presence of "foreign bodies" in the air. These included not just dust particles but "aqueous vapors" and "emanations" of various sorts. Aqueous vapors were beneficial to workers, he determined, because professions exercised in humid environments showed negative tuberculosis correlations. Similarly, "animal emanations" exercised a "protective" influence (butchers, for example, showed a negative tuberculosis correlation), but certain "vegetable" and "mineral" emanations were extremely harmful.[34]

Lombard found one of his strongest correlations to tuberculosis in the breakdown of professions by whether they were exercised indoors or outdoors. Seventy percent of outdoor professions correlated negatively with tuberculosis, and Lombard claimed that "consumption

[was] twice as frequent among workers confined to workshops [*ren-fermés dans des ateliers*] than among those who work outdoors [*en plein air*]."[35] Even within the category of indoor professions, however, space counted; "vast and open" workshops did not allow propagation of tuberculosis to the extent evident in more cramped working quarters. "Thus, one can consider the vitiated air of the workplace [*l'air vicié des locaux*] as the cause of the large number of consumption cases observed in certain professions, whereas pure and constantly renewed air is an excellent prevention against the disease."[36]

Here was Lombard's key finding: "vitiated air" caused tuberculosis, and air purified by ventilation and sunlight protected one from it. The elaboration of this concept marked a crucial step in the development of attitudes toward tuberculosis. It manifested an attitude toward the physical environment that laid the groundwork for later etiological theories, including the linkage of unsanitary housing and other environmental factors to tuberculosis. Lombard's fundamental conclusion—that occupations played a determinant role in the epidemiology of tuberculosis—was inherent in his method. A similar investigation in the same journal in 1831 took a slightly different approach to the same problem. Louis-François Benoiston de Châteauneuf's "The Influence of Certain Professions on the Development of Pulmonary Consumption" drew in factors such as sex differentials and the broader culture of poverty to the mix of pathogenic influences, but it too was as remarkable for the narrowness of its conclusions as for the breadth of occupations it considered.[37]

Benoiston had long felt that certain causes commonly linked with tuberculosis needed to be verified, so he compiled information from the entry registers of four Paris hospitals covering the period 1817–1827 and noted the occupations of 1,554 tuberculosis patients. Like Lombard, he grouped the occupations into categories—in this case, seven, based on the position of the body during work, the type of muscular activity involved, and particles or vapors to which workers were exposed. For example, category 5 consisted of "occupations which submit the body, and especially the lower body, to the effects of dampness." Unlike Lombard, Benoiston then calculated the ratio of workers with tuberculosis in each category to the total number of workers in that category represented in the registers for other illnesses. He then compared these ratios to the mortality rate from tuberculosis in the general population, to determine the relative susceptibility of workers in each category.

The way in which Benoiston chose to divide professions into categories predetermined to some extent the results of his investigation. No occupational conditions other than posture, muscle use, and particle or vapor exposure were considered. If certain occupations involved particular age groups, wage scales, work hours, types of housing, or other differential factors that might affect workers' health, such correlations would not appear in the study's findings. From the range of factors considered, Benoiston concluded—unlike Lombard—that those involving a hunched or bent over forward position (category 7, a curious mix of professions, including writers, shoemakers, and seamstresses) were the most dangerous, followed by those exposed to mercury vapors and "animal" particles. Occupations involving other particles and vapors were declared "innocent." Benoiston concluded by recommending that some kind of remedial action or regulation be undertaken to alleviate the hazards of occupations exercised while bent over forward.[38]

Benoiston's and Lombard's studies in the *Annales d'hygiène publique* are classic examples of the environmentalist style of medical thinking. This characteristic of pre-germ theory miasmatism sought the causes of disease in spatial relations and the exposure of bodies to weather conditions, vapors, particles, and other environmental factors. In the case of tuberculosis, environmentalism and essentialism were by no means mutually exclusive. Investigators often looked for local, spatial, and environmental correlations in the incidence of tuberculosis without denying the contributory role of an individual's heredity, temperament, or constitution in any given case.

In the course of his investigation, Benoiston noticed something that several other doctors and hygienists had pointed out but that none had truly analyzed: women died of tuberculosis at a significantly higher rate than men. His occupational categories caused him to comment on the different circumstances faced by women and men in various professions, and this discussion eventually led him into a full-fledged diagnosis of the fundamental pathology of women.

SEXUAL INEQUALITY BEFORE DEATH (THE
"GENTLE AND UNFORTUNATE BIRTHRIGHT"
OF WOMEN)

Benoiston had one simple and one complicated explanation for the over-representation of women among the victims of tuberculosis. The simple one was menstruation and pregnancy, or, as he put it, "phenomena particular to [their] makeup, which appear with puberty and whose periodic return ceases only with age." "The precautions that [these phenomena] always demand, the troubles they often go through, the storms of pregnancy, [and] the complications that follow it are enough to show why consumption is more frequent among women from age 15 to 50."[39] In fact, at least one scholar has credited exactly these factors, which can diminish the body's resistance to infection, for the greater female susceptibility to tuberculosis that was evident for the first two-thirds of the nineteenth century.[40]

A slightly different point of view emerged, however, when Benoiston remarked that occupational category 7—occupations necessitating a forward-leaning or bent over position of the body—exhibited an especially marked sex differential in tuberculosis mortality.

> This innate weakness of women, gentle and unfortunate birthright of their sex [*triste et doux apanage de leur sexe*], which when they work alongside men exposes them to more than their share of dangers, this same weakness has another harmful result: it also condemns them to lesser earnings, and thereby to a state of poverty.[41]

In other words, being female—and therefore burdened with an "innate weakness"—intensified all the regular occupational hazards, including poverty. This intensified poverty, Benoiston continued, prevented women from properly nourishing themselves, which added to their "natural weakness as women, and render[ed] their constitution less capable of resisting harmful influence[s]." This diminished resistance argument was remarkable enough for its time—it would later be a staple of germ theory analysis—but what followed was even more of a departure from what had come before.

> Thereafter . . . poverty extinguishes neither the taste nor the desire for life's pleasures—and even intensifies these desires while it deprives one of their fulfillment. . . . [T]hese continual and ardent wishes for a better state soon become an urgent need [and] push those [women] . . . into a series of imprudences and lapses whose sad effects end up destroying [their] organs, which were already impaired by painful labor and by even more painful privations.[42]

The reference to prostitution was barely veiled. This fate was the result, Benoiston implied, of the economic inability to satisfy one's desires and the concomitant intensification of those desires. Moreover, its effects added to the strain on "already impaired organs" that labor and physical hardships had set in motion. This chain of circumstances, Benoiston concluded, pushed women to an early death. "Thus, on the one hand, a weaker constitution, meager wages and the resultant poverty, and on the other hand, active passions and . . . excesses of all sorts, lead rapidly to the grave for these weak beings, led astray by deceptive dreams."[43]

This arresting segment of Benoiston's otherwise staid article oscillates without warning from the inherent pathology of women to a critique of economic and sexual disempowerment, from fatalism to moral condemnation. In the final analysis, fatalism and moral condemnation share center stage. Commenting on the fact that some occupational categories did not show such a high susceptibility for women, Benoiston invoked "a sort of fate, an inevitable destiny," which explained why certain occupations accounted for more *filles publiques* than others. Because this "fate" did not apply to men, men were less susceptible to tuberculosis than were women.[44]

Simply by means of this brief didactic narrative,[45] Benoiston managed to equate biology with destiny and reduce the sexual differential in mortality to a moral question—prostitution. In this respect, he echoed Laënnec and other doctors who implicated "venereal excesses" in tuberculosis, and he also reflected the early hygienists' preoccupation with prostitution.[46] Although Benoiston attenuated the blame that went along with such moral questions by lamenting the social circumstances that set poor women on the path to depravity, he did not do away with it altogether. He referred to "immoral behavior" (*l'inconduite*) as one of the causes of high tuberculosis mortality and formulated a conclusion that could serve as one of the central credos of the hygienic movement: "Of all the enemies that threaten man's existence, the most dangerous [and] the most inevitable will always be himself."[47] Like the widespread disgust at the filthy, overcrowded environment of the city, the moralistic attribution of blame to tuberculosis victims would survive to become a central tenet of the dominant etiology at the end of the century.

Immediately following Benoiston's 1831 article in the *Annales d'hygiène publique* there appeared a brief contribution by Pierre-Charles-Alexandre Louis entitled "Note on the Relative Frequency of Phthisis in the Two Sexes." Louis remarked on the paucity of literature on the subject and complained that previous authors "[had] not, as far as I know, resolve[d] the question, . . . at least not in a rigorous and comprehensive manner."[48] One of the most prominent clinicians of the so-called Paris school in the early nineteenth century, Louis was the pioneer of the "numerical method," by which systematic observation and statistics were used to assess the accuracy of theories and the efficacy of therapies.[49] True to his method, he approached statistically the question of women's and men's relative susceptibility to *la phthisie*. Among tuberculosis patients treated by him at the Hôpital de la Charité between 1822 and 1825, Louis found 23 percent more women than men (although his figures, 70 women and 57 men, do not add up to his total of 123 patients). In addition, he found tubercles in the lungs of two-thirds more women than men who had died of causes other than tuberculosis (out of a sample divided evenly between the sexes). These figures and data he collected subsequently led Louis to conclude that women were 37 percent more likely than men to get tuberculosis.[50]

After establishing this differential (based though it was on a fairly small sample), Louis addressed two factors traditionally thought to predispose women to tuberculosis. The first culprit was tight clothing, particularly corsets, which were then in vogue among Parisian women. Corsets inhibited chest development, it was thought, and thus invited tuberculosis. Most of the consumptive women Louis treated, however, grew up in the countryside, working in the fields, and did not wear corsets until after their arrival in Paris, when their chests were already fully developed and corsets would have had little effect on the dimensions thereof. Moreover, tuberculosis was more common among females even during childhood, when corsets were not generally worn. Louis therefore rejected the idea that tight clothing contributed to the onset of the disease.[51]

Louis seemed to be persuaded, however, by another characteristic traditionally thought to be associated with the incidence of tuberculosis. "Lymphatic temperament," the humoral orientation that was thought to make certain people languid and sluggish, had long been considered "favorable to the development of consumption" and was "incontestably more frequent among women than among men," even in childhood, according to Louis. While he did not explicitly endorse this view, he noted that the statistical evidence "supports" it. Furthermore, his discussion of lymphatic temperament is the last paragraph of his "note"; it therefore occupies the place of a conclusion, whatever the author's intent.[52]

This is a classic expression of essentialist medical thought: women died of consumption more often than men because of their lymphatic nature. In fact, all the various interpretations of the sexual differential in tuberculosis provide further evidence of the fundamental compatibility between medical essentialism and the hygienists' social perspective.

Neither contagionism nor any other particular etiology was a precondition for examining disease from a social viewpoint or for charting its ramifications through society. While the rise of germ theory changed the language in which tuberculosis was depicted and oriented preventive strategies toward a focus on microbes, many of the constituent elements of the early-century essentialist etiologies of tuberculosis (including heredity, overcrowding, filth, and vice) maintained their status in the heyday of contagionism decades later.

PIDOUX VERSUS VILLEMIN: THE CONTAGION DEBATE

Around 1865, the terms of discussion surrounding tuberculosis began to change; the old debates were engaged in a new way as they began to take on a different tone, and doctors aligned themselves on one side or another of a new controversy concerning the disease: contagion. In that year, Jean-Antoine Villemin, a military physician, announced that he had succeeded in inoculating tuberculosis into laboratory rabbits. By injecting tuberculous matter from a human cadaver into the rabbits, Villemin had produced the disease in the animals. If true, inoculability implied, though it did not prove, contagiousness.

Skeptical reaction was quick to follow Villemin's claims, particularly after he reported his findings to the Academy of Medicine, the nation's most prestigious medical body. The academy's members were not inclined to accept such a radical reversal of conventional wisdom without thorough proof and lively debate. For decades, the controversial doctrine of contagionism—with the quarantines and other restrictions on commerce that it implied—had been anathema in established European medical circles and among liberals in general, as Ackerknecht pointed out in a now-classic 1948 article.[53] At the time, contagion was seen less as a revolutionary new idea than as a relic of the past, a vulgar superstition kept alive by the uninformed masses. Many doctors committed to the optimistic outlook of positivism viewed contagion as a prejudice that inspired fear among the populace, pitted citizen against citizen, and stigmatized the sick as enemies of the healthy.

Michel Peter, known to posterity as a fierce anticontagionist and Pasteur's most dogged opponent,[54] responded to Villemin's experiments even before the issue reached the academy. "The idea of the contagiousness of tuberculosis is almost universally—and nearly without discussion—rejected by contemporary scholars." After describing Villemin's methods, Peter concluded that the rabbits' illness resulted from

the injection of "cadaverous matter" and from "purulent or putrid infection" rather than from the communication of tuberculosis per se; he
suggested that the results would have been different if tuberculous matter from a live patient had been used instead. Peter defended the tenets
of hereditarian essentialism in terms scarcely changed from the days of
Laënnec. Yet there was perhaps a slight trace in Peter's argument of
the hygienists' social investigations, as he briefly mentioned poverty,
malnutrition, overwork, and overcrowding as causal factors in tuberculosis.[55]

After Villemin presented his findings to the Academy of Medicine,
Jules Guérin—the originator of the term "social medicine" and an active participant in the republican revolution of February 1848—rose to
refute the new contagionist claims. Like other progressive liberals in the
crucible of mid-nineteenth-century medicine, Guérin refused to sub-
scribe to the fearful creed of contagion. "Let us posit as a fact," he
said in response to Villemin, "that in its essence, tuberculosis is not
contagious." It was enough to consider nonpulmonary forms of tuberculosis, he argued, for the very notion of contagion to "provoke a widespread smile of incredulity." If tuberculosis in other parts of the body
was not contagious, then it was impossible for what all parties agreed
to be the same disease to be contagious in the lungs.[56] Guérin suggested
that Villemin's results could be explained by the quasi-miasmatic "pu-
trefaction" emanating from the lesions of late-stage tuberculosis, which
was capable of reproducing the disease "by a sort of graft." The ensuing
"pure infection," like Peter's "putrid infection," had nothing in common with contagion, he insisted.[57]

Villemin's fiercest critic of all, however, was the academy's Hermann
Pidoux. His intervention in the controversy over the contagion of tuberculosis (in the Academy of Medicine debate and in his contemporary
writings) deserves detailed scrutiny, because its often intriguing perspective and rationale were lost to history when it went down in ignomini-
ous defeat. Like Peter, Pidoux came to be remembered for his opposition to germ theory, for expressing the "ardor . . . [and] indignation of
the old medicine which, feeling itself overtaken by an irresistible progress, clings with bitter desperation to its traditional ideas."[58] Of course,
at the time, Pidoux felt that he was *defending* progress against the assault of an archaic and fanciful theory. "It is truly far too simple to say
that disease has as its cause disease—that is, its seeds[—]just as rabbits
and cabbages have as their cause cabbage seeds and rabbit semen." Pi-

doux could not hide his disdain for Villemin's contention that the tubercle (the small nodular lesion that characterizes tuberculosis) was not the
agent of the disease but *contained* the agent (later identified as the tubercle bacillus). "This concept is at once naive and vulgar. It comes
straight out of the Middle Ages. It is an animist doctrine of viruses, in
which the specific agent is conceived of as a soul existing by itself. . . .
This is very pleasing to the imagination, but it is not serious."[59]

Today, more than a century after the triumph of germ theory, it may
seem more than a little strange that an entrenched foe of one of the
basic truths of modern medicine could pose as a fighter of medieval
fantasy. Pidoux was not alone, however, in this perception; he simply
went further than most in ridiculing the contagionists and burning all
bridges behind him. He could not understand how "all acquired notions" of tuberculosis could be "overthrown"; or that suddenly, in the
onset of the disease, "the subject, the constitution, hygienic conditions,
heredity, and diatheses are nothing." And if tuberculosis were contagious and each patient received it from another patient, Pidoux asked,
how did the first patient get it? One ended up with such speculative
questions when, like Villemin, one extrapolated unreasonably from animal experimentation "without consulting clinical experience, [which]
every day bears witness" that the disease is not contagious.[60]

The direction in which medicine *should* be moving, Pidoux argued,
was neither toward the dead end of contagionism (which posited as the
cause of disease an invisible being beyond the reach of medicine or public health) nor in Laënnec's voluminous description and classification of
the symptoms and manifestations of tuberculosis. Rather, he called for
a "medicine of the species above and beyond the medicine of the individual." This new medicine would have to come up with "more advanced and more *social* solutions" to the problem of tuberculosis.[61] At
the same time, he defended the traditional essentialist concept of "morbid spontaneity"—the spontaneous rise of disease conditions in the
body itself—with a twist. Pidoux's spontaneity did not exclude the action of intervening causes. He said, "When I speak of spontaneity . . . I
am considering the organism in its milieu, that is . . . surrounded by
agents of hygiene, . . . by stimuli that are sufficient or insufficient, regular or irregular, favorable or harmful, healthy or unhealthy."[62] He proceeded to identify the most important of these intervening causes. Few
were actually new to the medical literature, but the way in which he set
them forth in his impassioned speech to the academy was impressive in

its comprehensiveness and its social perspective. In light of the debates that were to take place thirty to forty years later concerning the social causes of tuberculosis, Pidoux's polemic was ahead of its time.

Consumptives, he said, fell into three categories: (1) those who contracted the disease upon the influence of "appreciable external causes"; (2) those who contracted it upon the influence of "appreciable internal or pathological causes"; and (3) those in whom neither external nor internal causes were apparent, who must have contracted it through a diathesis, or constitutional predisposition. The first two categories corresponded roughly to social position: the poor and the rich, respectively. In the *phthisie des pauvres,* the crucial role was played by "external poverty [or misery]" (*la misère extérieure*); in the *phthisie des riches,* it was "internal poverty [or misery]" (*la misère intérieure*).[63] It should be noted that like many medical writers of his era, Pidoux operated within what now seems a disconcerting semantic minefield, one laced with vague terms for the most common and familiar conditions. In this case, however, the field becomes negotiable when the notions of internal and external misère are explained.

External misère, the contributory cause of tuberculosis among the poor, meant "ignorance, overwork, malnutrition, unsanitary housing, [and] deprivations of all sorts," according to Pidoux. Internal misère, bane of the rich, consisted of various chronic diseases, "laziness," "habits of luxury and flabbiness [*mollesse*], excesses at table, [and] the torments of ambition." Both types of misère resulted in "organic depletion" within the body, and in both cases, the "most common mode of degeneration" was tuberculosis. In other words, the poor got tuberculosis from poverty itself—because of "work in factories," because they were "malnourished," because they were "redeemed from serfdom but not yet from wage labor." In contrast, the rich got tuberculosis from overindulgence in their own wealth.[64]

Pidoux bristled when contagionists claimed factors such as overcrowding among the poor as evidence for their case and when they recommended slum clearance to "extinguish the sources of tuberculosis." This was actually prominent in his own antituberculosis program, he explained, because overcrowding and unsanitary housing contributed greatly to external misère. "Therefore, we have a better right to this argument than do the contagionists," he asserted contemptuously. To pretend otherwise, and to invoke overcrowding in service of contagion, was to mistake "the effect for the cause" (that is, to attribute the frequency of tuberculosis in close quarters to the frequency of tuberculosis in close quarters).[65]

Perhaps more significant than his willing engagement in medical polemics, however, was Pidoux's call for concerted public action against tuberculosis. Existing associations devoted to "improving the lot of the masses" were fighting the right battle, but Pidoux felt that they were not enough. He called for new public–private "leagues" to be formed around the nation, specifically dedicated to combating "the causes and multiplication of tuberculosis." "In every city [and] in every village, there should be a permanent and active association for the extinction of Consumption. . . . The wealthy should use all the means at their disposal to help in this effort." All of the area's physicians would be involved, as would the local clergy.[66]

But Pidoux did not envision just another philanthropic project. In this case, the state would have to intervene. Encouraging the creation of local leagues, "protecting them," contributing money, even heading them directly was the state's responsibility. Government representatives would need to be actively involved in local efforts and report to departmental prefects and other authorities on the leagues' progress. To those who thought his proposals unrealistic or utopian, Pidoux replied angrily, "What I am proposing is less chimerical and less utopian than the search for new remedies against Consumption, [whose products] we see advertised every day and which are a disgrace to Medicine." Instead of mesmerizing the public by promising miracle cures for tuberculosis, he seemed to be saying, medicine should be *mobilizing* the public.[67]

Pidoux's plan was unusual in two respects. First of all, except for smallpox vaccination and temporary emergencies such as cholera epidemics, such associations involving state participation were not a commonly accepted public health strategy in the 1860s, as they would be several decades later. Pidoux was one of the first to call for a government-sponsored fight against tuberculosis. Furthermore, demanding public intervention on a collective scale was a peculiar stance for an anticontagionist dedicated to preserving medical essentialism and morbid spontaneity. As he took pains to point out, however, spontaneity was not incompatible with the influence of external causes, and it was these external causes that Pidoux sought to battle through collective action.

There was also a poignant moment in Pidoux's speech before the Academy of Medicine. It reveals one of the most elemental reasons for many doctors' opposition to contagionism. Emotionally, Pidoux simply could not bring himself to believe in contagion, even in the face of Villemin's evidence: "What a calamity such a result would be! . . . [P]oor consumptives sequestered like lepers; the tenderness of [their] families at war with fear and selfishness." The possibility was too horrible for him to contemplate. "If consumption is contagious, we must not say it out loud" (*Si la phthisie est contagieuse, il faut le dire tout bas*), Pidoux concluded plaintively.

> Let us believe, then, until there is proof to the contrary, that we are right . . . we partisans of the spontaneous degeneration of the organism under the influence of [various] causes that we are seeking out everywhere, in order to combat the disease at its roots.[68]

In retrospect, this was a turning point in French society's understanding of tuberculosis. Pidoux felt that contagionism entailed nihilism and helplessness in preventive efforts; later, in the heyday of Pasteurian medicine, the point was debatable. There was no shortage of plans to extinguish the tubercle bacillus, but they had little, if any, effect. He also felt that to admit the truth of contagion would unleash fear and prejudice against those who had or were suspected of having the disease; on this point, he would later be proven correct.[69]

On the etiology of tuberculosis—bacteriologically speaking—Pidoux was wrong. He ventured so far out on the limb of anticontagionism that when Koch finally identified the tubercle bacillus in 1882, thereby convincing nearly all the remaining doubters that the disease was contagious, every aspect of Pidoux's argument was discredited. Overwork, low wages, poor diet, fighting tuberculosis by fighting poverty—all fell by the wayside until resurrected much later by the political Left. There is no indication that Pidoux was any kind of political radical, and in fact much of his writing on tuberculosis (including his request that the clergy involve itself in the public campaign against the disease) exhibits the prevailing medical moralism of his age. Nevertheless, he prefigured in some ways the later leftist critique of tuberculosis, and his ultimate failure was by no means assured at the time of the contagion debate. Instead of overthrowing hereditarian essentialism, Pidoux attempted to modify it and expand on it, entering certain new variables into the etiological equation of tuberculosis. He seems to have been concerned with steering medicine into areas in which preventive strategies, public health, and the state could fruitfully intervene. That he failed—and that germ theory emerged triumphant—ensured that his perspective would be forgotten.

The contagion debate at the Academy of Medicine did not settle the matter once and for all; uncertainty over the etiology of tuberculosis persisted even after Koch's identification of the tubercle bacillus in 1882. Beginning in the 1880s, however, the terms of discussion changed dramatically. Some habits survived from the essentialist era, including the adoption by bourgeois investigators of a disgusted and moralizing tone in describing the urban poor. These observers continued to look at the working class as if it were another species, filthy and brutish. Hygienists carried on Villermé's method, examining the differential effects of tuberculosis in society and zealously collecting information without any corresponding imperative for intervention. But filth was henceforth dangerous in a new way, and the living conditions of the working class now contained the deadly menace of contagion. Furthermore, tuberculosis became not just a social disease but a national problem. Old worries were expressed in a new vocabulary of microbes and degeneration.

There was another facet to essentialism, however, that proved more resistant than Laënnec's or Pidoux's ideas to the emergence of new perspectives. In fact, in the history of perceptions and meanings surrounding tuberculosis, the mid-nineteenth century is primarily remembered neither for debates about contagion nor for the early hygienists' investigations. Rather, this period is remembered as the age of the consumptive literary heroine, whose illness and death were tragic yet beautiful, with both physical and spiritual dimensions. The significance of this phenomenon, which transcended medical knowledge and rendered it all but irrelevant, is the subject of the next chapter.

CHAPTER TWO

Redemptive Suffering and the Patron Saint of Tuberculosis

Mais j'ai compris. Je suis expiatoire.
. . . renonçant, priant, demandant à souffrir,
S'allonge pour se tendre, et mincit pour s'offrir!
. . . l'aiglon se résigne
A la mort innocente et ployante d'un cygne.

[I understand. I am the atonement.
. . . renouncing, praying, begging to suffer,
I lay myself out, emaciated, as an offering!
. . . the eaglet is resigned
To the innocent and docile death of a swan.]
    —*Edmond Rostand,* L'Aiglon, *1900*

God has deigned to make me pass through many types of
trials. . . . I am truly happy to suffer.
    —*Thérèse Martin (Saint Thérèse of Lisieux), 1897*

In the late 1890s, the legendary French actress Sarah Bernhardt capti-
vated theatergoers in France and abroad as few performers have before
or since. At the zenith of her popularity, the woman known as "the
divine Sarah" enjoyed unprecedented adoration, and her decisions regarding which works to perform and with whom made or broke the
reputations of playwrights and fellow actors. In the autumn of 1897,
after touring Belgium, Sarah returned to Paris and began a financially
successful and critically acclaimed run of *La Dame aux camélias,* the
work with which she is more closely identified than any other in her
long career. Her portrayal of Marguerite Gautier, the kind-hearted
courtesan doomed to an untimely death from tuberculosis, epitomized
to many of her admirers her brilliance on the stage.[1]

Meanwhile, also in the autumn of 1897, a young nun in the Carmelite convent of Lisieux was enacting her own death scene from tuberculosis—this one all too real, but no less staged. Twenty-four-year-old Thérèse Martin had led an uneventful and sheltered life, taking the veil at age fifteen. Her precarious health had deteriorated under the assault of tuberculosis, and she spent much of her last few years in the convent's infirmary. During her illness, Sister Thérèse began to keep a diary at the insistence of the mother superior. She continued to record her emotions right up until her death, after which the convent authorities decided to publish her writings as an autobiography, entitled *Story of a Soul*. With its simple, accessible spirituality and its exaltation of all things humble, the book quickly sold out of several printings and was translated into nine languages within five years; Thérèse soon became a cult figure among Catholics both in France and abroad. In 1925, she became Saint Thérèse of the Child Jesus and of the Holy Face, and during World War II, Pope Pius XII proclaimed her co-patron saint of France, along with Joan of Arc.[2] (In English-speaking countries, she is better known as "the Little Flower of Jesus," or simply as "Little Flower.")

What could possibly connect these two very different celebrities, Sarah Bernhardt and Saint Thérèse of Lisieux? After all, they seem to represent opposite poles of womanhood: one, perhaps the quintessential society figure of her time, was born into prostitution and saw her adult romantic liaisons become the object of public scrutiny; the other lived at a distant remove from society and died a virgin. However, there are intriguing ties of sorority that bind this unlikely pair, the worldly and the cloistered, the actress and the nun. Both played important roles in the elaboration of a versatile and long-lasting cultural vision that associated tuberculosis with a heightened state of creativity, emotion, and spirituality and that lent a tragic and redemptive quality to the disease.

Briefly stated, tuberculosis served as a key vehicle in the nineteenth century through which womanhood was associated with a kind of suffering that was morally and spiritually redeeming. Moreover, around the turn of the century, even as the French state and the medical and philanthropic communities were elaborating and actively promoting a new vision of tuberculosis as a *social* problem of the first magnitude, the older reading of the disease as a sign of redemptive suffering persisted and even thrived, in a sense complementing but also implicitly

contesting the new sociomedical orthodoxy. The association of womanhood with tuberculosis—and, through tuberculosis, with suffering and
redemption—survived in part because it addressed a cultural need that
medical discourse and organized social reform movements could not
fulfill. And although it may have done so initially and most memorably
through artistic media such as literature, theater, and opera, the ideal
of the suffering female consumptive operated in other realms as well.
Evidence of its power can be found in the real-life infirmary at the convent in Lisieux and on the pages of Thérèse's autobiography as well as
on stage in Sarah's unforgettable deathbed scenes. To understand the
allure of the suffering saint and the captivating actress around the turn
of the century, one must look back to the years before germ theory,
when medicine looked to passion, temperament, and individual essence
to explain illness. One must also take seriously the act of storytelling as
a means of understanding disease.

For much of the nineteenth century, making sense of the familiar
but little-understood scourge of tuberculosis—and making sense of life
through tuberculosis—involved, above all, telling stories. The stories of
tuberculosis that have survived from this era and are retold most often
are fictional ones, literary and artistic productions that stand as enduring portraits of suffering, love, and redemption. The sweet, agonizing
deaths of Fantine, Mimi, and Camille (in *Les Misérables, La Bohème,*
and *Camille/La Traviata*) are especially familiar today on page, stage,
and screen, and all originated in mid-nineteenth-century French novels.
Yet the use of narrative in representing tuberculosis is hardly exhausted
by novels, plays, and operas. Nonfictional narratives of the disease—in
texts ranging from diaries and memoirs to medical publications and
political debates—were equally central in efforts to make sense of life,
illness, and death in the nineteenth century. Certain ingredients in both
the content and the style of the various tuberculosis stories seem to
have made narrative a particularly compelling strategy in all of these
contexts.[3] Medical and political texts will provide the material for subsequent chapters; here stories (both fictional and otherwise) from the
worlds of literature, the performing arts, and religion will be examined
for their treatment of one particularly enduring theme: the association
of womanhood with suffering and redemption.

The image of the frail, consumptive heroine sanctified through illness
and death resonates throughout nineteenth-century French literature.
From Marguerite Gautier to the bohemian Francine/Mimi to Hugo's

desperate Fantine, tuberculosis seems to have been the preferred cause
of death for a certain type of female character. For the purposes of this
discussion, five novels (including two that became famous operas) and
one play manifest the most significant aspects of the consumptive ideal:
Dumas's *La Dame aux camélias* (later Verdi's *La Traviata*), Murger's
Scènes de la vie de Bohème (later Puccini's *La Bohème*), Hugo's *Les
Misérables,* the Goncourt brothers' *Madame Gervaisais* and *Germinie
Lacerteux,* and Rostand's *L'Aiglon.* Each of these works deals in some
important way with tuberculosis, as does the nonfictional story of Thérèse Martin, who appropriated the consumptive ideal in coming to
terms with her own disease. No choice of just six literary works covering more than a half-century of French culture can be truly representative, and there are many others that involve tuberculosis in some
way.[4] These six, however, exemplify several different ways of using tuberculosis to tell stories, all the while pointing to the predominance,
versatility, and enduring power of the redemptive-spiritual perspective
on consumption and womanhood. While this persistent literary theme
is commonly referred to as "romantic," the term is—like its counterpart
"romantic medicine"[5]—evocative but technically misleading: only Dumas *fils,* Murger, and Hugo can plausibly be associated with the literary
movement of romanticism, and they were on the cusp of realism. However, all the works under discussion here, in addition to dealing with
tuberculosis, share the preoccupation with sentimentality, passion, and
spirituality that characterized romanticism.

Most historians of tuberculosis have tended to treat the romantic
literary vision either as a quaint, entertaining sidelight to the medical
history of the disease or as support for the contention that the disease
sets in motion biochemical processes that actually heighten patients'
passion, sex drive, and emotional experience. A few have taken the consumptive ideal more seriously as a historical phenomenon of the early
and mid-nineteenth century; they argue that by the end of the century,
it was replaced or supplanted by the sociomedical view of tuberculosis,
and the tragic romantic heroine gave way to the specter of the contagious, working-class *semeur de bacilles* ("sower" or "disseminator"
of bacilli).[6] This chapter attempts to show, on the contrary, that the
redemptive-spiritual view persisted long after the sociomedical understanding arose and that (far from being mutually exclusive) the two
sets of meanings coexisted, at once complementing and contesting each
other, throughout the Belle Epoque.

SANCTIFYING THE FALLEN WOMAN:
DUMAS, MURGER, HUGO

La Dame aux camélias, best known to later audiences as Verdi's opera
La Traviata, stands as perhaps the consummate expression of the nineteenth-century consumptive ideal.[7] In the novel, first published in 1848,
Alexandre Dumas *fils* brings together all the elements through which
tuberculosis conveyed an idealized image of femininity in the nineteenth
century: the disease's wasting effect on the body is portrayed as enhanc-
ing feminine beauty; the fallen woman is paradoxically depicted as
more virtuous than the "respectable" citizens around her; the impossibility of pure love in an imperfect world propels the tragic inevitability
of the plot; and the heroine is finally redeemed through suffering and
death. The consumptive courtesan Marguerite Gautier comes to represent Everywoman, required to be both virtuous and alluring, and compelled to find identity in worldly suffering and the promise of other-
worldly redemption.

When Marguerite meets the young bachelor Armand Duval and finds
true love for the first time, she faces a dilemma: to maintain her extravagant and leisurely life in Paris, where her wealthy patron, the Count of
Varville, provides for her every material need, or to abandon that life
for her lover of more modest means. She chooses to follow her heart
and leaves for the provinces with Armand. This choice, however, immediately confronts Marguerite with her second dilemma, the problem at
the heart of the novel's tragic development. Even true love cannot
change her fundamental status as sinner against—and outcast from—
bourgeois morality. Armand's family cannot tolerate the couple's continued liaison, and his father pleads with Marguerite to end it. The relationship has sullied the family name and endangered the impending
marriage of Armand's sister. Marguerite feels the strong pull of emotional attachment, a feeling foreign to her previous life as a fashionable
prostitute, but realizes that her love for Armand is an impossible one
under the prevailing cultural circumstances. Forced to renounce her
love (and forbidden by his father to tell Armand of the real reason),
Marguerite returns to Paris and to prostitution. Before long, however,
emotional anguish and tuberculosis take their toll. In an emotional
deathbed scene, she is reconciled with Armand and with her fate; she
dies ennobled and at peace.

As much as any literary heroine, Marguerite embodies the classic
saint-and-sinner dichotomy imputed to woman's nature in nineteenth-

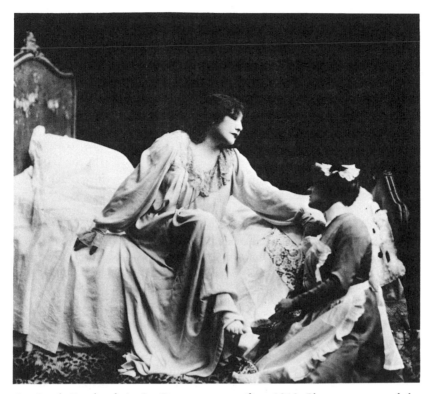

6.   Sarah Bernhardt in *La Dame aux camélias*, 1913. Photo courtesy of the Library of Congress.

century bourgeois society. She was "the virgin that a trifle [*un rien*] had made a courtesan, and the courtesan that a trifle would have made the most loving and pure virgin." [8] But this trifle made all the difference and sealed her fate. In the case of Marguerite, tuberculosis is more than an illness. It is her condition, her destiny, something to be resigned to, not to be cured. "Ah! There's no point in you getting alarmed," she reassures Armand after a coughing spell, "there's nothing anyone can do about this sickness." Like other tuberculous heroines, and like all martyrs, she accepts her destiny bravely and stoically: "Girls like me, one more or one less, what does it matter?" "Doomed to live a shorter life than others, I've promised myself to live a faster one." [9]

Like death from tuberculosis, Marguerite's fate is inevitable: she tries twice, once before and once after meeting Armand, to reenter polite society, but each time she is not accepted. On the novel's final page, Dumas wonders whether "all girls like Marguerite" (that is, all prostitutes) would be able to do what she did: "I only know that one of them felt in her life a serious love, that she suffered from it, and that she died of it."[10] Tuberculosis plays a crucial role as vehicle of both suffering and death. Yet the couple's love is impossible—and demands such harsh retribution—only because of social convention. As various critics have pointed out, society will not allow Marguerite to live; it cannot incorporate her type of woman, when social conformity is a higher imperative than love. "Happiness can only be realized," one critic has written, "in conformity with regular conditions of social life. . . . [I]n the name of society, [Dumas] condemns the courtesan."[11] Marguerite's redemption is real but is not based only on love.

> Marguerite is redeemed, not just because of the depth and sincerity of her love for Armand . . . but rather because of her heroic renunciation of this love for the sake of Armand and of society, and her acceptance of her punishment, because of her realization that she is wrong and the community right; so that, as she lies dying, all but excised from the social body, Armand may without fear of contamination return to her.[12]

Only renunciation and death could ultimately bring out the virgin in the courtesan.

With all of the sentimentality of *La Dame aux camélias* but somewhat less of the tragedy, Henry Murger's *Scènes de la vie de Bohème*[13] presents the death of a consumptive heroine in a minor key. The novel, a pastiche of episodes and portraits serialized in *Le Corsaire* between 1845 and 1849 and published as a novel in 1851, depicts the unstable and often comical existence of Bohemian writers, artists, and *grisettes* in Paris. The bulk of Murger's novel is concerned with the stormy relationship of Rodolphe and Mimi; the latter displays the pallid beauty and joie de vivre of the typical consumptive heroine but is not portrayed as ill. One chapter or "scene" concerns the ill-fated romance of Jacques and Francine, two friends of Rodolphe and Mimi; Francine is this novel's embodiment of fateful and beautiful suffering from tuberculosis.[14]

In both Mimi and Francine, Murger uses the physical type of the consumptive woman to signify beauty, youth, and carefree passion. Mimi is described as frail and delicate, "as pale as the angel of consumption." "The blood of youth [runs] hot and fast in her veins, and add[s] a rosy tint to her skin, [otherwise] transparent with the whiteness of a camelia."[15] It is unclear whether this description was written before or after the publication of *La Dame aux camélias,* although the camelia's echo is hardly coincidental. As a personal fetish, Marie Duplessis, the real-life inspiration for Marguerite in Dumas's novel, sur-rounded herself with camelias. Consumptive heroines up to and includ-ing Thérèse of Lisieux are often associated with flowers, a symbol of ephemeral beauty and the transitory nature of life itself.

The character of Francine develops even more clearly the mutual as-sociation of tuberculosis, womanhood, and ephemeral beauty. In her, as in most of her fictional counterparts, the essentialist perspective on disease assumes a literary, nonmedical form. The view of tuberculosis as part of one's essence and underlying identity, which led Laënnec and other medical authorities to seek the disease's causes in heredity, lym-phatic temperament, and "sad passions,"[16] led Murger and other nov-elists to depict it as the tragic, inevitable destiny of their heroines—a trait as fundamental to their identities as their femininity or their beauty. For Francine, it is "a vague premonition of her imminent pass-ing" (*un vague pressentiment de sa fin prochaine*) that leads her at age twenty to abandon herself completely to her love for Jacques. It soon becomes apparent to both young lovers that Francine is a *poitrinaire*, or consumptive, and shortly after their romance begins in the spring, a doctor friend tells Jacques that Francine will not live past the "yellow leaves" of autumn.[17] Francine's beauty is both timeless (in its purity) and ephemeral, and like the elemental, seasonal cycles of nature—like the falling leaves and the camelias—tuberculosis did not leave beauty much time to blossom before dying.

On her deathbed, knowing that she will soon die but wishing to shield Jacques from this fact, Francine asks him to buy her a fancy fur muff to keep her hands warm. The last yellow leaf from the tree outside her room then blows through her open window and onto her bed; the two lovers spend one last night together, and in the morning, on All Saints' Day, Francine dies, clinging to her muff for warmth. She knew that she was dying, "because God does not want me to live any longer," and her last words were "my God!" Through her illness, Francine is clearly sanctified in death, and when Jacques arranges her body for the casting of a death mask, the light "cast all of its clarity on the consump-tive's face," giving her a saintly glow, "as if she had died of beauty." At the funeral, Jacques cries out, "O my youth! It is you that we are bury-ing!"[18] Youth, pure beauty, and passion are not permanently of this earth in the romantic worldview; they express their purity and achieve transcendence only through death, thereby becoming celestial ideals that live on forever. Like Marguerite, though without the full weight of her social stigma, Francine was too pure and beautiful for her earthly existence; tuberculosis both proved these women's purity and purified them.

Ten years after Dumas and Murger, Victor Hugo used tuberculosis to tell quite a different story, but in so doing he reinforced the basic tenets of the redemptive-spiritual perspective and the consumptive ideal of womanhood. In his epic *Les Misérables* (1862), Hugo unremittingly attacks greed, callousness, and injustice in society. The story of Fantine—a case of "society buying a slave" and finally killing her—serves as a particularly effective vehicle for his social message. Yet it is significant that the means by which Fantine becomes a martyr to the cause of social justice all but replicates the treatment of such apparently nonpolitical heroines as Marguerite and Francine. It is above all the "grace, frailty, [and] beauty" of women in general and Fantine in particular that contain the feminine destiny: for Fantine, these qualities doom her to prostitution when she is unfairly fired from her factory job and must somehow find money to pay for her daughter Cosette's room and board.[19] Hugo echoes and amplifies Dumas in insisting on the thinness of the line between virtuous and fallen and in suggesting that women are imprisoned in this dichotomy that allows no middle ground.

Hugo also allows no uncertainty on the matter of the immediate origins of Fantine's illness; for example, "excessive work fatigued Fantine, and her slight dry cough got worse." Labor and poverty cause her tuberculosis, which worsens with her deteriorating material condition and improves only when she is given hope that she would soon be reunited with Cosette. In the end, Fantine's illness is both sign and vehicle of her martyrdom; on her deathbed, Jean Valjean even tells her, "I was praying to the martyr on high," then adds under his breath, "—for the martyr here below." As he makes his fateful promise to look after Cosette in Fantine's absence, Valjean reassures the dying mother that her suffering and death are necessary: "It is in this way that mortals become angels. . . . This hell you have just left is the first step toward Heaven. You had to begin there." When Fantine dies, Hugo does not skimp on the traces of her martyrdom and saintliness. Her body trembles as if "an unseen fluttering of wings" is preparing to take her away; "she looked more likely to soar away than to die"; "at this instant Fantine's face seemed strangely luminous."[20] The tuberculosis that originated in her poverty and fatigue serves to lift her above her earthly condition, and her martyrdom redeems not her own sins but the sins of an unjust society.

Fantine's demise recalls that of American literature's most saintly

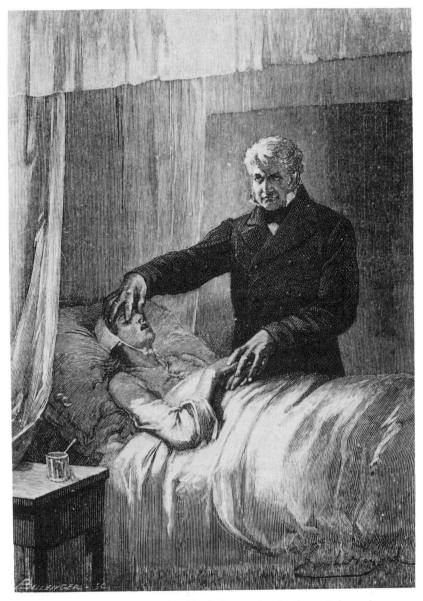

7.   Jean Valjean at Fantine's deathbed. Illustration by Bayard, from the
Hugues edition of *Les Misérables* (1879–1882).

tuberculosis victim, Little Eva of *Uncle Tom's Cabin*. Critic Jane Tompkins has argued that the sentimentality of such nineteenth-century women's novels—rather than providing escape from or even justifying "an oppressive social order"—served in its own way as an effective form of protest. In Tompkins's view, the common critical assessment of Little Eva's death as "nothing more than a sob story" ignores the ways in which extreme sentimentality can express "a theory of power."

> Stories like the death of little Eva are compelling for the same reason that the story of Christ's death is compelling: they enact a philosophy, as much political as religious, in which the pure and powerless die to save the powerful and corrupt, and thereby show themselves more powerful than those they save.[21]

The same can be said of Hugo's Fantine. The angelic aura surrounding her death and the circumstances of her life and illness certainly increase through sentimentality her image as socially redemptive martyr. But the same cannot be said of her fellow French literary victims of tuberculosis, whose suffering seems to redeem mainly themselves and women as a class. In this context, Fantine is exceptional in her political message but typical in her femininity, in the paradox of her purity and prostitution, and in her physical suffering. The most salient characteristic that binds all of these figures together, in short, is what it means to be a woman.

LATER VARIATIONS ON A ROMANTIC THEME

When romantic sentimentalism fell out of favor in French literature, the theme of women suffering from tuberculosis endured. Edmond and Jules de Goncourt, in two of their best-known novels, *Germinie Lacerteux* and *Madame Gervaisais,* managed to adopt the traditional literary usage of tuberculosis without endorsing it. Their occasionally cynical attitude toward their heroines implies that their handling of tuberculosis is meant to critique or even denounce the romantic tradition. However, in the final analysis, their treatment conforms so closely to that of their predecessors that the authors' intentions become irrelevant. They use tuberculosis to evoke a certain constellation of emotions and values; this evocation ultimately takes center stage, whether the Goncourts ultimately wish to project or reject these values.

Although the novel appeared only two years after *Les Misérables,* the title character of *Germinie Lacerteux* (1864) will never be confused with Fantine.[22] The unhappy domestic is continually beaten down by poverty and love, her attachment to an undeserving paramour leading her into a morass of self-destruction and despair. Germinie inherits the worst of both Marguerite and Fantine, devoted beyond reason to an impossible relationship, driven to drink and even a kind of prostitution. That tuberculosis finally claims Germinie testifies—on the surface— only to the depths of her self-abasement. "She sought to imagine the degree of humiliation to which her love would refuse to sink, but she could not find it. . . . [S]he would remain under the heel of his boots!" None of her acquaintances sinks so low in love; none invests the "bitterness, torment, [and] happiness in suffering" that Germinie puts into her liaison with Jupillon. It "killed her and she could not do without [it]." In stark contrast to Marguerite Gautier, Germinie goes to extraordinary lengths to maintain her impossible relationship, showering her lover with gifts that she cannot afford.[23]

Nevertheless, no matter how much the Goncourts depict Germinie's suffering as debased rather than exalted, she retains the fundamental qualities of woman's nature that qualify her for elevation to the status of consumptive heroine. When Jupillon is avoiding her and she stakes out his apartment in the rain, Germinie is wet and miserable yet strangely oblivious to her circumstances. She no longer feels anything "except the suffering of the soul." After Germinie eventually dies in the hospital, having sunk to the lowest depths imaginable, having lost money, love, sanity, and dignity, her employer (Mlle. de Varandeuil) is haunted by visions of her face in death. The horror is gone from the face in the apparition; "only suffering remained there, but [it was] a suffering of expiation, almost of prayer."[24] Finally, after plumbing the depths of humiliation, stripped of all but her last shred of humanity, Germinie is redeemed and purified. Of course, this redemption and purification takes place only in the imagination of the pious and moralistic Mlle. de Varandeuil. The authors appear to distance themselves from this exaltation of Germinie, if not ridicule it outright; yet they give her suffering and death no other meaning, no alternative interpretation. Like Marguerite, she dies as both sinner and victim, for whom tuberculosis provides deliverance and atonement.

If Germinie Lacerteux comes from the gray area where woman's nature meets the accident of social circumstance, the Goncourt brothers' other consumptive protagonist represents a hothouse variety of the spirituality contained in the French literary-religious reading of tuberculosis. Madame Gervaisais has scarcely any bodily existence at all; because

of her tuberculosis, every physical description of her downplays her cor-
poreality and highlights her asceticism. "Barely terrestrial," with the
"austere figure of a psychic creature," she lives a life that becomes with
each passing day more ethereal and less connected to her earthly surroundings. Starting a new life and convalescence with her young son in
Rome, the Frenchwoman falls under the influence of zealous clerics who
lead her into renunciation and fanaticism. Tuberculosis, which "softly
snuffed out the life of Mme. Gervaisais, . . . singularly helped steer the
mysticism . . . of this body that was becoming a spirit toward the super-
natural achievement of spirituality." [25]

Once again, self-abasement and love of suffering are essential elements of the female identity. As Madame Gervaisais's religious practices become more and more severe, her illness intensifies. First she
"cloisters" herself in her apartment, limiting as much as possible her
contact with the outside world. Then she begins to revel in humility and
privation.

> The more she absorbed the humility prescribed by her ascetic readings, . . .
> the more she heard herself repeating . . . that she deserved disdain and abjec-
> tion . . . that she was worthy of horror, damnation, anathema, execration—
> the closer she approached to the lowest depths of abasement and loss of
> personality.

Madame Gervaisais's "ambition" is to achieve a state of "holy everyday
torture." Her health deteriorates, but she accepts it with "that pious
fatalism that the exaltation of devotion often brings to women"; she
sees her illness as a matter "in God's hands," and "suffering bec[omes]
in her eyes a kind of spiritual advancement." [26]

The correspondence of themes between *Madame Gervaisais* and
Thérèse of Lisieux's autobiography (discussed more fully below) is
striking, as are their similar responses to suffering. The Goncourts'
novel can be read as a critique of religious attitudes that they considered
prevalent or at least a culturally significant phenomenon—attitudes that
Thérèse shared and developed even further in her life and writings. The
Goncourts obviously regarded such attitudes with a certain amount of
disdain. For example, they perceive in their novel a causal relation between Madame Gervaisais's tuberculosis and her spiritual excesses.

> The disease, the slow disease that extinguished almost softly the life of Mme.
> Gervaisais, *phtisis* singularly helped along [her] mysticism [and] ec-
> stasy. . . . [T]he gradual . . . death of the flesh under the cavernous ravages
> of the disease [and] the growing dematerialization of the physical being
> took her ever closer to the holy folly and hallucinated delights of reli-

gious love [*vers les folies saintes et les délices hallucinées de l'amour reli-gieux*].[27]

This ascription of mental and emotional symptoms to tuberculosis is part of the traditional romantic view, although the Goncourts clearly scorn these "hallucinatory" religious manifestations. More significant, perhaps, than their judgment of such "pious fatalism" and "exaltation of devotion" is their association of it—along with many other romantic and later authors—with womanhood and with the female condition. In other words, the Goncourts seem to share the romantic/Christian view of woman's essence, and they too use tuberculosis to express it, even though they ridicule rather than celebrate woman and her religious spirituality.

On the surface, a male tuberculous protagonist who captured the public imagination would seem to belie the contention that the redemptive-spiritual understanding of tuberculosis in the nineteenth century rested on a certain perception of womanhood. However, the Duke of Reichstadt in Rostand's play *L'Aiglon* actually reinforces the consumptive ideal by deviating from it. His character is feminized to such an extent—and his fate so closely linked to this feminization—that he becomes an appropriate exemplar of a traditionally female cultural role. In fact, Rostand wrote the part of "the Eaglet" expressly for his friend Sarah Bernhardt, and she inaugurated the role at the play's premiere on March 15, 1900.[28] *L'Aiglon* covers the last two years of the duke's life in the Austrian palace of Schönbrunn before his death from tuberculosis in 1832, at age twenty-one. The play focuses on the tragedy of his thwarted destiny as the frail and sickly son of the vigorous and heroic emperor; it follows his strained relationship with his mother and with the wily Prince Metternich, who is haunted by the first Napoleon, and it builds up to the climax of a nearly successful conspiracy to return the duke to France.

In one especially revealing scene, Flambeau, the loyal, incognito veteran of the Napoleonic wars, torments Metternich with convincing evocations of the empire. The terrified, delusional Metternich is taken in by Flambeau's ruse and half expects Napoleon himself to appear from the bedroom. Instead, it is a coughing young duke who emerges to find the cause of the ruckus distracting him: Rostand's stage directions describe his appearance.

> Instead of the terrible, short and thickset silhouette that [Flambeau] had almost made one expect to see, on the threshold is the unsteady apparition

of a mere child, too slim ... white as his gown ... rendered even more
feminine by his unfastened collar, under which the fabric of an undergar-
ment was visible, and by his blond hair in the lamplight.[29]

Throughout the play, the duke is portrayed as feminine both in appearance and in personality: he is highly sensitive, emotional, and indecisive
à la Hamlet, another of Sarah's famous roles.

As is the case with his female literary counterparts, the duke's tuberculosis is part of his tragic essence, and he realizes it. When he is asked
by a young Bonapartist conspirator, "Pale prince, so pale in your black
tie, / What makes you pale?" the duke replies, "Being his son!" Later,
he reflects on the meaning of his own death. "It is not from the crude
poisoning of melodramas / That the Duke of Reichstadt is dying: it is
from his soul! / . . . From my soul and my name!"[30] This essentialist
explanation fits the romantic pattern: his illness expresses his sensitivity
and his thwarted destiny, which in turn comes from his innate inability
to live up to his father. (Rostand traces this failing to the Hapsburg
bloodline of the duke's mother, Napoleon's second wife, Marie-
Louise.[31]) In the end, as also befits the consumptive ideal, the essential
affliction is redemptive. Coughing up blood as he surveys the plain of
Wagram, site of the emperor's glorious victory in 1809, the cries of the
battle's victims ringing in his ears, the frail duke envisions his suffering
and death as atonement for the blood spilled by his father's armies.

> I understand. I am the atonement.
> . . . renouncing, praying, begging to suffer,
> I lay myself out, emaciated, as an offering!
> . . . the eaglet is resigned
> To the innocent and docile death of a swan.[32]

When Sarah spoke these lines on stage, she reprised, in a sense, her
famous performance as Marguerite in La Dame aux camélias. (The
scene also links Sarah and the duke with Germinie Lacerteux and Thérèse of Lisieux, among others, who also "begg[ed] to suffer" from tuberculosis.) The duke's martyrdom expiates the carnage of Wagram,
and he dies a feminine death, "the innocent and docile death of a
swan." In the same scene, Rostand even puts in the duke's mouth words
spoken by Jesus on the cross, leaving no doubt as to the redemptive
significance of the duke's suffering.[33]

Thus, even with its male protagonist and referents, L'Aiglon evokes
the essentialist ideal of tuberculosis, feminine suffering, and redemption. To be sure, the real Duke of Reichstadt did in fact die of tuberculo-

sis, so Rostand did not simply choose the disease as a vehicle for a certain set of values. No account of the "Eaglet's" life could plausibly have ignored the cause of his untimely death. Nonetheless, Rostand did emphasize the disease—and the many cultural associations that went along with it—as both *sign* of his tragic essence and (in part) *cause* of his failure to measure up to his father. Like the Goncourts' satire, Rostand's deviation from the conventional redemptive-spiritual depiction of tuberculosis only preserved and strengthened its fundamental tenets.

THE CONSUMPTIVE HEROINE AS SAINT: THÉRÈSE OF LISIEUX

The consumptive career of Thérèse Martin is both simpler and harder to grasp than those of her fictional counterparts. The spoiled youngest of five daughters in a devout family, Thérèse entered the convent at fifteen, permission for which required special dispensation from the Catholic hierarchy. She lived there for nine years, before dying in the convent infirmary in 1897. As a result of her sheltered and cloistered existence, in contrast to most saints, Thérèse experienced and accomplished next to nothing in her entire life. Just before taking the habit, she prayed for the soul of a convicted murderer on the eve of his execution; it was later reported that the condemned man repented and kissed a crucifix after mounting the guillotine. This was the only instance of intercession or worldly works in her short life. (After her death, many miracles were attributed to her intervention, often involving wounds healed or illnesses cured after prayers addressed to her.) Although she never left Normandy except for a childhood visit to the Vatican, she was made patron saint of missions in 1927, two years after her canonization.[34]

Thérèse is a puzzle. The only thing she did that can explain her popularity and sainthood was write her memoirs—itself a strange undertaking for an adolescent girl who had little life experience. It is testimony to her unique brand of spirituality, to what she called her "little way," that when published after her death, her autobiography achieved such lasting popularity and inspired a cult that lasts to this day. Lisieux is perennially the second most popular pilgrimage destination in France, after Lourdes. Statues of Thérèse stand in thousands of Catholic churches around the world, objects of veneration especially for women and children. Her popularity sparked a kind of religious revival in early-twentieth-century France and forced the church to begin canonization proceedings despite the opposition of some ecclesiastical authorities.[35]

Simply put, Thérèse did little else in life but fall ill, suffer, write, and die. The hallmarks of her life were her suffering and her writing, and therein must lie the key to her extraordinary popularity. The inescapable conclusion suggested by *Story of a Soul,* Thérèse's autobiography, is that she wrote about suffering in a manner that closely parallels the fictional ideal of consumptive woman. Her "little way" touted self-effacement bordering on self-abasement and humility that verged on humiliation as the path to saintliness. In the convent, Thérèse shunned material comforts such as warmth and food and suffered everyday injustices and jealousies in silence. (Just one of the paradoxes of her autobiography is that she cannot communicate the importance of suffering in silence without breaking that silence in a detailed and sustained fashion; she dwells at length on petty episodes so as to urge that such matters not be dwelled on or complained about.) Thérèse deliberately sat next to the most annoying gossip in the convent at refectory and endured her torment silently; she even prevented herself from leaning back in her chair. In the early stages of her illness, she refused special treatment and insisted on going about her chores as usual.[36]

Tuberculosis was indeed the chief vehicle of suffering in Thérèse's life. No incident better illustrates the importance of the disease in her spiritual world than the Good Friday hemoptysis. After observing a rigorous Lenten fast in 1896, Thérèse went to bed on the eve of Good Friday and felt a joyous sensation.

> Oh! how sweet this memory really is! . . . I had scarcely laid my head upon the pillow when I felt something like a bubbling stream mounting to my lips. I didn't know what it was, but I thought that perhaps I was going to die and my soul was flooded with joy.

The morning of the sacred day brought confirmation of her fate, as she indeed found blood on her handkerchief.

> Upon awakening, I thought immediately of the joyful thing that I had to learn, and so I went over to the window. I was able to see that I was not mistaken. Ah! my soul was filled with a great consolation; I was interiorly persuaded that Jesus, on the anniversary of His own death, wanted to have me hear His first call.[37]

This hemoptysis, or coughing up of blood, meant tuberculosis, and tuberculosis meant death. It was Thérèse's first externally verifiable sign that she would soon be with her "Bridegroom," as "Jesus wished to

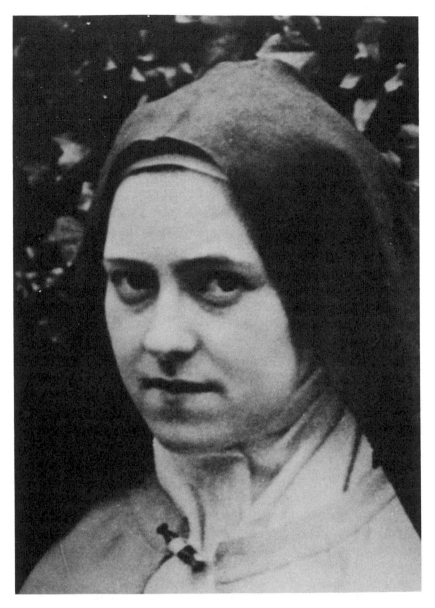

8.   Thérèse in June 1897, three months before her death. Photo courtesy of the Office central de Lisieux.

give [her] the hope of going to see Him soon in heaven." Again, as with Rostand's Duke of Reichstadt, the truth of real life intrudes on interpretation: just as Rostand did not invent the fact that the duke had tuberculosis, it would take the most extreme cynicism to doubt that Thérèse's first hemoptysis took place on Good Friday, whereas, for example, Francine's death on All Saints' Day, which carries a similar symbolic significance, is Murger's artful contrivance. However, the sense that she made of her experience was clearly culturally determined, and she called attention in *Story of a Soul* to this episode as a turning point in her life and faith.

The importance of the Good Friday episode cannot be overstated. The calendrical coincidence of receiving a sign of her impending death on the day commemorating the death of Christ does not exhaust its significance. Throughout her hagiography as well as within the structure of the autobiography, this 1896 incident stands out as a landmark in the progression of both her physical illness and her spiritual calling. This was the first crucial sign that death was relatively near, that Thérèse was materially different from her peers, and that her emotional idiosyncrasies (including her extreme sensitivity, her spoiled child's tendency to cry easily, and her penchant for self-abnegation) had a spiritual basis and needed to be taken seriously. The fact that it was tuberculosis and the fact that it happened on Good Friday called forth a strong link between the physical and the spiritual and suggested that Thérèse was destined to be out of the ordinary.

The young nun understood her fate immediately as the fulfillment of a long-standing wish. "I never did ask God for the favor of dying young, but I have always hoped this be His will for me." From that point on, the love of suffering that had been only one among her many distinguishing features became the focal point of her existence. "God has deigned to make me pass through many types of trials. I have suffered very much since I was on earth, but, if in my childhood I suffered with sadness, it is no longer in this way that I suffer. It is with joy and peace. I am truly happy to suffer." And she continued to suffer, through the sleeplessness, coughing, weakness, and difficult breathing brought on by her illness. Shortly before her death, when someone asked her what had become of her "little life," Thérèse answered, "My 'little life' is to suffer; that's it!"[38] With the fulfillment of death so close, the only meaning left in her life came through the experience of suffering—and in properly depicting the joy of suffering through her writings.

When her strength finally gave out and she could no longer bring herself to write, Thérèse continued her teachings through her conversations with those around her in the convent. The Martin sisters apparently felt that Thérèse's thoughts and writings would someday reach a wider audience (although nobody could have predicted at the time how wide the audience would become).[39] As a result, her last conversations were zealously recorded; some of them were published as part of her autobiography immediately after her death, and others were collected in separate publications. They carry her exaltation of suffering via tuberculosis through to the moment of her death. For example, on two separate occasions, Thérèse commented to her sister Pauline (then prioress of the convent) on the progressive emaciation of her hands, saying, "I'm becoming a skeleton already, and that pleases me," and "Oh, what joy I experience when seeing myself consumed!" As with the literary heroines, it is the wasting away of the body that allows the spirit to flourish. Near the end, when Pauline spoke of her wish that death would come soon so as to spare her sister further suffering, Thérèse replied, "Yes, but you mustn't say that, little Mother, because suffering is exactly what attracts me in life."[40]

Thérèse's conversations during her illness with her other sister and best friend, Céline, go even further toward explaining the relationship between physical suffering and religious fulfillment. Thérèse occasionally showed Céline her makeshift *crachoir*, a saucer in which she deposited her sputum. "Often she pointed to its rim with a sad little look that meant 'I would have liked it to be up to there!' " Céline answered jealously, "Oh! it makes no difference whether it was little or much, the incident itself is a sign of your death." Later, in the throes of late-stage tuberculosis, Thérèse experienced her pain as a trial sent by the devil and bore it accordingly. For a long time, her illness affected her right side in particular, she told Céline, until "God asked me if I wanted to suffer for you, and I immediately answered that I did." "At the same instant, my left side was seized with an incredible pain. *I'm suffering for you,* and the devil doesn't want it!"[41] A direct, one-to-one correspondence was established between spiritual desire and bodily symptom.

When the agony of tuberculosis made it difficult for Thérèse to breathe, she could not avoid expressing her pain. However, wanting to avoid at all costs giving the impression of complaining, she enlisted Céline in a poignant exchange to help her through the pain. Thérèse found herself repeating out loud, "I'm suffering," and told her sister to answer her every repetition with "All the better":

THÉRÈSE: *"Je souffre."* [I'm suffering.]
CÉLINE: *"Tant mieux."* [All the better.]
THÉRÈSE: *"Je souffre."*
CÉLINE: *"Tant mieux."*
THÉRÈSE: *"Je souffre."*
CÉLINE: *"Tant mieux."*

And so on, over and over.[42] There was not a trace of irony in Céline's reply, or in Thérèse's instruction to reply in this manner. She had come to desire suffering for its own sake, not just as a spiritual trial or as a sign of beatitude, although it was these things as well.

On her deathbed, her last words as recounted by her sisters maintained the exaltation of suffering until the end. Céline reported that Thérèse, in extreme pain, placed her arms in the form of a cross, and "our poor little martyr [looked like] a living image of Him." She then spoke through the pain.

> I am . . . I am reduced. . . . No, I would have never believed one could suffer so much . . . never, never! O Mother, I no longer believe in death for me. . . . I believe only in suffering! Tomorrow, it will be still worse! Well, so much the better![43]

Pauline's version differs slightly, adding an extra theological lesson to the passion of Saint Thérèse. After the phrase, "Never would I have believed it was possible to suffer so much! never, never!" Pauline reported that Thérèse added, "I cannot explain this except by the ardent desires I have had to save souls." All accounts agree on her last words: "Oh! I wouldn't want to suffer less! . . . Oh! I love Him. . . . My God . . . I . . . love You!"[44] (The ellipses here indicate pauses rather than omissions.) The last phrase appears on many of her statues. This deathbed coda serves to reiterate the basic theme of Thérèse's story: spiritual exaltation expresses itself through bodily suffering.

It is impossible to know whether Thérèse had read romantic novels or any of the literature that drew on the consumptive ideal of female suffering. She had certainly read the lives of the saints, in which suffering is similarly exalted. Whether her reproduction and reenactment of the ideal was conscious mimicry, subconscious role-playing, or merely coincidental resemblance makes little difference. Ultimately, what matters is that Thérèse learned how to be consumptive, whatever the sources of her inspiration. What she and the novelists had in common was the use of tuberculosis to express an age-old Christian attitude that exalted women's suffering as sublime, spiritual, and potentially redemptive. On the most basic level, of course, the Christian theology of redemptive suffering dates back to the Passion of Christ and the special need of women for redemption to Eve and Original Sin. Although the suffering of Christ redeemed all of humanity, the uniquely fallen state of womanhood caused many in the church to view the periodic reenactment of the Passion on a worldly scale as the lot of all women. Consciously or not, Thérèse drew on this attitude and acted out in her real life (as interpreted and retold by her and by those around her) the redemptive suffering of her predecessors, saintly and fallen alike. The theme was, if not timeless, centuries old. The nineteenth-century innovation was the expression of redemption through the suffering of tuberculosis.

In her pathbreaking history of anorexia nervosa, Joan Jacobs Brumberg has established the young woman's body as a nexus through which social, psychological, and religious forces have found expression throughout history. She has resisted the temptation to find in the "legendary asceticism" of medieval women such as Saint Catherine of Siena, or in the controversial "fasting girls" of the Victorian age, evidence of a transhistorical anorexic phenomenon that somehow explains present-day eating disorders. However, Brumberg has highlighted two particular historical patterns whose intersection may help to explain the appeal of Thérèse's story. The Catholic ideology of suffering and bodily renunciation has for centuries associated the wasting away of young female bodies with a heightened state of spirituality.[45] Furthermore, in the late nineteenth century, the new hegemony of medical authority in determining the truth of the body did not prevent many believers from invoking the religious tradition of saintly or pious abstinence to explain the behavior of young women who refused food.[46] "Deprived of many worldly sources of empowerment," Brumberg writes, "some Victorian girls chose to draw instead on the lingering tradition of anorexia mirabilis."[47]

This cultural legacy deserves attention not for any insight into etiology (whether of anorexia or of tuberculosis) but rather for the effect of persistent attitudes on the popular reception of a phenomenon such as Thérèse. Although Brumberg's nineteenth-century examples were drawn from Protestant cultures, France was also undergoing widespread secularization and wrestling with the question of women's proper role in society. Thérèse's wasting away from tuberculosis—or, more precisely, her portrayal and narration of her wasting away—paralleled the fasting girls' wasting away from self-starvation and appealed to similar cultural attitudes. In both instances, the decay of the body signaled the blossoming of the spirit and renewed in the traditionally feminine realm of religion and spirituality a traditional feminine ideal.

In the end, all of the nineteenth-century consumptive heroines succumb to the same fatal and fateful malady. Thérèse *is* Marguerite Gauthier, in a sense: though superficially opposites and though one redeems all of humanity while the other redeems only her own fallen self, both are fundamentally redeeming womankind through death from tuberculosis. As Marguerite on stage, Sarah Bernhardt (herself the daughter of a courtesan) portrayed the dying woman as worthy of Mary Magdalene's legacy, and theater critics praised her "ineffable sweetness," professing almost to "see the halo of a saint upon her forehead." [48]

Historians and other observers have made sense of these literary consumptives in various ways. Susan Sontag has denounced the tendency to romanticize and mystify disease, from tuberculosis to cancer and AIDS, as harmful and demoralizing to actual sick people. After carefully picking apart what she calls "the TB myth" and "the Romantic cult of the disease," Sontag concludes, "It is . . . difficult to imagine how the reality of such a dreadful disease could be transformed so preposterously." [49] This reaction raises several questions. Was, for example, Thérèse's account of her own illness a preposterous transformation of a dreadful reality? Perhaps so. But understanding the historical and cultural setting within which Thérèse produced the true story of her life and death hardly makes it "difficult to imagine" how she could perceive tuberculosis in the way she did. In Sontag's commendable effort to restore dignity to those who must contend with society's hostile or perverse metaphors for their illnesses, she imagines a "reality" of disease (dreadful or otherwise) outside of history and culture. Indeed, what is difficult to imagine is how a culture could understand or conceive of illness *without* metaphor. In a less polemical vein, Claudine Herzlich and Janine Pierret have perceptively analyzed the extent to which tuberculosis allowed the "sick person" to emerge as a cultural category for the first time. Because it did not kill its victims instantly but instead allowed them to languish, visibly afflicted but able to live lives whose quality and significance were transformed, tuberculosis can be credited with "creating" this modern figure on a large scale. [50] This circumstance, along with the gradual bodily decay that is symptomatic of the disease, helps to explain why it was tuberculosis in particular (rather than any other disease) that came to be freighted with these meanings.

Several historians, however, have contended that the last half of the nineteenth century saw the eventual rejection of the consumptive literary ideal and its relegation to the marginal status of a quaint antique, to be replaced by the social vision of the fearsome and contagious *cracheur de bacilles,* or "spitter of bacilli." Guillaume, for example, sees the romantic appropriation of tuberculosis under attack and losing its relevance from the 1860s on. Among other things, he calls *Germinie Lacerteux* and *Madame Gervaisais* (as well as Octave Mirbeau's *Journal d'une femme de chambre,* which features tuberculosis only peripherally) protests against the "hypocrisy" that associated death with exaltation. While the Goncourts may have quarreled with certain aspects of the romantic/Christian ethos, in both novels, tuberculosis is still intimately linked to the characters' spiritual condition. The progress of her disease measures Madame Gervaisais's spiritual temperature, in a sense, and Germinie's moral decline as well. Although it is true that Germinie's life is depicted in more "social" terms (complete with alcoholism, poverty, and other forms of material degradation) than any of the other heroines except Fantine, her decline is still the "fatal" result of her tragic and impossible love, recalling in this respect *La Dame aux camélias.* In her employer's view, moreover, Germinie redeems an entire class of "fallen" people with her death, in a socially didactic manner reminiscent of Fantine's demise.

At the close of the century, when Thérèse composed her memoirs in Lisieux and Sarah Bernhardt played Marguerite and the Duke of Reichstadt to the cheers of theatergoers, an explosion of sociomedical literature had begun to represent tuberculosis as a social and national scourge, a political threat that demanded political action. Yet the consumptive ideal of suffering womanhood was alive and well. Inasmuch as it concerned the individual experience of illness and focused obsessively and nearly exclusively on women as victims of disease, this spiritual mode of understanding tuberculosis could hardly serve as a comprehensive explanation of such a widespread social phenomenon. However, the converse is also true. The proliferation of medical, social, and political meanings that came to be attached to tuberculosis in the Belle Epoque could not achieve totality or exclusivity as an explanation of this common, everyday killer.

The so-called War on Tuberculosis that arose from the new sociomedical discourse at the close of the century all but erased women from public discussion of the disease, offering them only marginal roles as facilitators of transmission to the male workers and soldiers on whose health the nation depended. It could not fully satisfy society's need to make sense of the mysterious, dangerous, and threatening. Nor did it speak to the dominant cultural perception of woman's nature as not only pathological but also dichotomous—irreconcilably torn between the poles of virtue and vice. Historians and literary critics have long stressed the myriad ways in which "women haunt[ed] the imagination of nineteenth-century authors." As one critic has put it, the "woman as statue . . . muse and madonna . . . [was] raised up on a pedestal and sublimated. . . . [Authors] celebrate[d] this mysterious being, half-angel and half-devil, the oracle of Romanticism—woman."[51] The elevation of the consumptive woman to the status of archetype and ideal expressed this same obsession. Like the strategists of the War on Tuberculosis, authors from Dumas to Rostand to Thérèse saw the disease as an affliction with both moral and physical dimensions. Unlike the sociomedical authorities, however, these authors looked to the experience of illness itself for answers. They found the fundamental truth of tuberculosis not in the expert knowledge of medicine or public health but in the emotional and spiritual essence of women and in the redemptive possibilities of suffering. Ultimately, the dominant etiology of tuberculosis could explain the meaning *of* disease but could not find meaning *in* disease. It could not fully supplant or displace the forms of meaning so powerfully evoked by the likes of Sarah Bernhardt and Thérèse of Lisieux.

Because of its frequency in society and its physically consuming quality, tuberculosis in nineteenth-century France came to stand in for all illnesses and occupied a cultural space in which it redeemed humanity in a diffuse, spiritual sense. In the essentialist cultural reading of tuberculosis, the disease expiated and explained, giving otherwise senseless or random suffering a meaning and a purpose (just as, in general, narrative imposes moral sense and causality on otherwise random sequences of events).[52] This reading arose when essentialism still predominated in medical circles, but it persisted long after the rise of contagionism. When Thérèse wrote in her diary and when Sarah played Marguerite or the Eaglet, fiction and nonfiction converged, and the literal truth of the particular stories became irrelevant. The underlying tale of redemption through slow, wasting—and feminine—suffering and death resonated in churches and theaters alike. Individual sins and human frailty demanded expiation, and frailty's name was woman. Throughout the century, tuberculosis gave that spiritual redemption a material shape.

Around 1900, the suffering of Thérèse Martin in the convent or of Sarah Bernhardt on stage could be read as an alternative way of understanding tuberculosis. A few decades earlier, before the final victories of contagionism, essentialism, both literary and medical, was the *only* established means of explaining the disease. Hygienists had begun to consider tuberculosis a social phenomenon in its incidence, but etiologically and in other respects, it remained largely a matter of personal experience and circumstance. By century's end, the disease would become not just a social problem but a national crisis as well. The following chapters discuss these developments in the realms of medicine and politics during the Belle Epoque.

CHAPTER THREE

"Guerre au bacille!"

Germ Theory and Fear of Contagion in the War on Tuberculosis

Playwrights, novelists, and nuns were not the only ones in nineteenth-century France making sense of tuberculosis by telling stories. Indeed, the use of narrative as a strategy to give meaning to disease seems to have been one of the few traits common to all parties in the public discussion of the tuberculosis problem. Within the framework of the dominant etiology during the Belle Epoque, narrative played an important role in the production and communication of medical knowledge. Housing conditions and immoral behavior were prominent among the social causes of tuberculosis that were denounced in the War on Tuberculosis; yet one cannot understand any of the various social factors implicated in the spread of the disease without first examining the concept of contagion itself, with its various social and political ramifications.

For the first two-thirds of the nineteenth century, essentialist explanations of tuberculosis predominated in France, from Laënnec to Hugo and the Goncourts. After Koch's 1882 identification of the tubercle bacillus, the rising tide of contagionist medical opinion in France gained considerable momentum. Debate over the transmissibility of tuberculosis continued sporadically throughout the 1880s, but the few remaining anticontagionists were on the defensive; in the ascendancy of the Pasteurian revolution, they were so isolated as to appear backward-looking and resistant to change rather than as serious contenders for scientific legitimacy. Yet while the basic notion of contagion as it applied to tuberculosis was widely accepted, not everybody in the medical community agreed on just what contagion meant or how it operated.

This chapter explores the implications of contagion as it became the cornerstone of the dominant etiology of tuberculosis around the turn of the century. Doctors and hygienists close to the government and affiliated with the leading medical schools and periodicals pursued the notion of contagion to remarkable lengths and targeted spitting as the principal vehicle of tuberculosis and a fearsome threat to public health. Some doctors—mainly outside the profession's dominant institutions and publications—hesitated to follow the doctrine of contagion quite so far and denounced what they saw as its excesses.

Yet zealous campaigns to eliminate or neutralize the tubercle bacillus prevailed, at least in the theory and propaganda of the antituberculosis crusade. The extent to which they were put into practice is less clear, but the dispensary movement provides some clues. Although antituberculosis dispensaries, which sprang up around France in the years before World War I, were ostensibly aimed at bringing preventive health care to the needy in their neighborhoods, much of the dispensary literature displays a different impulse at work. *Dépistage,* or tracking down those infected with the bacillus to render them harmless to the community, seems to have been a major motivating factor behind the dispensary movement. Many hygienists and public officials militated for mandatory declaration of tuberculosis cases, a highly controversial issue among doctors; some prominent figures went so far as to propose the forcible isolation of all infected individuals in *tuberculoseries,* or modern leper colonies, for the protection of the rest of society. While such proposals were extreme and marginal relative to the medical mainstream, they arose out of the same contagionist impulse that led the crusade against tuberculosis to focus its energies on isolating and containing the spread of the bacillus rather than on the strengthening of bodily resistance or the improvement of overall standards of living.

THE SPREAD OF TUBERCULOSIS: SOIL AND SEED

A fundamental tenet of the dominant etiology of tuberculosis around the turn of the century was the need to consider the importance of both "soil" (or terrain) and "seed" in the spread of tuberculosis. The body's state of receptivity or resistance, in other words, deserved as much attention as did contagion or the tubercle bacillus itself. It eventually became obligatory and formulaic, in the parlance of the time, to invoke both soil and seed in any discussion of the disease's causes or prevention. However, most texts gave far from equal treatment to exposure and resistance. In the mainstream of French medicine, the tubercle bacillus and how to avoid coming into contact with it preoccupied most of the antituberculosis crusaders. Typically, a speech, article, or other text would begin with the ritual invocation of both soil and seed and mention in passing the importance of moderation, rest, and nutrition in maintaining organic resistance to infection. The remainder of the argument or discussion would focus exclusively on the various means of transmitting or receiving bacilli, as would the concluding remarks and practical recommendations. In this manner, the formulaic references to the equal importance of soil and seed were belied by the disproportionate weight of argument on the side of seed.

An apparent exception to this pattern was the "moral etiology" of tuberculosis, in which immorality—via alcoholism and venereal disease—contributed to the spread of tuberculosis by diminishing the body's ability to fight off infection.[1] This moral theme obviously depended for its validity on the soil side of the etiological equation; in fact, it was not uncommon for the perfunctory nod toward bodily resistance to consist of a denunciation of alcoholism. However, because of its moral and political content, even this conspicuous exception to the rule of "bacillocentrism"[2] tends to reinforce rather than contradict the defining trait of the dominant etiology: the central role of social and political anxieties in the development of medical knowledge in France concerning tuberculosis.

Even before Koch's experiments succeeded in isolating the tubercle bacillus as the living microorganism responsible for tuberculosis, the groundwork was being laid in France for a contagionist, bacillocentric strategy against the disease. Although Villemin's 1865 inoculation experiments on rabbits were not absolutely conclusive, they eventually convinced many French doctors that tuberculosis was transmissible; the identification of the bacteriological culprit, they felt, was only a matter of time. Among these doctors was Louis Landouzy, at one time dean of the Paris medical faculty and one of the leading authorities on tuberculosis during the Belle Epoque. Landouzy presented a series of clinical lectures to medical students at the Charité hospital in 1881 entitled "How and Why One Gets Tuberculosis." The lectures carefully allow for a divergence of opinion on the question of contagion but finally come down on the contagionist side of the argument.

In the Charité lectures, Landouzy established the pattern for his later career, in which he insisted repeatedly and forcefully on the dual importance of soil and seed while subtly steering discussion (and especially policy considerations) toward bacillocentrism. To the medical students, he "insist[ed] at length on the question of soil" "because it dominates the entire tuberculosis question." "To fight against the likelihood of the seed falling on soils that would allow it to germinate; [and] to modify [soils] so that . . . they become unsuitable for the development of tuberculosis—this must be the doctor's ideal."[3] While this may have been Landouzy's "ideal"—to concentrate on rendering contagion harmless by fortifying the soil—it was not reflected in the thrust of his work or the work of other mainstream hygienists.

Most of the lecture series consisted of an examination of various current theories and experiments concerning the possible transmission of tuberculosis. According to some German experiments, Landouzy noted, respiration "seem[ed] to play the preponderant role" in introducing the disease into the body; furthermore, the same experiments highlighted the spittle of tuberculosis patients as an "agent of transmission" by showing that dogs forced to breathe air containing such spittle contracted the illness.[4] This attention to spittle was significant, as it would later occupy a privileged place in the dominant etiology of tuberculosis.

Landouzy left open, however, the possibility that tuberculosis could be transmitted via other avenues. In fact, he went out of his way to suggest the myriad ways in which the *agent morbifique* might enter the body.

> Who knows if the contaminating agent does not enter, simultaneously or successively, by dust from tuberculous expectoration, by tuberculous meat, by milk from tuberculous cows, perhaps even by water that is considered potable but might have been polluted by contact with the waste of consumptives?

This passage is curious in several respects. Its syntax, beginning "Who knows if . . . ," appears to violate the scientific demand for testing and proof of hypotheses (and thus to undermine the authority of the hypotheses that follow). Moreover, it seems at least to counterbalance, if not actually to contradict, Landouzy's insistence on soil and its "domination" of the tuberculosis question. Finally, the casual mention of tainted milk, meat, and even drinking water could not help but contribute to a quite unscientific reaction—possibly leading to panic or hysteria—among the general population concerning the possibility of contracting tuberculosis. Perhaps Landouzy himself sensed these peculiarities, for he immediately followed this sentence with the defensive assertion, "I do not underestimate the enormous gravity of the questions I am raising." It was better, he maintained, to "agitate" such matters publicly and thereby "shed light" on them than it would be to "leave these questions in the shadows."[5]

Another common feature of what later became the dominant etiology that is evident in Landouzy's Charité lectures is the core narrative. To illustrate their arguments, doctors and hygienists (or indeed, politicians, labor organizers, and novelists) often made use of archetypal stories that explained in lay terms the origin and spread of tuberculosis in a given social context. Often, through a simple tale, they offer a glimpse of the ideology at the core of a scientific explanation. Typically, there is a before-and-after quality to the narratives, in which an idealized past or state of grace is followed by transgression and tragedy. Whether they were hypothetical stories or purported to be factual reportage or case histories, the core narratives served the same essential function: to make moral sense of a fearsome and seemingly random killer.

The nature and function of narrative have always been subject to various interpretations, and the relation between narrative and "historical reality" has recently become a contentious topic of debate among historians. At the same time, humanists in the world of medicine have been investigating related matters, including "the art of the case history" and "the narrative structure of medical knowledge."[6] One of these scholars, Kathryn Montgomery Hunter, sees a special connection between medicine and literature that sets these two endeavors apart from other studies of humankind. The medical case history resembles literary narrative, she argues, not just in form but also in that both genres "can be about only one set of circumstances at a time." Through their use of narrative, in other words, medicine and literature are linked in their particularism and uniquely individual meanings.[7] This may be true for the specific genre of the medical case history as it evolved in clinical settings, but it hardly applies to the cloudy mixture of fact and fiction that constitutes much medical narrative. Some of the nineteenth-century tuberculosis narratives purport to be factual case histories of real patients; others present themselves strictly as fictional parables or as generalizations from years of experience; still others amalgamate bits from each of these categories. What unites them all and gives them their representational power is precisely their transcendence of the particular—their universal applicability, or at least their *social* applicability in a given context. Through these stories, individuals become archetypes.

The historian and cultural critic Hayden White has distinguished three styles of recording sequential events, which he calls "annals," "chronicle," and "narrative."[8] Each befits a particular worldview and epistemology. Of the three, only narrative manages to represent reality in such a way as to impart moral significance, order, and causality to otherwise disconnected or meaningless facts and events. "Narrativity, certainly in factual storytelling and probably in fictional storytelling as well, is intimately related to, if not a function of, the impulse to moralize reality, that is, to identify it with the social system that is the source of any morality that we can imagine."[9] Modern readers, as White points out, find annals and chronicle frustrating and incomplete as historical representations precisely because they lack the "plot" and narrative closure that tie significant events together in a causal order and make moral sense of them. This explanation (the theoretical details of which White lays out with admirable clarity but are beyond the scope of the discussion here) fits the core narratives of tuberculosis quite well. The style of these stories contrasts sharply with the detached, empirical, neutrally observant tone of standard medical writing, which is couched in the universal scientific present tense. (For example, "HIV infection is a risk factor for tuberculosis," or "The tubercle bacillus is transmitted from person to person by inhalation of dried sputum particles.") Medical or sociomedical narrative, in contrast, was indispensable in giving tuberculosis a coherent social and moral meaning. The ostensible universality of the core narratives contributed vitally to the dominant etiology's efforts to speak to all of society.

In the 1881 Charité lectures, Landouzy's featured core narrative concerned spousal contagion: a wealthy young man, with a history of tuberculosis in his family, married a "magnificent young girl," with no such family history. Eighteen months after giving birth to their first child, the wife died of pulmonary tuberculosis. Two years later, the widower remarried into a family whose robust health history promised to "compensate" (in the words of the husband) for his own fragile heredity. After the birth of two children, the second wife also died of tuberculosis. "As for the husband, he died only later, of a slowly developing tuberculosis."[10] Landouzy followed this with several more stories of household and/or spousal contagion, a theme that later became a leitmotiv within the dominant etiology. These narratives may have been chosen to respond to the legion of instances, often cited by anticontagionists, in which spouses or others continuously in close contact with tuberculosis patients remained perfectly healthy. Landouzy's story certainly contained implicit moral lessons concerning contagion, marriage, and ethical responsibility; one always needed to be vigilant against the possibility of contagion. Even at this embryonic stage of organized antituberculosis efforts in France, such narratives added a vital dimension to the sciences of medicine and public health, which in these years aspired increasingly to treat the social body as well as the individual body.

Landouzy concluded that even if the contagiousness of tuberculosis could not be proven, "it is our . . . strict duty to conduct ourselves as if the matter were definitively established." One reason for this was that "often families will anticipate certain preventive measures, which you will be able to institute tactfully, without revealing the theoretical preoccupations that dictate your conduct." [11] Once again, scientific caution was uncharacteristically thrown to the winds, and doctors were advised to follow an unproven doctrine in their everyday practice. Landouzy's reasoning seemed to be that patients' families would take certain "contagionist" measures regardless of what the doctor said; therefore, it behooved the responsible physician to guide the families and to use his "tact" to make sure that they did not go too far.

Landouzy was not moved by the anticontagionists' ethical argument (espoused most notably by Pidoux) [12] that even if tuberculosis were contagious, it would be necessary to keep that fact quiet (for fear of panic and ostracism). Citing the example of widespread tuberculosis in the army, he asked, "Is it really an affront to our nature to be afraid of a coughing bunkmate[?] [S]hould this cougher be removed from the barracks as soon as possible, and sent to the hospital?" What would be unethical, in his view, was to do nothing in the face of mounting contagionist evidence. He concluded the lecture series by calling for doctors to "preoccupy themselves" with the issue of contagion rather than avoid it.

> We must seek the truth and, if we sense it, we must not shout it from the rooftops but rather make it inspire our behavior, conform our practice to it, allow our patients to benefit from it, and make it filter into the thinking of the various officials who are responsible for the public health. [13]

By the end of the five-part lecture series, the insistence on equal consideration of soil and seed was gone (or at least momentarily forgotten). The burning issue of the moment was contagion; the seed was everything, or nearly so.

Contagionism enjoyed one of its finest hours the following year, in 1882, when Koch identified the tubercle bacillus. Germ theory was reaching triumphant maturity, and none in the medical profession could ignore its power any longer. By the late 1880s, even the cautious within the profession had been won over to some extent, and hygienist Jules Rochard was able to write in 1888, "Today, the contagiousness of phthisis is admitted by nearly all doctors." Nevertheless, many elements of prior etiologies continued to survive in these years. Rochard himself, for example, wrote in his hefty and influential *Traité d'hygiène sociale* that heredity was responsible for roughly half of all cases of tuberculosis and that "instances of contagion [were] extremely rare." Given that he allowed for only two modes of "transmission" for the disease, heredity and contagion, the two assertions seem to contradict each other. Later theorists would cast this relationship in terms of an inherited soil that the contagious seed would or would not find receptive to its implantation. Indeed, Rochard discussed the importance of soil in his book, though not in connection with heredity; until at least the mid-1890s, heredity remained a looming, independent disease-causing presence. In the matters of both contagion and heredity, Rochard advocated gently persuasive education rather than strict, repressive regulations to persuade the general public to avoid contagion and to discourage tuberculous patients from marrying and procreating.[14]

The rise of germ theory profoundly altered discussion of tuberculosis in France, and it is significant that bacillocentrism carried the day. Yet the appearance of unanimity or consensus can sometimes hide a more nuanced reality in which dissent and uncertainty persist. Somewhat lost in the increasingly contagionist atmosphere of the eighties and nineties were the protests of a few isolated figures who did not share the belief that the discovery of the tubercle bacillus had irrevocably altered the outlook and tactics of the fight against the disease. Some of these doctors, including Michel Peter, were veterans of the Villemin debates of 1865–1868. Peter had compromised his prominent position in the French medical establishment by taking the lead in opposing Pasteur and germ theory, thereby securing for himself permanent obscurity and discredit.[15] Nonetheless, Peter continued to speak out against contagionism for the rest of his life. The 1893 edition of his *Leçons de clinique médicale* revived the notion of "morbid spontaneity," citing the body's "spontaneous" ability to prevent germs or other contaminants—constantly absorbed into the body in various ways—from causing illness. The fact that most of these hundreds of thousands of germs never resulted in disease, Peter reasoned, rendered "contagion" all but irrelevant. The relative rarity of various illnesses among doctors and others who were constantly exposed to them proved the same point. Koch's discovery, in Peter's view, had little practical value.

> Koch's discovery was a scientific conquest. . . . It is an interesting fact from the point of view of pathological anatomy and semiology; but there ends its importance and its scope. . . . [T]he Koch bacillus has expanded the limits of our anatomical knowledge without advancing therapeutics in the slightest.[16]

Peter did not deny that microbes existed; rather, he believed that they became "noxious" only when the body underwent "internal or external modifications," such as through fatigue, malnutrition, or other debility.[17]

Isidore Straus showed more caution in criticizing contagionism; in fact, he dedicated his 1895 masterwork, *La Tuberculose et son bacille,* to his former teacher, Louis Pasteur. Yet Straus too argued that in tuberculosis, "the intervention of the microbe is not everything." Like Peter, Straus emphasized the "powerful" role of "predisposing and adjuvant causes," including fatigue and privation as well as poverty, "sorrows," alcoholism, and certain debilitating diseases. The absence of these factors, he held, explained the fact that autopsies of those who died of other causes routinely revealed the presence of "healed" tubercles or tuberculous lesions. References to this phenomenon were quite common in later medical literature on tuberculosis: some accounts reported this result in half of all corpses, others in 90 percent or more.[18] Straus attributed such signs of "latent" tuberculosis to early childhood exposure to the bacillus; the infection would remain latent unless "awakened" later in life by the various "adjuvant causes."[19]

Straus and Peter were in a distinct minority in the 1880s and 1890s, when contagionism was on the rise. By the turn of the century, even equal attention to both soil and seed was more of a slogan than a practice. During the decade 1898–1908, when the War on Tuberculosis reached its peak, discussions of the disease were much less likely to include such qualms as Peter's and Straus's than the following sorts of injunctions: "the fear of contagion is the beginning of good health"; "it is . . . toward the *destruction of the bacillus* that our efforts should be directed." In the words of Albert Calmette, the physician who later earned fame as one of the originators of the BCG tuberculosis vaccine, "The enemy is the *tuberculeux* who is spitting bacilli." Indeed, the identification of the victim as "enemy" and a preoccupation with spitting were two of the most significant new features of the bacillocentric perspective on tuberculosis.[20]

In 1903, the hygienist Edouard Fuster testified to the victory of contagionism when he summarized the War on Tuberculosis at a meeting of the Société de médecine publique.

The prevention of tuberculosis as a social disease includes . . . all measures destined to remove recognized vectors of contagion—the sick—from still healthy milieus; consequently, to *search them out* in all human communities, and then to *isolate* them as soon as they are a threat.[21]

The various means proposed to fight tuberculosis by searching out and isolating the dangerous "vectors of contagion" will be discussed below. Before doing so, however, it is worth exploring in more depth the denunciation of spitting and human contact as conducive to the transmission of tuberculosis as well as some misgivings that were expressed regarding the inevitable consequences of sounding the contagionist alarm.

SPITTING AND THE DANGER OF CONTACT

"Spitting, that is the enemy!" (*Le crachat, voilà l'ennemi!*)[22] If medical literature is any indication, spitting was a common and disgusting habit in Belle Epoque France.[23] Furthermore, it was known that pulmonary tuberculosis significantly increased expectoration; its victims could therefore be expected to account for more than their share of this everyday practice. Doctors and hygienists tirelessly preached the antispitting gospel to anyone and everyone. "Each crachat," one periodical told its working-class readership, "is, alas! a veritable army of billions of vigorous microbes, that [one] sends to attack the health of [one's] wife, children, friends, and neighbors."[24]

Although they were commonly blamed for careless spitting, workers were not the only intended audience for antispitting propaganda. Maurice Letulle, speaking to an employers' association in 1902, insisted that "terror of the crachat is the beginning of hygienic wisdom" and repeatedly stressed the importance of keeping the workplace spittle-free.

A single sick worker can contaminate an incalculable number of his comrades, the foremen, and even the bosses; since bacillus-laden crachats are lying on the ground everywhere! woe to the shoe sole that picks them up. In the street, on stairways, at home . . . in all places, the hideous homicidal crachat will be there [*le hideux crachat homicide trouvera place*].[25]

The message was an urgent one, full of fear and loathing: no matter where one went, the "hideous homicidal crachat" would be waiting. Letulle's unrestrained, almost frenzied tone suggests that sheer revulsion contributed as much as germ theory to medical concern about spitting.

Letulle's comments also point to a crucial class distinction; the spitter is a worker. Furthermore, the practice is all the more nefarious because, through contagion, "even the bosses" are at risk. When the antispitting crusaders told of even respectable bourgeois men indulging in the habit, their indignant and surprised tone suggested that, in fact, spitting was considered a vulgar working-class practice. The negligent worker coughing, spitting, and infecting innocent bystanders—even the wealthy—was a recurrent motif in the antituberculosis literature.[26]

In his 1908 medical thesis, Roger Reveillaud went so far as to observe the spitting behavior of passersby on the Parisian *grands boulevards*. On just one sidewalk, between the Opera and the rue Montmartre, he counted 875 crachats of various sizes lying on the ground. "And this does not count," he added,

> those that may have inundated the café terraces, where one quite often sees clean and polite people spitting up veritable lakes. . . . [O]n the terrace of the Théatre-Français café, we noticed a gentleman coughing continually and covering the ground, utterly shamelessly, with I don't know how many five-franc pieces, which the waiter came over twice to cover with sand.
> Is not a law necessary here?[27]

Presumably, Reveillaud was referring to sputum globules the size of five-franc pieces; like Letulle's, his tone conveys as much repugnance as concern for public health.

It is not necessary to take issue with the scientific proposition of droplet infection to see that the antispitting forces were influenced to some extent by a kind of visceral revulsion. The history of disgust is still largely uncharted territory, but the pathbreaking work of historians such as Norbert Elias and Alain Corbin has revealed some turning points and zones of particular anxiety in the development of modern mores. In the late nineteenth century, three nodes of disgust assumed preeminence in the official antituberculosis campaign: unpleasant smells, the "promiscuous" crowding together of bodies, and bodily fluids and excreta. Corbin has described the process by which, beginning in the late eighteenth century, the smell of excrement and other types of refuse came to be considered intolerable and disgusting.[28] The power of these particular objects of horror and concerns about disease helped constitute each other: disgust fueled the War on Tuberculosis, in a sense, while efforts to improve public health directed increased attention toward the living conditions of the poor and intensified bourgeois disgust at them.

Elias has shown that far from being frowned on, spitting was encouraged in etiquette manuals as late as the mid-eighteenth century, when it was thought "ill-mannered to swallow what should be spat ... [as] [t]his can nauseate others." One hundred years later, by 1859, manners had changed in polite society to the extent that spitting was viewed as "a disgusting habit." As Elias has pointed out, this change was entirely unrelated to medicine and the rise of germ theory. "Rational understanding of the origins of certain diseases, of the danger of sputum as a carrier of illness, is neither the primary cause of fear and repugnance nor the motor of civilization, the driving force of the changes in behavior with regard to spitting."[29] Disgust preceded and eclipsed science, for even after spitting came to represent the transmission of disease, an underlying sense of revulsion often pervaded the medical outcry against the practice. It also provided the strategists of the War on Tuberculosis with a means of getting their message across. Fuster, for example, suggested that spitters could be shamed out of the practice and advocated an education campaign "insisting on the fact that the habit of spitting is repugnant."[30]

Spitting was most often depicted as spreading tuberculosis in the victim's home and workplace, via dried-up particles dispersed through dry sweeping and other unhygienic practices. Yet many observers insisted that the danger was even more widespread than that. Any public space was a potential arena of contagion; as one doctor put it, "It is primarily in public meeting places that the ... contagiousness of tuberculosis is exhaled to the highest degree." These dangerous spaces included theaters, post offices, omnibuses, government or administrative offices, train stations, train cars, workshops, department stores, hotel rooms, military barracks, and schools.[31] Several studies, finding high rates of tuberculosis among laundresses, sounded the alarm over contagion through laundry. Negligence was found at *blanchisseries* in the handling of both clean and dirty laundry (the two often came in contact with each other), and no effort was made to disinfect laundry coming from tuberculous households.[32]

The medical column of the Parisian daily newspaper *Le Matin* called yet another contagion menace to its readers' attention in December

1905: reading books. The columnist, "Doctor Ox," claimed that an average book from a circulating collection or library could contain forty-three bacteria per square centimeter of printed surface, which, for a 300- or 400-page book, "represents a worrisome number of bacilli and micrococci." Who could know, Doctor Ox wondered, how many book borrowers or library readers were ill or convalescing and handled pages after coughing or sneezing on their hands? "Have you ever thought," he asked his readers, "about the number of volumes a consumptive can infect during the long months of his illness?" Many people, he suggested, probably never thought about such things until it was too late.

> Bacilli . . . are preserved quite well between the pages of a novel, just as plants are preserved in a botanist's herbarium. And when this bacteriological herbarium comes into your hands, can you be surprised that you or a family member comes down with scarlet fever or diphtheria of unknown origin[?][33]

It would be difficult to imagine the lay readers of *Le Matin* not being panicked, or at least disturbed, by such alarmism.

Doctor Ox went on to relate a recent case of "reading contagion" from the Ukrainian city of Kharkov. An outbreak of tuberculosis among city hall employees was found on investigation to be largely confined to those who worked in the city archives. Bacteriologists determined that the archival documents were "literally covered with tubercle bacilli."

> Where did these bacilli come from? The investigation . . . revealed that, some years before, an employee assigned to the archives died of consumption, and that this employee was in the habit (a quite common one) of moistening his fingers with saliva when turning the pages of documents.

The infected employee had "tuberculized" his documents and posthumously contaminated his successors through the *"archives bacillifères."* One peculiarity of this story concerned the fact that in scientific experiments, the tubercle bacillus had never been known to survive for very long, whereas the Kharkov archivists fell ill "several years" after the death of their careless predecessor. Doctor Ox even cited a maximum life span of 103 days for the bacillus under laboratory conditions; instead of casting doubt on the veracity of the story, however, the doctor concluded that the Kharkov incident proved the experiments wrong.[34]

As this column in *Le Matin* shows, sputum-related contagion was thought to involve more than mere spitting. The chain of contamination and the vicissitudes of the bacillus seemingly extended into every realm of daily life. One could not be too careful, hygienists warned. "You should not think that it is . . . the hideous crachat alone . . . that constitutes the great danger." Spitting into handkerchiefs or napkins, for example, and letting them dry on beds, pillows, or nightstands was likely to coat those furnishings (as well as the room's occupants) with bacilli. Similarly, even those patients who took care to use spittoons were warned not to leave them uncovered, lest unwelcome creatures bathe in them. "I must note in passing the open spittoon that the fly dips its legs in before wiping them off in the sugar bowl[,] for the fly is one of the great traveling salesmen of tuberculosis." The same doctor went on to warn against intimate *talking*.

> In the same bed, on the same pillow, when we talk to each other mouth to mouth, so to speak, the column of air breathed out carries with it infinitesimal bits of bacillus-laden spittle and reaches the person to whom one is talking, or the child to whom one is telling a story—like a poison arrow that makes him smile.[35]

As will be seen below, such extreme prohibitions were not allowed to go unchallenged, even within the medical community. Yet the point remains that even the most apparently innocent activities in daily life at some point became charged with bacteriological significance.

Given the range and diversity of practices condemned as hazardous to public health, it is perhaps surprising that there were only two concrete preventive measures on which doctors widely agreed: a prohibition against spitting on the ground and distribution of hygienic *crachoirs,* or spittoons. Even spittoons caused some controversy and debate, however. Fixed spittoons installed in public buildings were the subject of an exchange at the 1905 International Tuberculosis Congress in Paris. Jules Héricourt argued that the sight of such spittoons constituted a "solicitation to spit." Passersby then spit in the general direction and often missed the target, causing a greater mess than if there were no spittoon at all. As head doctor for the postal service, Héricourt consequently had spittoons removed from all post offices. Landouzy disagreed, contending that Héricourt's objection applied only to old-fashioned spittoons situated at ground level. Landouzy argued that the absence of spittoons in public buildings was certainly no disincentive to spit, as the most cursory observation would show; nor was the "habitually filthy" condition of most post offices. Furthermore, he asked, how could hygienists prohibit or discourage spitting on the ground without providing spittoons as an alternative?[36]

Hygienic spittoons also came in individual, portable models, though some patients considered them a nuisance. Even those who were very conscientious about using spittoons in the sanatorium, in the hospital, or at home would not think of doing so outside, according to one doctor. Some refused to spit into the apparatus to avoid revealing the nature of their illness in public; others complained that the spittoon was pointless, since they would have to use their handkerchiefs to wipe away the spittle that clung to their lips or beard anyway. The indignity of washing out one's own spittoon was also used as an excuse, as were the revulsion of servants at performing that task and the inconvenience, when riding a bicycle or horse, of stopping, dismounting, and retrieving the spittoon from one's pocket.[37]

A flat prohibition against spitting in public may have seemed a simpler strategy, but it too encountered obstacles. Fuster complained that "liberty is understood in such a way that our democracies, even while claiming to be guided more and more by science, seem more and more incapable of imposing such restraints on themselves." He advocated a tireless effort to educate people, to achieve piecemeal local restrictions, and eventually to approach as nearly as possible the complete suppression of spitting, which would "in theory, render unnecessary all other measures" in the War on Tuberculosis.[38] More ambitious, the medical student Reveillaud called for parliament to pass a law against spitting on the ground. "The crachat being the primary vehicle of the bacillus, we would like to see it, and only it, be the main target of our energies. . . . No matter what they might say, tuberculosis will disappear with it [the crachat]."[39] Reveillaud's "No matter what they might say," likely referred to the advocates of soil-related prevention, who often pointed to poverty, slum housing, and other general social ills as causal factors in tuberculosis and as arenas of possible intervention. Hard-line bacillophobes such as Reveillaud would have none of it.

Meanwhile, hygienists and national and local authorities covered walls in public places with placards and posters warning against spitting on the ground or floor. Many dispensaries and other organizations published and distributed antituberculosis instructions aimed at lay audiences. The "recommendations" published by the prefecture of the Seine were fairly typical in their focus on spitting. "It is expressly recommended that you not spit in public," they read. After explaining in simple language how bacilli could be transmitted from person to person, the tract added, "Every crachat is suspect, because, at a glance, nothing proves that it does not contain bacilli." Then, as if to defuse any panic that such a frightening concept might engender, it immediately added the reassurance that tuberculosis, "despite its gravity," was curable at every stage of its development—a misleading yet apparently necessary addendum that became a commonplace in the War on Tuberculosis. (Although no effective medication or other treatment existed at the time, "cures" were claimed when, typically after a period of rest and abundant nourishment, a patient's symptoms disappeared, whether temporarily or permanently.) Also like other examples of the genre, the Seine prefecture's instructions went on to recommend practical measures against contagion such as the use of spittoons, disinfection, wet mopping instead of sweeping, boiling of milk, and "sufficient" cooking of meat.[40]

Of all the possible objections to antispitting propaganda, there was one that rarely surfaced in public, although it may help explain the official insistence on curability. Sooner or later, even the least scientific-minded layperson would realize that in order for sputum to present a danger, the spitter must *have* tuberculosis. The acknowledgment of this condition would amount (in the minds of most people, according to contemporary observers, and in statistical probability) to a death sentence and was therefore something to be avoided. (And those who knew for certain that they had the disease could hardly be expected to keep the protection of others uppermost in their minds.) The conscious mental leap from "spitting spreads tuberculosis" to "*my* spittle might actually be dangerous to others" was almost literally unthinkable. After all, the nontuberculous person who spit was guilty of nothing, unless it was of setting a bad example.

It may have been in response to this unspoken objection that antituberculosis crusaders repeatedly asserted that one could have tuberculosis without being aware of it, that a diagnosis of tuberculosis was not a death sentence, and that patients could harm *themselves* by spitting (through reinfection that could aggravate their illness). As Reveillaud put it, "We must convince him of the idea that he is not marked for death because he is consumptive, and that Tuberculosis does not necessarily equal Death." One popularizing pamphlet imagined a healthy person interrogating a hygienist, "What? you want to prevent me from spitting as I wish, when I do not have tuberculosis?" The hygienist's response was brutal in its simplicity: "I hope you are right, and that you do not have it, but you just don't know."[41] The apostles of public health seemed to be caught between the need to fight complacency and to stress the ubiquity of tuberculosis, on the one hand, and the desire to reassure the sick, promote the powers of medicine and hygiene, and avoid panic, on the other. Each individual assertion seemed to err on one side or the other and had to be counterbalanced (without being contradicted) by another.

The perceived danger of exposure to contagion led some people outside of the medical community to reject the presence in their neighborhoods of certain facilities intended to diagnose, treat, or house tuberculosis patients. Henry Fleury-Ravarin, a deputy from the Rhône, even introduced a bill in parliament to outlaw such establishments "in the vicinity of residential areas."[42] In 1901, city employees in Nantes wrote a letter to the mayor protesting a proposal to temporarily install an antituberculosis dispensary in the city hall, where they worked. On the heels of recent reports of widespread contagion in public buildings, including the main post office in Nantes, the employees could not accept the implantation of a new *foyer de contagion* in their midst. Some of them, they wrote, had even seen "crachats streaked with blood" on the stairs and in the hallways of the city's health department. The following year, the neighbors of the newly proposed site for the dispensary, on the rue Voltaire, petitioned the municipal authorities to prevent its installation. The city was forced to solicit a legal opinion on the applicability of laws against unsanitary establishments, as well as medical advice from Paul Brouardel, France's preeminent hygienist who held the chair in legal medicine at the Paris medical school; all of the advice encouraged the city to go ahead with the dispensary, which opened as planned.[43]

Brouardel was called on for an expert opinion again in 1906, this time in a dispute over the location of a facility outside of Tours. The Count de Lafont, a landowner whose property was situated across the road from the *cure d'air,* or fresh-air rest home, of the local antituberculosis league, sued the league, contending that the proximity of so many tuberculosis patients constituted a contagion menace and, moreover, depressed his property's value. The league's lawyer, Maître Henri Robert, argued that the presence of the home (which was not, he insisted, a sanatorium, contrary to the count's contention), far from being a public health danger, probably represented an improvement in the overall hygiene of the area. Instead of catering to the fear and prejudice that would treat the victim of a contagious disease as the ancients had treated lepers, the Ligue contre la tuberculose en Touraine enforced strict rules on hygiene and distributed brochures discussing the true circumstances under which tuberculosis could be spread. Any spitting by a patient outside of a crachoir would result in immediate expulsion from the cure d'air, and other precautions kept the home in an exemplary hygienic state, providing a model for its neighbors.[44]

"Tuberculosis is only contagious if there is direct contact or absorption of the Koch bacillus," Robert maintained, and "as long as the spitting *tuberculeux* takes certain precautions, one can live with him without danger and without appreciable risk." In pleading his case, he even called on the nation's most eminent hygienists, through the government's Permanent Commission for the Prevention of Tuberculosis, to bolster his argument. Brouardel sent a report in the committee's name to the court supporting the local league's position. Even a sanatorium, Brouardel wrote, was not "a danger for the surrounding area." "The precautions taken in [such] an establishment to prevent the propagation of tuberculosis seem to be, on the contrary, a lesson [on prevention] for residents of the surrounding area." While the "free" tuberculosis victim was indeed a "social danger," according to Brouardel's report, "the consumptive [who is] taken in, educated, treated, [and] kept in check . . . becomes totally harmless." Under such strict discipline, there could be no danger of contagion at the rest home; without some sort of proof that the patients had ignored the rules against spitting outside the crachoirs, the Count de Lafont's fears—and his lawsuit—were groundless. The court agreed.[45] However, even if lawsuits and organized protests were exceptional and generally unsuccessful, they suggest the considerable extent to which the hygienists' propaganda and educational efforts penetrated the public consciousness. Other types of evidence, including scattered accounts of ostracism and hysteria related to tuberculosis, point to the same conclusion.

DEMURRALS FROM BACILLOPHOBIA

Bacillocentric alarm occasionally became so widespread and reached such a paranoid pitch that it caused some doctors to caution against overreaction and panic. Often, this took the form of casual references in the "official" antituberculosis literature[46] to the exclusion or rejection commonly experienced by victims of the disease. Yet even in such instances, the strategists of the War on Tuberculosis rarely shifted emphasis away from contagion as the key etiological issue at stake; they simply denounced superstitious or cruel tendencies "in certain circles composed of overly simplistic people."[47] Other doctors, most often from outside the powerful institutions of French medicine, took issue with what they saw as an overemphasis on contagion in the etiology of tuberculosis. These doctors blamed the instances of ostracism and rejection on constant warnings against the ubiquitous danger of germ transmission.

The "official" doctors and hygienists often recommended discretion in the implementation of certain measures against contagion because, in Fuster's words, "it is essential that we not forget that the *tuberculeux* ... is already considered a pariah [*un pestiféré*], denied work and shunned." A sensitive bedside manner would be needed to confront popular prejudices, which manifested themselves in various ways. Brouardel himself, who insisted on the harmlessness of "disciplined" tuberculosis patients, reported several distressing incidents: a worker thrown out of his Paris boardinghouse after returning from the sanatorium at Angicourt; a domestic servant who stopped going to the dispensary for fear of his illness being found out by his masters; a chambermaid "brutally" dismissed and called a "plague infecting the house"; and a patient whose own family threw him out on the street after he was discharged from the hospital.[48]

Residential disinfection, touted by many doctors as a practical means of combating contagion, had its drawbacks as well. When a program of systematic weekly disinfection was tested on a group of one hundred tuberculosis patients, their neighbors threatened to move out. The angry landlords finally evicted "those mangy, scabrous types who caused all the trouble." The program had to be abandoned. Albert Robin, one of the leading medical proponents of solidarism,[49] told of a day laborer in the early stages of tuberculosis, still vigorous and strong enough to work. No sooner did a disinfection team show up at his lodging house than the man found himself out on the street, homeless.[50]

But the odyssey of a young maid, as reported by Dr. Jules Lancereaux, may be the most poignant and revealing story of contagion paranoia. When she came down with bronchitis and began to cough, she was fired by her masters and forced to rent a room in a boardinghouse. There, showing signs of tuberculosis, she was promptly asked to leave. Fleeing to the countryside, where her prospects for recovery might have been greater, she sought refuge with her sister. There were young children in the household, however, and the sister refused to have her. The young woman's last resort was the hospital, but even there, the doors were closed to her, because all of the beds were full.[51] Obviously, whether through posters and official propaganda or by more informal channels, a great deal of bacillocentric medical theory had filtered through to the general population.

There were some doctors who fought back, not just against popular prejudice but against the excesses of contagionism in medical and public health circles as well. While neither particularly numerous nor influential, these peripheral figures challenged official medicine by drawing a clear causal link between the mainstream etiology of tuberculosis and popular contagion paranoia. Perhaps the clearest example of this controversy surfaced in the pages of *La Médication martiale,* a minor medical journal, in 1904.

Paul Cuq, a doctor from the Hérault, wrote the journal to warn against the role of kissing in the spread of tuberculosis, particularly where infants were concerned.

> Physicians should undertake a veritable crusade against the common habit of kissing children. The nicer they are, the more we smother them with kisses, without noticing that in our affectionate folly we might kiss the corner of the [child's] mouth or even the whole mouth, thereby inoculating the tuberculosis that we could be carrying without knowing it.

The slightest abrasion or ulceration on the baby's face, Cuq maintained, could be enough to allow the "perfidious microbe" to penetrate the delicate organism. On such "frail" terrain, the seed would multiply rapidly.[52]

Cuq embellished his argument with the obligatory didactic narratives. One concerned a family in which both parents enjoyed superb health, yet saw two children die of tuberculous illnesses. Their search through the household and among the staff for clues turned up nothing, with the exception of an old servant woman in poor health who had been employed by the family for generations. A favorite of the parents, she spoiled the children and loved to kiss them while she played with them. The parents hated to part with her, but when a third child succumbed to tuberculosis, they relented and fired her after a doctor diagnosed a slowly evolving lesion in her lungs.[53]

Even more remarkable was a case on which Cuq himself was consulted, involving the children of another robust and healthy family. When a relative arrived in the house for an extended convalescence from tuberculosis, the family took all proper precautions to prevent contagion, including housing the relative in a separate wing. Nevertheless, the two previously healthy children both eventually came down with tuberculosis and died. Cuq discovered the unexpected means of the disease's transmission. "My research on the etiology of their illness led me to note that the vehicle of the bacillus was a lovable little dog who ran throughout the house, played with the children and kissed them in his own way, even licking them on the face and mouth." The same dog, it seemed, had free access to the convalescing relative's room, where it "licked and swallowed the bits of meat chewed and spit out by the patient, and doubtless sputum as well, particles of which it carried on its tongue back to the children." The immediate moral of the story— limit pets' intimate contacts with people, and keep a close watch on children's apparently innocuous play—was not the only lesson Cuq drew from the incident.

> I will finish my plea—or rather my indictment—against kissing by pointing out that there are legions of young married couples who inoculated each other with tuberculosis by kissing on the lips. . . . Conclusion: Beware of kissing in general and above all, try to protect your children from it.[54]

Cuq's final admonition, "Beware" (*Méfiez-vous*), could well have served as a motto for the bacillophobes who dominated the official campaign against tuberculosis.

The next issue of *La Médication martiale* carried a response to Cuq's piece from another provincial physician, A. Mirabail of the Cher. In an exceedingly sarcastic tone, Mirabail ridiculed the lengths to which Cuq was willing to go in the effort to prevent contagion. "After forbidding us to spit on the ground or even in our handkerchiefs, after condemning us to breathe only at a distance of a meter and a half from each other, now my excellent colleague . . . takes kissing away from us." Mirabail pleaded for his readers not to fall for the contagionist alarmism. "At the risk of Doctor Cucq [*sic*] casting lightning bolts full of millions of expectorated bacilli in my direction, I urge the public not to submit to such a draconian measure!" He complained that the "fears" so common in the population, as well as among doctors, were largely unfounded, because they "forgot only one thing: the notion of terrain." Citing 90 percent as the proportion of cadavers who did not die of tuberculosis and showed healed or cretaceous tubercles on autopsy, Mirabail argued that exposure to the disease was nearly universal. Since only a small percentage of people ever actually developed symptoms or full-blown, "open" tuberculosis, exposure could not be a decisive factor in the disease's incidence. "[I] do not deny contagion—quite the contrary, because I recognized that we are all exposed to contagion—but must we attach so much importance to this fact? I think not."[55]

Instead of hunting down microbes wherever they might lurk and attempting to prevent any of them from entering the body, Mirabail reasoned, it would make more sense and yield better results to try to fortify the body itself, making it inhospitable to infection. Preventing contagion, he wrote, was as "ridiculous" as covering a field with a net to combat weeds. "We start by proscribing the kiss; where then will we stop? Will we find a well-intentioned doctor to prohibit conjugal relations and replace them by fertilization without contact?" In fact, Cuq *had* warned against contagion among newlyweds through kissing on the mouth, and some doctors had suggested the possibility of genital transmission of tuberculosis. But Mirabail would not hear of it. "Let us continue to kiss each other: if kissing gives us a few extra microbes, we will forgive it, considering the sweet joys it brings."[56] Beneath the sarcasm, Mirabail's quarrel was really with the dominant etiology of tuberculosis as a whole, to the extent that it was ignoring its often stated promise to deal equally with soil and seed.

There are some signs that disaffection with bacillocentrism may have extended beyond the occasional sarcastic letter writer in medical journals, although it never seems to have had a major impact on the official War on Tuberculosis. Another of the newspaper medical columnists, Lucien Descaves in the daily *Le Journal,* spoke out in 1906 against the danger that the battle against one scourge (tuberculosis) might lead to one even worse: fear. Descaves strongly opposed recent proposals for the mandatory declaration of tuberculosis cases, saying it would make the lives of patients and their families "intolerable." He went on to ridicule what he saw as the excesses of contagionist hygiene. "We are seeing sources of contagion everywhere: in the kisses that children give or receive; on their fingertips that they put in their noses; in old books . . . ; in meat, milk, and I don't know what else! We are positively terrifying the public." Mandatory declaration, Descaves wrote, would cater to the "blind pretentions" of those who would treat people with tuberculosis like plague victims. Patients would be forcibly estranged from family and friends "on the pretext" that they pose a threat of contamination. Descaves finished with a bit of hyperbole: "These practices will soon return us to the leper colonies of the Middle Ages."[57] He was probably unaware of the degree of truth in his rhetorical flourish; as early as 1905, as will be seen below, at least one prominent Parisian doctor had begun to propose in all seriousness the revival of leper colonies for tuberculosis victims.

In 1908, the same year that Reveillaud's ultracontagionist thesis was published, another medical thesis with quite a different message appeared. Xavier Jousset aligned himself with the partisans of soil and advocated fortifying the body instead of preventing the entry of the bacillus as the appropriate means of fighting tuberculosis. Unlike some of his fellow combatants in this debate, however, Jousset explicitly mentioned class as the key variable in society's contagion paranoia. "Tuberculosis being principally a disease of the poor, those unfortunates who must struggle to earn their livelihood are becoming, for the rich, horrible sources of contagion, and . . . are doomed to the worst, most inhuman measures of ostracism." Jousset also attempted to explain the bacillophobia of mainstream medicine in terms of overreaction to or misinterpretation of individual experiments or incidents. Doctors had too easily extrapolated, he claimed, from transmission of tuberculosis under laboratory conditions (including Villemin's inoculation of rabbits) to "social" transmission under the conditions of everyday life. Furthermore, certain terrifying stories with little or no basis in fact—according to Jousset—were repeated so often that they became part of the medical lore of tuberculosis, and their veracity became immaterial. For example, he cited the case of the boarding school in Chartres which caused a commotion at the Academy of Medicine when it was first reported. Thirteen girls had died of tuberculosis at the boarding school in a two-year period, and their deaths were attributed to drinking milk from a diseased cow. At the academy's next meeting, the member who had reported the case was forced to retract it; on investigation, it was found that not only was milk from the cow in question served only to the school's staff but all of the milk at the school was boiled before being consumed. This retraction, Jousset complained, received little attention, and the original story continued to make the rounds among hygienists. As long as it was repeated and used to illustrate the perils of contagion, its accuracy no longer mattered.[58]

Sparks flew when mainstream bacillophobia was confronted with an aggressive opponent in a series of meetings of the Société médicale du IXe arrondissement in late 1905 and early 1906. Dr. Adolphe Leray, head of the X-ray laboratory at the Saint-Antoine hospital in Paris, presented a paper attacking the doctrine of contagionism and its consequences. His arguments were not significantly new, but his coverage of the history and range of contributions to the debate was thorough and the force with which he delivered and defended his thesis in front of a largely hostile audience was remarkable. Poverty and poor hygiene, Leray contended, not only prepared the soil for tuberculosis; they were, in fact, its primary determinant causes. The very omnipresence of the bacillus that so worried many hygienists proved that contagion could not account for who got tuberculosis and who did not. He restated at length the favorite argument of the early anticontagionists, namely, that contagion violated common sense and everyday observation: with so many thousands of consumptives spreading germs everywhere they went, why was not the entire population of Paris, for example, struck down by the disease within a matter of a few years? Why did physicians so rarely contract the disease, when they spent much of their lives exposed to its victims and their crachats?[59]

Neither did Leray spare his opponents their share of ridicule. He accused them of promoting "the most detestable of tyrannies," worthy of "the little despots" of past centuries. He quoted Emile Duclaux, Pasteur's close collaborator, as wondering what would happen if all those suffering from tuberculosis could be exiled to a desert island. "This measure would be as beneficial," Duclaux was reported to have said, "as eliminating within a few days all rabid dogs." After citing this comment, Leray could only exclaim incredulously, "Comparing poor tuberculosis victims to rabid dogs!!!" His reaction to the antispitting campaign was little different, as his comparison to Don Quixote shows.

> The war on spitting takes us back to more heroic times, when a certain illustrious knight, clad entirely in iron and accompanied by his faithful squire, also went off to war. Spittoons and disinfecting equipment have replaced swords, armor, and shields, which are outmoded weapons today.
>
> Alas! nothing new under the sun.[60]

Not surprisingly, the response to Leray's paper at the Société médicale du IXe arrondissement was vehement and defensive. Leading the charge was M. Francon, who denied that contagionists sought a "brutal sequestration" of tuberculosis victims, or any kind of "tyranny." He insisted that they only wanted to make obligatory what Leray called "rules of hygiene," a task that would be made easier the more doctors were able to "educate the masses." Francon threw back at Leray the example of the Œuvre Grancher, which temporarily placed children from at-risk urban backgrounds with families in the countryside to protect them from all of the influences that predisposed to tuberculosis. He asked sarcastically if this philanthropic venture was yet another "cruelty, a torture revived from the age of barbarism" because the children were taken away from their families. On the contrary, Francon said, such measures were in the best interests of all concerned.[61]

However, not all the reaction to Leray's polemic was negative. Several speakers rose to endorse his position and to reinforce one or another of his points. One supporter deplored the "exaggerations committed by overly absolute and authoritarian hygienists" and lampooned the obsessive attention paid to different varieties of spittoons at the recent International Tuberculosis Congress in Paris. "If the Koch bacillus has not yet been killed by sheer ridicule, this is certainly due to its great resistance!"[62] Leray himself finished with a plea for compassion rather than isolation, and material aid rather than quixotic fantasies.

> Pity for those who go hungry! Pity for those who are cold! Fresh air for those who lack it; [a]nd finally, sunlight, to chase away mites and myths at the same time.[63]

While few would have argued with such sentiments, the participants certainly believed that there was a fundamental disagreement involved. Two particular characteristics of the War on Tuberculosis stand out from this exchange: first, the representatives of the dominant etiology, who tenaciously held to the soil-seed duality and defended their humanitarian sensitivity, consistently confined their practical recommendations to the field of contagion prevention; second, the rough balance between Leray's defenders and his opponents which prevailed among those who intervened at these meetings in no way reflected the distribution of power in the broader arenas of medicine and public health.

In the antituberculosis literature as a whole, these demurrals from bacillophobia represent a small fraction of the opinions expressed. They are summarized and quoted at length here to illustrate that bacillocentrism was not the inescapable, automatic product of a given set of circumstances. Rather, it was a contingent phenomenon, predominant during a given period despite the efforts of a few dissenters to discredit it. To oppose this scientific dogma was not unthinkable.

DISPENSARIES AND *DÉPISTAGE*

Notwithstanding these vociferous but marginal protests, the hypercontagionist influence prevailed in the official antituberculosis campaign. Several different strategies were contemplated—and, to various degrees, put into practice—to identify and isolate potential vectors of contagion. The antituberculosis dispensary was the first line of defense in the War on Tuberculosis; it was to be the state's hygienic eyes and ears in France's remotest urban neighborhoods as well as the crucial vehicle for distribution of primary health care and philanthropic assistance. Although the dispensaries themselves stressed their care-giving and charitable aspects, their strategic role in the national campaign against tuberculosis was first and foremost one of *dépistage,* tracking down those who might be infected.

Dispensaries, it should be emphasized, aimed their intervention at one specific clientele: the poor. After all, this was where tuberculosis found most of its victims. Between 1901 and 1905, adult residents of the poor twentieth arrondissement of Paris were over six times more likely to die of tuberculosis than those in the wealthy eighth arrondissement. Annual adult tuberculosis mortality rates in those districts, 78 per 10,000 population and 12 per 10,000, respectively, suggest the degree of inequality before death that prevailed in the capital. Even if one discards the city's low and high extremes for 1901–1905, one still finds an annual tuberculosis mortality for adults of 60 per 10,000 in the thirteenth, fourteenth, and fifteenth arrondissements compared to 28 per 10,000 in the affluent sixteenth arrondissement—a ratio of more than two to one.[64]

While tuberculosis showed a marked preference for those on the lower rungs of the social ladder, the bourgeoisie was certainly not immune from the disease. Even the comparatively low death rates cited above for the city's wealthy neighborhoods amounted to approximately 120 and 260 tuberculosis deaths per year in the eighth and sixteenth arrondissements, respectively[65]—not all of which can be accounted for by domestic servants. Patients of means, while not the population with which the War on Tuberculosis was primarily concerned, confronted their own dilemmas and uncertainties when they found themselves ill. Those who could afford to do so, of course, sought treatment from private physicians. But seeking medical treatment for tuberculosis at the turn of the century was not as straightforward as it would become after the advent of streptomycin, rifampin, and isoniazid.

Even after medical science knew increasingly minute details about the nature, behavior, and transmission of the tubercle bacillus, it could still do nothing to treat tuberculosis. Germ theory by itself did not end the era of therapeutic impotence. The treatment regimens recommended by physicians for their tuberculous patients changed little with the bacteriological revolution. Commonly used treatments included goat's milk, cod liver oil, lichen (ingested in teas and jams and applied to the skin in pastes), antimony, tannic acid, creosote, arsenic, and the inhalation of tar vapors. Occasional innovations such as the administration of formaldehyde gas with currents of static electricity vied for attention in the pages of medical journals and popular newspapers with advertisements for myriad patent remedies claiming miraculous curative powers. A "cure" could be claimed, it seemed, with every sign of improvement in a patient's condition, or whenever a patient regained strength over a period of several months. The symptoms of tuberculosis could disappear even for years at a time—for example, when the patient was removed from the milieu or circumstances in which the illness appeared—only to return with equal or greater severity in times of stress or weakness.[66]

Medicine's inability to find a specific, reliable cure for tuberculosis in the nineteenth century merely underscores the remarkable presumption on the part of physicians to "treat" the disease socially by pronouncing on the most intimate matters of personal conduct and the most complex issues of social organization. That they did so owes less to the accumulation of knowledge about tuberculosis than to the increasingly prominent social and political position of medical doctors in nineteenth-century France. The degree to which physicians participated in government on both the local and national levels—not to mention philanthropy and other areas of social influence—made France unique among industrialized and "medicalized" nations. The pathbreaking discoveries of the Pasteurian revolution in microbiology and the promise of science to cure not only the individual's but society's ills allowed French medicine to arrogate the authority to prescribe social reform as well as medication.[67] Such authority, however, did not add to the doctor's therapeutic arsenal. In the absence of a "magic bullet" for tuberculosis, the only systematically reliable treatment in the years before antibiotics was what doctors described as *la cure d'air, de repos, et de suralimentation* (the fresh air, rest, and overfeeding cure): a well-fed vacation. Only with ample nutrition and rest in a healthful environment, it was observed, could the body withstand the ravages of tuberculosis.[68]

These were, above all, cures for the bourgeoisie, and they could not have been universally prescribed even if the medical profession had wished to do so. Whatever the therapeutic value of the various treatments for tuberculosis, the working-class clientele of the dispensaries did not have the luxury of trying them, and they certainly could not afford to leave work and family to seek a rest cure in the countryside. The dispensary, therefore, could not reasonably be expected to cure disease. It could only attempt to alleviate some of the effects of poverty and to prevent the spread of tuberculosis by observing and reforming the local population.

The annual reports of French dispensaries for the years before World War I are replete with statistics on the monetary value of linen, meat and milk coupons given away, laundry washed, home disinfections, and other aid offered to the poor and indigent. This real material assistance was an important part of dispensaries' day-to-day functioning, and it should not be disdained simply because many of the theorists and strategists of the War on Tuberculosis were preoccupied with dépistage. Nevertheless, it would be naive to accept uncritically the dispensaries' self-representation and not to distinguish between strategic raison d'être, on the one hand, and the noble intentions or deeds of individual participants, on the other.

The model for all antituberculosis dispensaries in France was the Préventorium Emile Roux in Lille, established by Calmette in 1901. The phrases "modeled on the Lille dispensary" and "of the Calmette type" recur frequently in annual reports and proposals for the creation of new dispensaries.[69] Calmette himself conceived of the ideal "preventorium" as a combination "recruiting office and practical school of hygiene." First among all of its duties, he wrote, had to be recruitment: "to *seek out,* to *attract,* and to *retain* . . . workers who have, or are suspected of having, tuberculosis [*les ouvriers atteints ou suspects de tuberculose*]." This was the function that Calmette and others came to refer to as "dépistage." The second major role of the dispensary was educational, to instill in its target population the elementary notions of personal and domestic hygiene.[70]

Auxiliary to these two primary functions were others that complemented them in various ways. Dispensaries could serve as "filters" or triage centers for sanatoriums (assuming that enough of the latter could be created and made accessible to the poor), referring only patients who were "almost surely curable." For the majority of patients, who for whatever reason could not go to a sanatorium and were not ready for the hospital, the dispensary could attend to their material needs by distributing food, clothing, bedding, and medication. For hopeless cases, it could at least protect family members and others from contamination. "It will give them the means to finish their lives without harming those close to them, without spreading contagion and misery all around them."[71]

Still, despite this variety of goals and activities, dépistage seemed to remain foremost in the minds of hygienists and public officials, who promoted the dispensary as a practical and inexpensive alternative to the sanatorium in the War on Tuberculosis. It would be unsatisfactory for dispensaries simply to offer their services and material aid to the public, as Calmette apparently understood.

> I think that instead of waiting for the consumptive worker to go to the doctor . . . , we should adhere in principle to the necessity of going to him and giving him assistance, even before he notices that he is gravely ill. I would like for us to be able to track down [*dépister*] tuberculosis in the patient at the very beginning of its development.[72]

This may have been the crucial difference between medicine and public health or hygiene: medicine waited for patients to come to it, whereas hygiene went out to find patients—even when patients did not know they were ill. Camille Savoire, another early and outspoken advocate of dispensaries, agreed with Calmette that "we must not wait for the patients to come to the doctor" and felt that dépistage had to go beyond haphazard and piecemeal efforts. He called for a "permanent and periodical medical inspection of all public and private organizations and groups," which would constitute "a very fine-meshed net that will in passing filter out *tuberculeux* from various social milieus in order to give them the care that their state demands, to render them incapable of harming the community, and to ensure an early diagnosis."[73] At the very least, the fine-meshed net was meant to prevent patients from harming others (by contagion) as much as it was meant to single out potential recipients of medical care.

Governmental authorities were also quite receptive to the dépistage that dispensaries could offer in the struggle against tuberculosis. Paris city councilman Ambroise Rendu, for instance, reported in 1908 on signs that the disease might be on the decline in Paris: "Among the means employed effectively in the fight against this scourge, we must give special priority to dépistage through dispensaries, and to the cooperation that has been established between them and the casier sanitaire."[74] It is revealing that Rendu not only singled out dépistage in praising dispensaries but also linked them to the casier sanitaire, the municipal administration's office that monitored the city's housing stock from the point of view of tuberculosis mortality. (See chap. 4, below.) Both aimed at extending the eyes and ears of the state (or its partners in the medical profession) into the neighborhoods, homes, and daily lives of the working class. Both relied more on observation and administrative knowledge than on material improvement or intervention.

The importance of administrative knowledge—the official registration and integration of a person into a network of aid, surveillance, and obligations—is suggested in other discussions of dispensaries as well. For example, the director of a Paris dispensary explained to a correspondent in 1903 that patients had to undergo three types of examinations before being registered: "clinical" tests, involving observable symptoms; "bacteriological" tests of sputum, blood, and urine; and a "social" inquiry into their housing and work conditions. Finally, "the patient, known [*connu*] from this triple point of view—clinical, bacteriological, and social—is admitted into the dispensary."[75] Without these fundamental and far-reaching *connaissances,* in the medical and administrative context of France at the turn of the century, the dispensary strategy would have been unthinkable.

The second great aim of the dispensary movement was hygienic education. Along with pocket spittoons, every dispensary gave patients printed "catechisms," or lessons for avoiding tuberculosis, which were reviewed in person during visits as well. They admonished patients to wash themselves every day, to boil their milk, to cook their meat thoroughly (except for horse meat, which could be eaten raw because horses were not susceptible to tuberculosis), to beware of dust and, of course, of spittle too. "Be sober," the catechisms advised, disinfect new lodgings with bleach when moving in, and breathe through the nose rather than the mouth, as one such sheet recommended. "The nose is a microbe-killer. A closed mouth preserves health, says the English proverb."[76]

All of the measures commonly found in the dispensary catechisms, except for sobriety, involved avoiding contagion. This is strange, given the fact that the only patients likely to get to the catechism stage of dispensary treatment were already designated as infected. Yet the instructions were generally phrased as contributing to the patient's own protection, rather than the protection of family and friends.[77] Such instructions were presumably intended to shield the as yet uninfected from contagion, but dispensary officials apparently did not deem it acceptable to admit as much openly. Perhaps it was feared that only self-interest could motivate a patient to follow the recommended regimen, or that at least some hope needed to be held out to the suffering patient.

With education came surveillance. Once admitted to treatment at the dispensary, "the *tuberculeux,* along with everything that concerns him, is never lost from sight," as one legislator put it. Even if the patient was referred by the dispensary to a sanatorium or hospital, "as soon as he returns . . . the dispensary again assumes certain powers over him [*le dispensaire reprend certains pouvoirs sur lui*], always in his own interest and in the interest of those around him." Fuster also emphasized that "the improved patient remains a suspect, from the social point of view, and for his own sake has a pressing interest in staying under observation." [78] In other words, no matter what the circumstances that led patients to the dispensary in the first place, the treatment and charitable aid they received there was not strictly voluntary. The patient who had been *dépisté* was from that moment onward a "suspect," a potential danger to all those around him or her. At that point, individual rights were subordinated to the right of others to be free from contagion. As far as dispensaries were concerned, such issues rarely arose in public debate; but they came out into the open when attention turned to the mandatory declaration of tuberculosis and to proposals for the isolation of consumptives.

MANDATORY DECLARATION AND ISOLATION

Mandatory declaration—the legal obligation of doctors to report cases of tuberculosis to the authorities—represented the ultimate form of dépistage. Like the dépistage of dispensaries, it was inherently a preparatory measure, one that would have made little sense if not followed up by other measures. It is possible that advocates of mandatory declaration and other ways of tracking down those afflicted with tuberculosis intended to follow up with basic health care, residential disinfection, and education. However, the theme of forced or semiforced isolation arose often enough in discussions surrounding the War on Tuberculosis to suggest that at least some authorities considered it a corollary to mandatory declaration.

The most enthusiastic champions of mandatory declaration tended to be the nondoctors among hygienists and public officials. The medical profession was deeply divided over the issue, since it violated the *secret médical,* the almost sacred obligation of doctor-patient confidentiality. Some observers such as Fuster (who was not a medical doctor) treated ethical considerations as more of an annoyance than anything else. He called mandatory declaration of tuberculosis "the only serious resource with which the public powers could arm hygienists." He envisioned declaration as obligatory not only for doctors but also for parents, employers, public assistance offices, and heads of schools, hotels, and other establishments. However, Fuster complained, "certain habits of liberty will no doubt long prevent us from giving hygienists the satisfaction on this point that their logic demands."[79] On one level, it is noteworthy that Fuster thought of objections on moral grounds as bothersome obstacles to progress. Yet on another level, one must wonder why he referred to "certain habits of liberty," rather than specifically to the *secret médical,* for example. The only reason for which anyone would have raised such an objection would be that the "hygienists' logic" would undermine personal freedom in some way—for instance, isolation of a less than voluntary nature—once mandatory declaration had become law.

Official calls for the quarantine of consumptives dated back even to the time of the contagion debates before the discovery of the tubercle bacillus. In 1880, when Dr. Adolphe Lecadre of Le Havre went before the Conseil d'hygiène publique of the Seine-Inférieure to argue that tuberculosis was indeed contagious, he called for its victims to be isolated within hospitals to prevent them from infecting others. In reporting Lecadre's proposal, along with another that would keep children with tuberculosis from attending school, the *Revue d'hygiène et de police sanitaire* called them "premature," since the contagiousness of the disease had not yet been conclusively proven. "Mandatory isolation always implies a certain infringement on individual liberty; in this case, the infringement would not be justified in the general interest, because the contagiousness of phthisis has not been proven."[80] The journal implied, however, that isolation would be justified when the disease was proven to be contagious.

By the time the dominant etiology had been fully elaborated and had achieved hegemony within the French medical community around the turn of the century, a consensus had developed on the proper roles of various institutions in the War on Tuberculosis. Whereas dispensaries were needed for dépistage and acted as the first line of defense, sanatoriums—to the extent that enough money could actually be raised to create them in sufficient numbers—were to be reserved for patients in the early stages of illness, who were eminently "curable." The more hopeless cases, many hygienists agreed, were to be isolated in "asylums," where they could "die tranquilly" without contaminating others.[81]

This last category of patients, "who can no longer render society any more than intermittent services, or who will be a permanent drain [on society's resources] until their imminent end," were of interest to the authorities only in their capacity as vectors of contagion. Only patients with the potential to be useful to society in the future could be allowed to occupy scarce beds in sanatoriums. With both sanatoriums and asylum hospitals, Calmette wrote, "We will achieve as much as possible the *isolation* of the bacillus-spitting *tuberculeux*." [82] During the solidarist era before World War I, when private philanthropy was expected to fund all such institutions, this strategy was never put into practice extensively. Yet some historians have in fact argued that when sanatoriums came into more widespread use in France during the interwar period, they served a carceral function and that this function took precedence in practice over therapeutic goals. [83]

The hard-liner Fuster drew a sharp distinction between isolation and effective treatment: the latter was rarely a realistic expectation, yet the former was vital. To fulfill the hygienist's objectives, that basic truth had to be hidden from patients. In calling for the institutionalization of contagious cases, Fuster made it clear that treatment was not the primary aim. "[It would be] fortunate if our therapeutic resources could enable us, in addition, to cure this individual socially, that is, to bring him to a state of health in which he would no longer be contagious!" Improvement in the patient's condition would be an added bonus, from the hygienic point of view, because he or she would no longer pose a threat to society. This was as true of the sanatorium as it was of any other institution; although it offered mild cases of tuberculosis "a few chances of spontaneous cure," it also offered "the immediate advantage of removing from the family or social milieu persons who would soon be contagious." [84] From Fuster's point of view, the harsh truth was that the treatment of sick individuals was not the goal of the War on Tuberculosis. The hygienist's responsibility was to the healthy majority of the citizenry, to protect it from contagion.

Fuster cautioned, however, that isolation would be difficult to put into practice without unforeseen help from legislators. The tuberculosis patient, he explained, often enjoyed prolonged periods of improvement in symptoms and rarely lapsed into the "resignation of the infirm." These episodes of remission gave sick persons renewed hope and made them unlikely candidates for the role of "the good asylum patient, condemned but calm." Under these circumstances, without a law enabling forced internment, convincing the patient to volunteer for isolation would be all but impossible:

> It is essential to always speak to him of possible treatment, if we want him *to allow himself to be isolated* [and] interned. Because, ultimately, no law authorizes us to take him away from his lodgings and his habits. . . . To isolate them, we will therefore have to open small asylums where dispensar-

ies and other *dépisteurs* can send them, leaving them the illusion that they are going there to recover.[85]

It was up to the "dépisteurs," then, to feed enough false hope to patients that they would be obedient and allow themselves to be "interned" under the pretext of medical care. Fuster's views on these issues were almost certainly not typical of all those who aligned themselves with the War on Tuberculosis; after all, not being a physician, he did not have to deal with patients on a personal, everyday basis. Yet he was honest enough to state baldly what he probably saw as uncomfortable truths. Much of what he admitted may have underlain, unstated, the positions of others who elided the distinctions among such concepts as dépistage, isolation, and treatment.

One doctor who matched, and at times even exceeded, Fuster's brutal candor was Jules Héricourt, who unabashedly championed forced isolation of tuberculosis patients throughout his career. Héricourt reasoned, just as Fuster did, in terms of the relative value and danger to society of sick and healthy individuals and concluded that one group had to be protected at the expense of the other. The cold logic of his argument merits a close reading, to explore a point of view that pushed at the outer limits of the acceptable even in the heyday of germ theory.

Héricourt advocated the creation of *tuberculoseries,* modern-day leper colonies, to eliminate tuberculosis by removing its victims from society. His premise was that the consumptive represented a reduced (if not null) social value:

> From the social point of view, the sick man is obviously of less interest than the healthy man. His value is reduced, if not annulled, from the point of view of production, and he constitutes a danger to the community, whereas the healthy man retains all his present value and, through his family, represents the future.

For these reasons, the hygienist was obliged "to protect the healthy man." To do so, Héricourt suggested that the twentieth century could learn something from the Middle Ages, when "our ancestors . . . had the genius to eliminate leprosy by eliminating lepers, that is, by confining them in leper colonies." The medieval example was all the more admirable in that, "several centuries before Pasteur," it succeeded in implementing "on a vast practical scale" what the great microbiologist achieved in the laboratory by separating diseased silkworms from their healthy counterparts.[86]

Héricourt's solution to the tuberculosis problem was a revival of *léproseries* as tuberculoseries, where the infected would be confined to prevent contagion. In 1905, he believed that the idea's time might finally have come. "It has now been fifteen years since I first dared to speak of tuberculoseries. Since then, the idea has progressed, and the word now appears fairly frequently in speeches. Let us hope that some day it will be put into action." His optimism seems to have been unjustified. In fact, the only speeches in which the word *tuberculoserie* occurred to any noticeable extent were Héricourt's own. As shown above, even when doctors and hygienists spoke of "isolation" as a means of combating tuberculosis, they usually qualified their endorsement by acknowledging that such measures were unrealistic in the context of prevailing mores and concerns about "individual liberty." More typical than Héricourt's solution was his lament about what would happen if drastic action was not taken soon: "as long as *tuberculeux* continue to circulate, they will spread contagion in the streets and in public places, and through their coughing, they will continue to breathe contagion into the atmosphere."[87]

Héricourt's extreme positions did not necessarily represent the mainstream of French medical opinion, and his plans were never fully realized. Some present-day readers may find his recommendations harsh and repressive. (Nevertheless, even in the 1990s, public health experts still consider incarceration a viable weapon in the fight against tuberculosis. In 1993, New York City reopened an old hospital ward on Roosevelt Island for the forcible detention of patients who had repeatedly failed to complete their full course of antituberculosis treatment.[88]) Was this doctor articulating what his peers felt but were afraid to say, or was he simply a bizarre extremist? While there may be no clear answer to this question, it is certainly true that Héricourt was an influential and well-connected figure in the world of French science at the turn of the century. He served as editor of the prestigious *Revue scientifique*. He collaborated closely for many years with Charles Richet, the 1913 Nobel Prize winner in medicine and physiology, who wrote the preface to one of his books. The same book was dedicated to "my learned friend" Gustave Lebon, the famous crowd psychologist.[89] Whatever else he may have been, Héricourt was no mere crackpot; whether his colleagues shared his views on tuberculosis prevention or not, he clearly enjoyed an influential and respected place in French medicine.

Héricourt's tuberculoseries, along with the dépistage and surveillance functions of the dispensary, recall Foucault's discussion of the "carceral archipelago" in *Discipline and Punish*. In the context of the history of prisons and penology, Foucault described the vast network of institutions and practices that contributed to the dual functions of discipline and normalization as follows:

> The judges of normality are present everywhere. We are in the society of the teacher-judge, the doctor-judge, the educator-judge, the social-worker-judge; it is on them that the universal reign of the normative is based; and each individual, wherever he may find himself, subjects to it his body, his gestures, his behaviour, his aptitudes, his achievements. The carceral network ... with its systems of insertion, distribution, surveillance, observation, has been the greatest support, in modern society, of the normalizing power.[90]

It is not difficult to see Héricourt's tuberculoseries and the strategies of some sanatorium proponents as fundamentally disciplinary and carceral in nature. But can the same be said of public health programs, such as the dispensary, that purport to be strictly philanthropic? Certain institutions and their advocates may have been preoccupied explicitly with punishment and incarceration, yet it is important to recognize the extent to which auxiliary, facilitative policies also contributed to a general environment of "the 'carceral' with its many diffuse or compact forms, its institutions of supervision or constraint, of discreet surveillance and insistent coercion."[91]

The disciplinary and carceral aspects of the War on Tuberculosis did not necessarily operate as conscious motivations for the medical men and politicians who participated in these debates. This would be a far too instrumental and conspiratorial reading of the actors and texts involved. Héricourt certainly must have known that his proposals bore a close relationship to the penality of the prison; but even if he had been less straightforward, and even though some of his colleagues may have been less self-conscious in their appeal to the carceral impulse, the power of that impulse should not be underestimated simply because it remained unacknowledged. During the nineteenth century, as Foucault took pains to point out, the various forms of discipline and surveillance became less easily identifiable and less distinguishable from one another as they became more sophisticated. The "great carceral continuum" also constituted "[a] subtle, graduated carceral net, with compact institutions, but also separate and diffused methods." The judgments that resulted were subtle and continuous rather than sharp, conscious, and distinct.[92] The principles of dépistage and isolation were triumphant precisely to the extent that they appeared both *necessary* and *natural* to nineteenth-century reformers. Once the key notions of hygienic urgency and social danger were accepted, the progression from assistance to surveillance to confinement was just a small logical step.

No single factor can explain the powerful and enduring appeal of bacillocentrism in the French response to tuberculosis. The dramatic success—and dramaturgical power[93]—of Pasteur's experiments with wine, silkworms, rabies, and anthrax no doubt encouraged in many observers first the hope and then the conviction that salvation from all manner of ills lay in controlling microbes. Yet there must have been more to it than that, particularly where tuberculosis was concerned. Germ theory explained the disease and in so doing conferred blame for it; rather than blaming the individual victim for his or her own illness, as other facets of the dominant etiology did, contagion blamed victims as a class for spreading the disease. On occasion, participants in the War on Tuberculosis attributed blame directly, as when one doctor urged patients not to spit on the ground. "What moral responsibility [would be yours] if, by your negligence, you contaminated a relative, a friend, [or] any one of your compatriots." The patient who ignored this injunction was guilty of "sinning against his brothers [and] against society."[94]

Through spitting, the spread of tuberculosis was associated with a practice perceived as disgusting and uncivilized. Spitting also brought with it a class dimension. The warnings of Paul Juillerat, a hygienist and director of the Paris municipal *casier sanitaire*, highlight the perceived danger of interclass contagion. Juillerat went to great lengths to convince all Parisians of the need to fear the germs of tuberculosis. Millions of "murderous bacilli" were distributed every day in the streets, the offices, the workshops, and the lodgings of the city, he cautioned, by coughing and spitting consumptives.

> One shudders at the permanent danger to which one is exposed. Who can pretend, *whatever his social position,* that he will never receive at his residence someone with tuberculosis, visitor or servant, who will deposit the fearsome germ in his home?[95]

Perhaps unintentionally, this statement expressed with unusual clarity the respective social ranks of the vehicle and victim in the archetypal transmission of tuberculosis. Even the bourgeois had something to fear, if only because he had daily contact with his servants.

Even without considering the statistics (widely quoted at the time) that showed the working class to be far more susceptible to tuberculosis than the rest of the population,[96] it is clear that tuberculosis was generally considered to be a disease of the poor, to which others also occasionally fell prey. Contagion allowed hygienists to sound the alarm among the wealthy and powerful that even they were not immune; it also served to embody the threat in a human (working-class) form. The resulting bacillophobia turned casual passersby into suspects, and patients into potentially murderous coughers and spitters.

CHAPTER FOUR

Interiors

Housing and the Casier sanitaire in the War on Tuberculosis

Too often, the slum is only a slum by the fault of the tenant—negligent, slovenly, misinformed of his own interests.
                                    —*Edouard Fuster, 1903*

It is clear that the supreme goal of the bill's authors is to . . . forge a link which will tie all of our domiciles to a central point, and this central point will be Paris. . . . [D]o you not fear . . . arming the representatives of state power with the right to penetrate whenever they wish . . . into our domestic interiors; . . . to wage the war against microbes even into the privacy of our homes?
                     —*Senator François Volland,*
          arguing against health inspection law, 1897

In the years around the turn of the twentieth century, as government officials and doctors in France attempted to make sense of tuberculosis as a "social scourge," their attention was immediately drawn to the deplorable condition of working-class lodgings in the cities. Slum housing took its place alongside contact with microbes and moral deviance in the interlocking trinity of the dominant etiology. The integration of housing into both the medical understanding of tuberculosis and the official response to the disease's spread involved not only the appropriation of some familiar, pre-germ theory attitudes toward disease but also the beginnings of a newer, more characteristically "modern" reaction.

The impulse to attribute blame for illness—and particularly to blame the victim—is doubtless as old as humankind. The fact that blame was sought for the prevalence of tuberculosis in nineteenth-century France, then, should not be surprising, but the intensity and variety of its manifestations are representative of a unique social and political context.

The "moral etiology" of tuberculosis was, of course, the primary vehicle for the attribution of blame, but the impulse is evident even in the discussion of housing and its role in spreading the disease.

Also inherited from an earlier era was the desire to explain disease in terms of geography, and to control disease by controlling space. What Alain Cottereau has called the "*glissement écologique*" (ecological slide),[1] the expression of social relations in terms of relations with the environment, was typical of the early-nineteenth-century French hygienists' understanding of tuberculosis, but it reappeared in new germ theory garb through the integration of housing into the dominant etiology.

The more historically novel features in the housing-tuberculosis connection included a strategy based on administrative inventory and surveillance of housing stock. In particular, the casier sanitaire des maisons, a tool used most comprehensively in Paris, represented a remarkably ambitious effort to see into the obscure corners of the capital's pathologies. This municipal government office assembled files on every residential building in the city, recording each death by contagious disease (noting the exact cause and date) so that the most dangerous sources of contagion could be identified.

The government's approach to the housing connection also owed much to another late-nineteenth-century phenomenon: the new ideology of solidarism, championed by Léon Bourgeois, which came to dictate the contours of the official War on Tuberculosis in France before World War I. In fact, a detailed analysis of the housing aspect of the *lutte antituberculeuse* reveals the central contradictions of solidarism, a political movement that existed largely in theory and never fully translated its tenets into practice. The principle of collaboration among all sectors of society to address social problems resulted in a partnership more rhetorical than material.

This mixture of old and new strands combined to form a coherent understanding of (and the basis for a response to) the role of housing in tuberculosis. This understanding emerged through a commonsense transition from investigative description to medical and administrative response. The two steps of this transition are examined here in turn, with emphasis on the disgust and moral outrage of the descriptive genre and on the Paris casier sanitaire as an exemplar of the official response. Finally, the curious role of women in the housing narratives—chiefly as negligent wives and dangerous *domestiques*—is examined as a significant undercurrent in the exposure of the domestic interior.

DARKNESS, FILTH, AND PROMISCUITY

The late-nineteenth-century shift in sanitary anxiety over the pathological urban center has been aptly described by Ann-Louise Shapiro in her history of French government housing policy. "Not only were the garbage heaps and wastes surrounding workers' housing seen as a serious public hazard, but contemporaries had come to understand the very walls, ceilings, furniture, and clothing of the worker as presenting a danger."[2] In other words, the preoccupation of miasmatic theory and Haussmann-style public works with *external* causes of disease moved indoors. Cleaning up the interior of urban dwellings replaced sanitizing the city's exterior as the main task of hygienists when the War on Tuberculosis began to take shape in the Belle Epoque.

The most striking feature of the attacks on slum housing is the priority given to graphic description. Mastery of a certain naturalistic genre of reporting seems to have been almost obligatory, a prerequisite for addressing the role of housing in tuberculosis. Knowledge of the details of urban squalor contributed as much to this branch of medical literature as did knowledge of the tubercle bacillus and its properties. There were four primary characteristics of working-class housing that riveted the attention of bourgeois observers: lack of sunlight, poor ventilation, filth, and overcrowding.

Interestingly, these four characteristics were scarcely ever disconnected from one another or examined individually. Rather, they formed a chain in which the presence of each link strengthened the others and gave the slum descriptions a unique, synesthetically repellent quality. The following excerpt gives a good idea of the structure and workings of the genre; it is taken from a two-part series on the War on Tuberculosis in the *Annales des sciences politiques*.[3]

> We know in a general way that the unsanitariness and uncleanliness of housing in the poorer quarters of large cities are one of the principal factors of all microbial diseases. But we can scarcely imagine the true degree of this overcrowding [and] this filth.

Already the authors have made a claim for the enhanced status of their own detailed knowledge, as if to justify on epistemological grounds the abundance of unpleasant detail that follows.

> In order to understand it you have to have seen up close these houses with their thin walls of plaster-coated brick, where the winter cold makes itself cruelly felt; these interior courtyards ... onto which face the windows of

innumerable lodgings which contaminate each other with their stench; these abominable water-closets—if one can call them that without irony—where never a drop of clean water flows . . . whose odor spreads throughout the building.

Three of the four major elements of the standard slum description—lack of sunlight, poor ventilation, and filth—have by this point been mentioned in the text, and the fourth follows soon after. "One finds single rooms occupied by 9, 11, 14 people, with only two cubic meters of air per person." The authors then allow another voice—that of Dr. Gabriel Séailles in a much-cited 1897 article in *La France médicale*—to finish the description, with the same tone of disgust.

> Whoever has not served as a charity-bureau doctor, whoever has not at all hours of day or night crossed the threshold of these single rooms, without ventilation or sunlight, cannot have any idea of the disorder and repulsive filth that reigns in these dim recesses of our cities.

Still in Séailles's voice, descriptive revulsion turns soon to medical etiology and the first mention of tuberculosis.

> In these rooms, they do everything: they cook, they eat, they sleep. This is where our patients cough, where they spit, where they waste away, and where they die. . . . The consumptive is left alone all day: he coughs, he spits on the ground; it is easy, then, to understand the danger faced by the children coming home from school or the workers coming home to rest. This is the time when they pretend to clean the room. They sweep, and from the dried sputum, the microbe is lifted up and suspended in the air.

The transition is seamless. Read as a whole, the description leaves the impression that the totality of appalling conditions contributes en bloc to the proliferation and transmission of microbes. An analysis of the constituent elements of this description and of similar passages reveals some of the persistent attitudes and associations underlying the slum–tuberculosis connection.

Despite the impression of overall congruence between slum conditions and the causes of tuberculosis, it is important to note the specific factors that the dominant etiology explicitly cited as facilitating the disease's transmission. Because direct sunlight had been shown to kill the Koch bacillus, an apartment with little or no exposure to sunlight was considered dangerous. Ventilation could not only clear microbe-laden particles out of a room but also renewed "stale air," which interfered with proper respiration. Dust (and, by extension, dirt or particles of any kind) provided the bacillus with a home—and a pathway into human lungs. (Therefore, sweeping the floor rather than wet mopping was continually denounced as an extremely hazardous method of cleaning.) Finally, overcrowding increased the risk of direct contagion, and also resulted in stale air when the volume of air per person in a given space was inadequate.

Yet all of these ingredients of slum housing were *disgusting,* too. Séailles emphasized the "at times repulsive disorder and filth" of the slums. Others described the "horribly vitiated air" of overcrowded rooms. Nearly every bourgeois observer took pains to evoke the smell of working-class housing. In a room occupied by many people for long periods of time, one doctor wrote, exhaled air "is an excrement, and, as such, it smells bad and is toxic." The description quoted above lingered on the "abominable water-closets" whose odor permeated the entire building.[4]

"Vitiated air" and putrid smells were the stock in trade of miasmatic theory in the pre-Pasteurian age of medicine. The doctors and hygienists of the antituberculosis crusade would certainly have scoffed at any comparison of their scientific work with the outdated dogma of the era of anticontagionism and spontaneous generation. Yet visceral aversions survived such paradigm shifts. As Corbin shows in his pioneering history of smell in France, the period between 1750 and 1880 saw the triumph of a bourgeois ideal of cleanliness that entailed a rejection of the foul-smelling (and eventually, on a social level, of the working class) as uncivilized, unsanitary, and pathogenic. In medicine, "pre-Pasteurian mythologies" about miasmas and decaying matter sanctioned and reinforced this trend, until germ theory discredited them. However, as Corbin points out, even doctors retained many of the old ways of thinking—and smelling.[5]

One word that often appeared alongside *encombrement* in discussions of overcrowding was *promiscuité.* While the latter's meaning has different nuances in French than in English, its frequent use betrays a deep-seated fear of uncontrolled proximity in any context—another reaction characteristic of the nineteenth-century bourgeoisie. One doctor condemned the arrangement of domestics' quarters on the sixth floor of a building "in a promiscuity as immoral as it is unsanitary." In a similar vein, another wrote of "entire families of *tuberculeux* succumbing to the ravages of cohabitation."[6] The explicit reason for these sorts of denunciations was the danger of contagion, but both moral judgment and gut-level disgust underlay them.

Each of the four factors that bothered bourgeois observers about working-class housing (lack of sunlight, poor ventilation, filth, over-crowding) could be denounced on etiological grounds, and each was to some extent an object of aversion. The ability of sunlight to kill tubercle bacilli had been irrefutably demonstrated in laboratories; other links on the "medical" side of the chain seem to have been less well established, although widely assumed to be true. The point is that the degree of their proof or even provability was irrelevant to their place in the housing–tuberculosis connection. As long as there was a chain of factors commonly associated with each other within the descriptive genre, the medical validation of even just one of them validated the whole chain. Even if observation or statistics failed to show any correlation between one of the factors and tuberculosis (as in fact happened in some studies of over-crowding), that element could (and did) continue to appear in the descriptions. Darkness, filth, and promiscuity owed their presence in the antituberculosis campaign as much to disgust as to medical science.

THE CASIER SANITAIRE DES MAISONS IN PARIS

The name *casier sanitaire* itself evokes the *cordon sanitaire,* the policy of quarantining an area or limiting the entry of outsiders during epidemics. Indeed, the administrative tracking of tuberculosis mortality by house represented in a sense an updated version of attempts to confine disease to a particular area. Yet the word *casier* offers a deeper insight into the impulse behind the institution. A pigeonhole or compartment—and by extension, a grid of compartments—the word *casier* suggests the need of hygienists and administrators to understand the problems of slum housing and tuberculosis by classification and compartmentalization. Officialdom's knowledge of the dangers and pathologies lurking in the dim recesses of the capital could only be complete if each constituent element of the diseased city was placed—and observed—in its proper casier.

While the casier sanitaire system of housing surveillance represented a departure in many ways from past administrative practice, it was not without its precedents. Since the ancien régime, the French cadastral survey had kept records on all real property for taxation purposes. These records included files on every residential building in Paris, with a brief description of the size and shape of each dwelling unit and the gross rental income of the entire building. In the nineteenth century, several European countries instituted systems of housing inspection, and the 1848 law on *logements insalubres* gave France a legal framework under which local commissions could enforce certain minimum standards for residential upkeep and sanitation.[7]

The cadastre, however, was never used to actually "look inside" lodgings; and housing inspectors as well as *commissions des logements insalubres* only responded to complaints, rather than relying on prior classification based on "objective" criteria such as mortality statistics. Perhaps the most significant analogue of the casier sanitaire—and testimony to a similar current in the science of public health—were city maps showing the geographic distribution of mortality by cause of death. Some of these maps showed neighborhoods or administrative units in graphic shadings or patterns corresponding to the statistics, while others showed each case or death as a dot on the precise location of the victim's residence. (See chap. 6, below.) The casier sanitaire refined this concept to the point where each dot was, in effect, magnified into an entire file, a window into the dwelling that produced the disease. This strategy represented a qualitative leap in sanitary fact-finding in several respects. The inspection system of the commissions des logements insalubres was reactive, responding within the limits of its resources to the complaints concerning individual properties. Likewise, "spot maps" of disease incidence prior to the late nineteenth century were temporally limited and responsive, produced in the context of epidemic emergencies. The casier sanitaire, in contrast, was predicated on regularity and permanence; it envisioned the constant surveillance of all lodgings, informed by both medical and social knowledge, backed by the authority of the state and the possibility of official intervention.

The first European casier sanitaire was created in Brussels in 1871. In 1876, M. Lamouroux of the Paris city council invoked the example of Brussels in proposing a "sanitary file of houses" for the French capital. His proposal never reached fruition. Three years later, Mayor Jules Siegfried of Le Havre succeeded in establishing France's first municipal health department (*bureau d'hygiène*) in his city. One of the Le Havre board's primary responsibilities was the maintenance of a casier sanitaire, although budgetary constraints periodically interrupted its functioning. Prefect Poubelle of the Seine renewed the call for a casier sanitaire in Paris in 1892 and commissioned a report by Dr. A. J. Martin on the information that should be included in its files. Early the next year, all health-related services in the prefecture of the Seine were reorganized, and the new Bureau de l'assainissement de l'habitation was charged with the creation and upkeep of the casier sanitaire.[8]

The office's first director was Paul Juillerat, who subsequently spent his entire career as France's leading hygienic missionary for two parallel causes: the prominent role of housing conditions in the pathogenesis of tuberculosis, and the importance of the casier sanitaire as an arm of local government. The office's beginnings were somewhat slow, as the logistical difficulties involved in assembling detailed files on every residential building in a city of over three million inhabitants apparently took their toll. Eleven years passed before all the relevant information was collected and filed. By January 1, 1905, every single death from pulmonary tuberculosis in Paris since January 1, 1894, had been cataloged by street address and by story within each building, along with a description of the residential unit, its layout, and sanitary condition. Whenever possible, files contained further information on the professional, personal, and family history of the deceased. The files were constantly kept up to date and periodically analyzed after January 1, 1905.[9]

Once the arduous initial task of assembling the files was completed, Juillerat began to study them and compile statistics. A special committee was formed by the prefect in 1905 to deal with the role of housing in the spread of tuberculosis, and Juillerat reported regularly both to the prefect and to the committee. The numbers contained in the files, he argued, were unequivocal: there was a clear correlation between substandard housing and tuberculosis in Paris. "We are forced to conclude that the houses in which the most people die are always the same." The 5,200 buildings singled out by his office as *maisons tuberculeuses* or *foyers de tuberculose* accounted every year for nearly one-third of the deaths from pulmonary tuberculosis in Paris. Three quarters of a century after Villermé had pointed out the vastly unequal death rates in rich and poor Parisian neighborhoods, the next step had been definitively taken. The object of study had shifted from mortality in general to tuberculosis, its leading constituent factor; moreover, the general pathology of poor neighborhoods had become the specific pathology of slum housing. The etiological role of the maisons tuberculeuses was the chief problem to be addressed, Juillerat reported, "if we really want to curb the distressing progress of tuberculosis."[10]

Insufficient sunlight and ventilation chiefly accounted for the frequency of tuberculosis in the deadly houses.

> The saying "tuberculosis is a disease of darkness" was confirmed as we advanced in our investigation. Each of the houses noted for its excessive tuberculosis mortality contains rooms without air and light. That is where the Koch bacillus is stored up; it is from there that it spreads throughout the neighboring population.[11]

In other words, the ill-lit, dank dwellings of the Parisian poor that so disgusted bourgeois visitors provided an ideal home for the tubercle bacillus. From these incubators, the lethal microbes emerged to threaten the rest of the population. Thus, the linkage of disgusted description with medical etiology was achieved, the voluminous statistics were explained, and a rational basis for intervention was set forth.

Intervention was, of course, the logical corollary of the casier sanitaire. The time and expense of maintaining such comprehensive records could not be justified without practical results. Once a building had been identified as a foyer de tuberculose, there were three possible remedial responses: disinfection, structural modification, or demolition. Microbicidal disinfection—treatment of an apartment's walls, floor, and furniture with various solutions, most often bleach or lime water—was performed during a resident's illness, during a stay in the hospital, and/ or after a death from any contagious disease. The Paris Bureau d'hygiène disinfected lodgings on request or on a doctor's recommendation, within the limits of its resources. According to official figures for the years 1893–1905, the health board performed between 7,000 and 11,000 disinfections for tuberculosis in the city each year (including multiple visits to many apartments).[12] This number is roughly equivalent to the number of deaths from tuberculosis per year in Paris (although not close to the total number of those ill), but few doctors or functionaries ever claimed that a vigorous disinfection policy would significantly reduce tuberculosis mortality. The conditions that originally brought about illness, most observers reasoned, quickly reappeared in most apartments (if indeed they were affected at all) after disinfection.

For structural modification, in contrast, at least one observer—Juillerat—voiced high hopes and impressive claims. From the time in late 1905 when the casier sanitaire personnel began investigating buildings and making recommendations to the end of 1910, they visited 2,112 maisons tuberculeuses. Roughly half of them (1,012 buildings) were assainies—"made healthy" or "sanitized"—by the end of 1910, while work on the remaining buildings was "under way" at that time.[13] Juillerat claimed in his 1910 year-end report that the improved buildings were, in fact, sanitized to such an extent that tuberculosis mortality among their inhabitants had fallen 22 percent from the corresponding rates in 1908.[14]

Demolition was not, in Juillerat's view, a viable option for the casier sanitaire. Only forty-one maisons tuberculeuses were demolished in the first five years after the office began investigating buildings and making recommendations for *assainissement*. All were torn down voluntarily by their owners, to be replaced by new structures. Juillerat believed that his office did not have the legal authority necessary to expropriate buildings for sanitary reasons—a view not shared by some critics, as will become clear below. In his reports, he repeatedly called for passage of a law that would give the government that authority. Meanwhile, the casier sanitaire office limited itself for the most part to persuasion in its dealings with landlords over housing improvements.[15]

In all of his lengthy and comprehensive reports, curiously, Juillerat rarely mentioned one of the central dilemmas of the working-class housing problem: how to keep rents down while accomplishing the necessary renovation of the city's housing. If rents rose in proportion to the physical improvements, the old residents who had been easy prey for tuberculosis would presumably be forced to look elsewhere for shelter—to other low-rent, unsanitary units. Juillerat alluded to this difficulty on one occasion, in discussing the voluntary demolition of buildings classified as maisons tuberculeuses. The property owners took this step "to erect in their place modern buildings [that would bring in] more income."[16] Why would any landlord who undertook *travaux d'assainissement* at the urging of the city health authorities *not* raise rents to compensate for the added expense? Juillerat did not address this practical question in his reports, although he called for "the multiplication of cheap, sanitary housing" as the ultimate remedy for tuberculosis. There is no indication that the casier sanitaire attempted to limit rent increases or otherwise attenuate the likely consequences of capital improvements in the city's housing stock.

In fact, there are signs in Juillerat's reports that the driving force behind the casier sanitaire was not the execution of housing improvements at all. The constantly recurring imperative in all of the reports is information gathering rather than policy implementation. There is no suggestion of any kind of triage that would orient the office's resources toward pursuing intervention in the most serious *foyers* at the expense of further data collection, even once the building mortality files were up to date. There appears to have been a continual push to convince doctors, dispensaries, and other philanthropic institutions to share all of their tuberculosis-related records with the casier sanitaire. As Juillerat wrote in his 1907 report, "The precious information that our office [expects] from the cooperation of dispensaries and doctors . . . strengthens the conclusions that we [can] draw from the casier sanitaire documents and helps reveal ever more fully the evolution and the ravages of the terrible disease." In the same report, Juillerat castigated the Paris *bureaux de bienfaisance* (public charity offices) for their lack of cooperation in data sharing and expressed the need for "the progressive extension of our information networks."[17] Often, this seems to have been the bureau's primary concern.

The casier sanitaire's reports are filled with dozens of charts and statistical tables cataloging everything from the professions of the parents of children with tuberculosis to the departmental origin of tuberculosis patients. Many of the charts are never commented on in the report's text or conclusions, nor were any of the casier sanitaire's policy recommendations based on them. They appear to have been displayed for the sole reason that the information was available. Detail made official knowledge objective and true, and where the "dangerous classes" (who now represented not just a political threat but a contagious biological threat as well) were concerned, no detail was superfluous. The surveillance motive need not necessarily have been planned or conscious to have operated on a fundamental level and played a pivotal role in the functioning of the casier sanitaire.

Although the casier sanitaire was widely praised by hygienists and politicians alike, there were occasional rumblings of disagreement, even from within mainstream French medicine. It is quite significant that few if any of its opponents cited the danger of extending the state's tentacles into the most private spaces of working-class life. The desirability and utility of modern administrative surveillance methods seem to have been widely taken for granted. The warnings of Senator François Volland, cited in an epigraph to this chapter, apparently fell on deaf ears. Arguing against legislation in 1897 that would have required local authorities to certify all residential buildings as sanitary before they could be occupied, Volland asked his colleagues, "Do you not fear . . . arming the representatives of state power with the right to penetrate whenever they wish . . . into our domestic interiors, . . . to wage the war against microbes even into the privacy of our homes?" As with so much French social welfare legislation, *obligation* was the rub; Volland's opposition carried the day on the 1897 bill, and sanitary inspection remained possible but not mandatory. Obligation represented an unacceptable infringement on the rights of private property. Following this same pattern, the casier sanitaire anchored itself firmly in the domain of information gathering, never threatening the rights of landlords.[18]

Yet some observers remained less than fully convinced that housing conditions played a crucial role in the spread of tuberculosis in the first place. In November 1905, Professor Victor-Henri Hutinel of the Paris medical faculty gave a lecture on tuberculosis in which he argued that the role of housing in the etiology of the disease had been exaggerated by the likes of Juillerat. Hutinel admitted that poor housing often drove workers to the cabaret, where alcoholism would lead them inevitably to tuberculosis, but he doubted its direct influence.

> It is often because he is poorly housed that the worker takes up the habit of the cabaret. So unsanitary housing is one of the etiological factors of tuberculosis. Its role has been exposed these past few years—and perhaps a bit exaggerated—by the work of M. Juillerat.

Hutinel saw other factors, including poverty and overcrowding, as more directly related to the spread of tuberculosis.

> Some have tried to make phthisis a matter of housing and said that tuberculosis mortality was directly proportional to the number of stories in the building and inversely proportional to the size of courtyards. Certainly, the hovels of certain poor neighborhoods, with their blackened facades and their walls oozing moisture, are well suited to harboring morbid germs; however, if we moved the tenants who live there to housing that was more sanitary but just as crowded, would tuberculosis not follow them? [19]

Hutinel cited recent German statistics supporting the claim that tuberculosis rates were higher on the upper floors of apartment buildings—where sunlight and ventilation were more plentiful—than on the lower floors. "Is it because these floors are occupied by domestics who were contaminated on the lower floors?" Hutinel asked. "You must admit that it is not so in workers' houses; it is rather because poverty takes refuge in the highest and least costly stories." Poverty caused overcrowding in working-class apartments, he contended, and even the cleanest, most well-ventilated apartment became a nest of tuberculosis when overcrowded. Therefore, the social remedy for the disease would have to address all of its causes: "lodgings would have to be comfortable, spacious, and well ventilated, diets would have to be nourishing, workplaces would have to be healthy, and labor would have to be limited and amply remunerated." [20]

Oddly, Hutinel's argument reinforced the housing etiology by ostensibly refuting it. The importance of conditions inside the working-class home was not diminished at all in his account. Rather, one aspect of the official housing-tuberculosis connection (lack of sunlight and ventilation, emphasized by Juillerat) was pushed aside in favor of another (overcrowding, downplayed by Juillerat). Furthermore, Hutinel endorsed a third aspect, the dismal domestic interior pushing the worker out to the cabaret, which linked housing with the rest of the dominant etiology. Nevertheless, even this mild criticism of the casier sanitaire was quite rare within the boundaries of the official War on Tuberculosis.

On the Left, objections were not so hard to come by, although they were far from uniform. From the socialist camp came cries that Juillerat and the casier sanitaire were being too soft on landlords. In 1911, the *Revue socialiste* published an exposé of the bureau's operations by Ernest Lepez. Lepez praised the administration for its tireless efforts to track down those lodgings that were habitual hosts of tuberculosis and to document the appalling sanitary conditions that made them so. Yet he faulted Juillerat for his failure to exercise all the powers potentially available to him under the law. Lepez dismissed Juillerat's frequent claims that new legislation would be necessary for his office to be able to take over and improve many of the problem buildings.[21]

The casier sanitaire, Lepez charged, was not at all as powerless as its director pretended; or rather, it was "disarmed because it wish[ed] to be so." An *interdiction d'habitation* was not the same as an expropriation and did not require indemnification of the owner. Such an interdiction, or even demolition of a building, could be accomplished under municipal police powers when the building presented a danger to the health of occupants and neighbors. By pleading impotence, Lepez contended, Juillerat proved himself to be "more concerned about the interests of selfish landlords than [were] the laws and regulations themselves." Despite his goodwill and diligent investigations, he ultimately represented the interests of capital rather than those of the working class, Lepez wrote. Socialists could not count on Juillerat or others like him to take the necessary steps.

> It is up to socialist municipalities to enforce the law on landlords' selfishness, and it is up to socialist representatives in parliament to hasten a vote on the expropriation bill. . . . Experience has shown that no party has earned more glory and benefit than the socialists from its campaigns for legality and for the public interest.[22]

Perhaps the most significant feature of this criticism is that it completely accepted the general policy of the casier sanitaire and the social etiology of tuberculosis it represented. Lepez quibbled only with the details of the policy's implementation. This approach typified the socialists' overall stance toward the mainstream War on Tuberculosis.[23]

From the extreme Left came a quite different response to the housing–tuberculosis connection. Fernand Pelloutier and other revolutionary syndicalists, in keeping with their rejection of both liberal and socialist solutions to social problems, dissented from the view that the
incidence of tuberculosis in the various neighborhoods of Paris could
be attributed to housing conditions. Pelloutier compared the Temple
quarter in the central Marais district, which he maintained was
crowded and unsanitary but populated principally by bourgeois Parisians, with Ménilmontant, a less crowded but poorer neighborhood on
the outskirts of the city. The fact that tuberculosis mortality was far
higher in Ménilmontant, Pelloutier argued, disproved the housing thesis.[24] It is worth noting in passing that in his 1908 report, Juillerat used
the same neighborhood comparison tactic to support the importance of
housing which Pelloutier had used in 1900 to deny it. The report contained a table listing the annual tuberculosis mortality per thousand
inhabitants of the twenty arrondissements and eighty *quartiers* in Paris
between 1894 and 1908. Juillerat compared the quarters with the lowest and highest annual mortality figures, Champs-Elysées and Saint-
Merri, respectively. "The social differences in the populations of these
two quarters surely are not enough to explain the enormous difference
in tuberculosis mortality; in contrast, an examination of housing conditions explains it overabundantly."[25]

Still, Juillerat knew that comparing wealthy Champs-Elysées with
working-class Saint-Merri did not further his case much. In an attempt
to find a more apt contrast to Saint-Merri, he chose Javel in the fifteenth
arrondissement as representative of working-class neighborhoods with
low population density and lodgings receiving sufficient sunlight and
ventilation. With 3.81 tuberculosis deaths per thousand inhabitants per
year, Javel ranked well below Saint-Merri's 6.74, the highest in Paris.
Juillerat then concluded that the difference between the Champs-Elysées
mortality figure (0.67) and that of Javel represented the "maximum effect produced by social differences" in the incidence of tuberculosis.
Therefore, the substantial difference between the Javel and Saint-Merri
figures could only be attributed to the effect of housing. It is possible,
however, that these statistics could have been made to "prove" quite a
range of theories about tuberculosis. For example, although Juillerat
did not mention it, his table showed Pelloutier's sanitary, working-class
area (the twentieth arrondissement, containing Ménilmontant) with a
mortality figure of 5.26, while the third arrondissement (the Temple,
unsanitary and bourgeois) ranked much lower at 3.91.[26]

The experience of the casier sanitaire exemplifies a relationship between the public and private sectors typical of the War on Tuberculosis as a whole. Essentially, the solidarist ethic of public-private partnership evaporated into a sea of words when put into practice. The public sector mobilized medical experts, mapped out a national strategy in tandem with them, and urged the private sector to come forward with the money to pay for implementation. Meanwhile, private philanthropists founded high-visibility charitable works that followed the guidelines of the national strategy but could never hope to reach more than a tiny fraction of the population at risk.

Juillerat's efforts to obtain cooperation from private dispensaries and other institutions in information collection have already been noted. One of his associates, Alfred Fillassier, gave a speech to the Academy of Moral and Political Sciences in 1905 on the need for private-sector collaboration with the casier sanitaire. Fillassier characterized the relationship as an *"entente nécessaire."*

> It has always been the doctrine of the academy to call for state intervention when it is legitimate and necessary but to reserve the greatest role for private initiative. Is the latter enough in this area? In an absolute sense, we think not, but it remains no less true that we should resort to private initiative whenever it manifests itself, and even solicit it.[27]

And solicit it they did. Fillassier proposed that the casier sanitaire make public its findings (a step that would almost certainly violate medical confidentiality) and that charitable works use the information to orient their efforts strategically. In fact, he described a relationship so close that it almost amounted to a merger—but it was far from an equal partnership. All information would flow through the casier sanitaire, which would be responsible for collecting and organizing it, while actual intervention (and its funding) would be left to the charities.[28]

The municipal service in charge of disinfections also looked hopefully toward philanthropy, in this case to take on the lion's share of tuberculosis-related disinfections. The service found its resources strained to the limit just by disinfections involving illnesses other than tuberculosis. To even pretend to cover tuberculosis cases comprehensively would be impractical, as one official noted in a 1906 report. "Here is a problem that could be resolved someday when we are able to meet its pecuniary demands; for the moment, it is better to help and subsidize the private philanthropic works which are striving in this direction."[29] The attitude that encouraged reliance on philanthropy until some unspecified time in the future, when public powers would have the resources to act decisively, was a common one in housing policy circles. Juillerat adopted a similar stance in opposing state regulation of residential overcrowding. "Only the multiplication of sanitary low-cost housing will remedy the problem; any regulation would be, *at the present time,* vexatious and above all impotent." [30]

It is quite possible that these public officials took such positions less out of conviction than necessity—and frustration at their limited budgets. However, the tendency to rely on the private sector to finance the government's War on Tuberculosis reached into the upper echelons of its strategists in the medical community as well. Few voices were more respected on the question of tuberculosis than that of Dr. Louis Landouzy, the dean of the Paris Faculty of Medicine. Landouzy was a major strategist of the War on Tuberculosis, known as much for his poetic oratory as for his medical expertise.

In a 1901 speech to civic leaders in Lille on the subject of "La Lutte contre la tuberculose," he set forth the dominant social etiology of tuberculosis in detail and made an impassioned plea for all citizens to join in the battle against the disease. Working-class housing, of course, was an important part of the battle, and Landouzy urged the formation of an alliance among all forces in society to improve its quality.

> It is up to city officials [*édiles*], administrators, legislators, economists, employers, and mutualists to pursue and achieve the elimination of unsanitary housing, just as they have been able to achieve the drainage of marshes or ponds and the demolition of ramparts, when the former threaten the city's salubrity and the latter stand in the way of its commercial or industrial expansion!

Obviously, Landouzy was appealing to capitalist self-interest, as he continued his appeal with visions of a healthy and disciplined workforce.

> It is up to city officials, mutualists, and philanthropists [*Aux édiles, aux mutualistes, aux philanthropes*] to push for the construction of sanitary housing which . . . we know will so greatly benefit the health as well as the morality of workers and artisans. [31]

On their surface, these remarks seem to be primarily about the potential long-term benefits to employers of investment in the antituberculosis crusade. But on close inspection, this latter passage in particular also reveals the imbalance inherent in the practical application of the solidarist partnership. "Aux édiles, aux mutualistes, aux philanthropes" is Landouzy's version of the ritual invocation of solidarist spirit, but it is telling. Why would these be the three entities called on, if not because the *édiles* organizing the campaign needed the money that the mutual aid societies and the philanthropists controlled? The three forces were to "push for the construction of sanitary housing"; one can only conclude that it was the task of the *édiles* to "push," while it was up to the mutual aid societies and charities to "construct"—and pay.

This was the essence of solidarism, in which government (in conjunction with experts) drew up the plans for resolving social problems and tried to convince private citizens of the necessity and merit of financing the plans. In the case of tuberculosis, evidence that existing private initiatives were inadequate to the scale of the problem did not change the orientation of the strategy. On the contrary, such evidence was taken as proof of the need to step up the intensity of the appeals for help. Rarely was there any suggestion of a role for government beyond planning and "pushing"—for example, appropriation of the needed funds from the same private sources through taxes or bonds. In the age of solidarism, resources for addressing social problems could be actively solicited but not compelled.

THE WIFE AND THE *DOMESTIQUE*

"Le taudis est le pourvoyeur du cabaret": the slum is the purveyor of the cabaret.[32] So went one of the commonly cited maxims of the antituberculosis movement. The dismal, filthy state of working-class apartments, it was believed, drove men to seek comfort and sociability in the local drinking establishment. This inevitable result meant that slum housing was doubly implicated among the causes of tuberculosis, inasmuch as alcoholism was a key ingredient of the dominant etiology. The preference of cabaret over hearth not only linked two of the three principal strands of that etiology but also brought women into the narratives and polemics of the War on Tuberculosis.

As noted above, doctors and hygienists often explained the spread of tuberculosis to lay audiences (and even among themselves) by means of core narratives.[33] And women rarely figured in any account of the disease's causes except as careless wives, dangerous domestic servants, or prostitutes. On the rare occasions when women were portrayed as *victims* of disease, that status was usually secondary to their role as vehicles of transmission or contagion (endangering males). Two of the more common types of core narrative relating housing to tuberculosis involved the wife/mother who failed to keep house properly (upon which either the husband sought refuge in the cabaret or the household was overrun with microbes, or both); and the *domestique* who became infected in the kitchen or in her garret, thereafter threatening the health of her respectable bourgeois employers and their children.

Philanthropists used core narratives of tuberculosis both to orient and to explain their intervention in working-class neighborhoods and households. The wife and mother in poor families kept an unhygienic house not out of sloth, according to these stories, but out of ignorance and lack of time. One bourgeois woman used a conversation with a "decent" but less fortunate mother of her acquaintance to illustrate a lesson in good housekeeping. The family met misfortune when the father and two of the three children fell ill, coughing and losing weight. When a doctor friend expressed the view that the patients were not beyond hope but could not afford to be properly taken care of, the bourgeoise paid a visit to her working-class counterpart. The visitor was greeted with a sincere expression of worry: "Am I going to see them all cough themselves to an early grave, one after the other?" (*Est-ce qu[e] [je vais] les voir s'en aller tous de la poitrine, tous, l'un après l'autre?*) The dialogue that followed between the mother, Madeleine, and the visitor, whom Madeleine refers to only as "Madame," bears all the hallmarks of paternalistic charity, as the reform-minded bourgeoise enlightens the ignorant *ouvrière*:

—Let's see, Madeleine, are you prepared to follow my advice?
—Yes, of course, Madame.
—Well then, start by opening the window—we're suffocating in here.
—Oh, it's just a little stuffy [*C'est seulement une odeur de renfermé*], shot back the good woman, a bit piqued.
—But the smell of stale air is a smell of infection.[34]

The conversation continued in this vein, with the visitor gently rebuking the woman who was unknowingly endangering the health of her family. Madeleine should have opened all the windows in the apartment as soon as everyone left in the morning, she was told, and aired out all the bedclothes. She should have cleaned the tile with a damp cloth, put away the dirty laundry, tidied up the various objects lying about, and, above all, immersed in boiling water the handkerchiefs into which her loved ones had been coughing and spitting. As it was already midafternoon (Madeleine had been out working earlier in the day), everything in the apartment had been absorbing for seven hours the germs released into circulation overnight.[35]

Given the family's limited means and the need for the extra income that her work brought in, Madeleine certainly did not have the luxury of cleaning house from top to bottom every day. However, even with little time available, there were certain essential precautions she could take to guard against the invasion of microbes, as her visitor demonstrated.

—What are these crusty clothes doing hiding behind the door, as if they were ashamed to show themselves?
—Those are my little girls' skirts. I haven't brushed them off yet because the hems need to be changed and I haven't had the time.
—I'll grant you that you haven't had the time to fix them completely, but you can at least get rid of . . . this layer of mud . . . and the false-hem, which is a receptacle for dust. . . . You have no idea of the horrors that people bring back with them from the street and the workshop![36]

Madeleine grabbed one of the skirts and vigorously ripped off the filthy hem, raising a cloud of dust and the ire of her visitor.

I raise my hands in protest and cover my face with a handkerchief against the asphyxiating cloud that envelops us.
—No! . . . but . . . aren't you at all afraid of microbes?[37]

Receptive to instruction and full of goodwill, Madeleine had committed only the sin of ignorance. Her hygiene-savvy mentor went on to teach her about microbes, the "sales bêtes" who threatened her family and had found such a welcome home in her apartment.[38]

Others echoed the claim that proper construction and sufficient space was not enough to make housing sanitary. One doctor lamented that "an unclean working-class family, ignorant of the elementary principles of hygiene, will soon render insalubrious the most hygienically built lodging."[39] Ignorance and lack of free time, most observers agreed, were the primary reasons that "these unfortunates [could not] properly maintain their crowded homes."[40] At least one of these two problems had a ready solution.

What the working-class wife needed was education. Landouzy was among the many antituberculosis crusaders who called for a mandatory program of éducation ménagère for girls in school. "Every girls' class should receive lessons in HOUSEHOLD EDUCATION, teaching the child: how to clean the body, the laundry, and the house; [and] the importance of soaking household linens in boiling water as an effective and economical means of disinfection."[41] The young girl would take the lessons she learned back to her parents' home and later to her own home as wife and mother. Landouzy quoted Jules Simon on the efficacy of this teaching method: "Every time you teach a woman, you are founding a small school." [42] The woman who had been exposed to such a program would know the importance of sunlight and ventilation in preventing tuberculosis; she would never again disperse microbe-laden dust throughout a room by dry sweeping the floor; and she would protect her children from "the breath and caresses of coughers." [43] Another hygienist proposed that municipalities award "prizes for good housekeeping" and suggested that household education might also cause cabarets to lose some customers, further depleting the ranks of potential tuberculosis victims. [44]

Household education need not only take place at school, however. Lessons could also be given to adult women in the home itself, as Madeleine found out in the anecdote above. Several charitable works seized on the idea as a way of encouraging community involvement in the War on Tuberculosis. Ideally, as in Madeleine's case, the teaching was to take place from woman to woman, because certain female affinities could cross class lines and because home was the woman's domain. It was always assumed that those in need of instruction were working-class women, while those with the knowledge and the time were bourgeoises.

One female doctor who helped to organize such programs in Paris, Madame Edwards-Pilliet, spoke to an audience of three hundred *"dames du monde"* in 1902 and sounded the call of social duty: "Show solidarity with us." Each woman would be responsible for a certain number of underprivileged households in her neighborhood or arrondissement. She would enter the dwellings of tuberculous patients, bringing medication, food, and, above all, advice. The goal was to teach "these people" cleanliness and hygiene, "because they have not the slightest notion" of these concepts. [45] The initial contact would be difficult, Edwards-Pilliet warned, and the bourgeoise might be greeted with more than a little mistrust.

> Well! this is easy to understand: if they receive you poorly, [it is because] they are not well off, they are miserable, they are deprived, they are ill, and when one is ill one is not disposed to receive people who are healthy and who come to tell you: "Now open your windows." Well then, no! That is not the way you must go about it.

The way to establish trust was to *be a woman,* to stake out a common ground of shared femininity in motherhood and housekeeping.

> If the woman has a sick child, you must tell her: "I too have a child who was sick, and we treated him in this or that way." *It is not the scientific notion that she will accept, it is what I have come to call your womanly advice [vos conseils de bonne femme]*; she might accept it with a bit of defiance, but when she sees that your advice is at least as good as that of the corner *mercière . . .* she will accept you, since a mother is always very attentive when someone comes to help her treat her child.[46]

Eventually, after receiving help in changing the baby's diapers properly, perhaps after accepting an offer of toys for the children or some household items that she might be lacking, the poor woman would begin to trust her benefactor. The crucial hygienic advice—to leave the windows of the apartment open all day, not to sleep in the same bed with the child, and the like—would then be listened to and followed. Later, when the bourgeoise saw the poor family's child, rosy-cheeked and healthy, she could say to herself with relief, "There is one that won't have tuberculosis when he plays in the public parks; there is one who won't be coughing next to my [child]."[47]

Although the language was designed to be comradely rather than condescending, there is more than a hint of paternalism in Dr. Edwards-Pilliet's lecture. Indeed, much of the mainstream War on Tuberculosis in France involved the bestowing of wisdom from above on the ignorant masses, that is, from the bourgeoisie to the working class; to some extent, this is an inescapable structural feature of most charities. The women's antituberculosis outreach can also be seen as part of a broader effort in the nineteenth century to civilize the working class, to tame it and render it harmless. Of course, there is another, simpler explanation that must be taken seriously: that hygienists and philanthropists were merely trying to help the working class and to save lives, however myopic or paternalistic their methods may seem today. It must be emphasized that this straightforward interpretation of reformers' conscious motivations is by no means incompatible with a critical analysis of the underlying social and cultural structures that conditioned all such reform efforts.

At this point, the claim that the War on Tuberculosis "ignored" women needs to be nuanced. Both the dominant etiology and reform efforts *involved* women in several respects. This chapter points out that working-class wives and domestic servants were implicated in the spread of tuberculosis through slovenly housekeeping and direct contagion. Nevertheless, they were rarely, if ever, the ultimate targets or endpoints either of social etiologies or of charitable intervention. Women were portrayed primarily as vectors, not victims, of disease. Likewise, in the world of philanthropy, women were actively involved in antituberculosis efforts. In the case of Madame Edwards-Pilliet's lecture, the medical expert giving advice, the audience, and the recipients of intervention are all women. However, the purpose of the lecture is not so much to prevent women from getting tuberculosis as it is to prevent them from causing or spreading it.

The key to such intervention was the notion of *conseils de bonne femme*. The female perspective was necessary, reformers believed, if charities truly expected to reach the working-class family and change its habits. Only a new kind of interaction, based not only on paternalism but also on the personal interaction of women with each other, would allow the open communication of hygienic and other teachings. Charitable work, in the War on Tuberculosis and in the service of many other causes, was a central aspect of the social world of bourgeois women in nineteenth-century France. More specifically, causes that concerned women, children, and families were the particular province of charitable ladies.[48] With education, visits to their homes, and conseils de bonne femme, it was felt, workers might eventually be remade in the self-image of the bourgeoisie: disciplined, healthy, and industrious. Moreover, in the case of tuberculosis, every poor child saved from the disease meant one less child coughing in the vicinity of one's own children in the park. Fear of interclass contagion also explained, at least in part, the power of the *domestique* as a symbol in the literature on housing and tuberculosis. More than any other figure, the domestic servant represented contact between social classes and therefore became the object of profound anxiety and curiosity on the part of many in the bourgeoisie. Tuberculosis crystallized the vague fear of contact with the working class and gave it a terrifying immediacy.

Yet the domestic servant occupied a prominent place in the dominant etiology for other reasons as well. For the doctors and other strategists of the War on Tuberculosis, evoking the danger that lurked in the very households of the rich and powerful no doubt caught many people's attention, stirred awareness of the tuberculosis problem, and bolstered support for an energetic campaign against the disease. At the same time, the domestic "explained" the incidence of this *maladie populaire* among the wealthy by serving as a target for blame.[49] Her sex as well as her class worked against her in this respect. (Although there were certainly male domestic servants, the figure in tuberculosis narratives was always female.)

On the administrative level, the *domestique* also provided an explanation for occasional anomalies in the statistical distribution of tuberculosis, because she lived "upstairs" but spent most of her time "downstairs," and lived amid affluence but in poverty. For example, if the upper stories of certain buildings (which had greater exposure to sunlight) failed to show the low tuberculosis mortality that the theory would lead one to expect, the answer could be found in the unique circumstances of a domestic servant's existence. The same would be true for unexpectedly high numbers in a wealthy neighborhood or arrondissement.

In its simplest form, the story of the domestic and tuberculosis fit neatly into the standard housing connection.

> In the rich quarters, it is in the concierges' apartments and in the domestics' rooms under the eaves—just 2 to 2-1/2 meters wide, with an insufficient volume of air—that tuberculosis originates, and it is from there that the disease gains access to the masters' apartments.[50]

The servant's presence alone, then, could account for cases of tuberculosis in well-to-do homes where none of the more familiar components of the dominant etiology was present.

Juillerat, who agreed that the domestic was a common source of contagion among the bourgeoisie, traced the domestic's illness to the kitchen rather than to her cramped living quarters. The nuance was significant, because to implicate the *chambre de bonne* under the roof would have weakened the general "sunlight" model that associated lower risk with dwellings on the upper stories of a building. In a 1907 lecture to a group of bourgeois women, Juillerat warned his audience that most kitchens were dangerously unsanitary. Lack of light and the mutual proximity of sink, garbage can, stove, and larder made the kitchen especially hospitable to microbes.

> If a tuberculous domestic has spent time in a dark kitchen—and there are very few of them who have not—the bacilli that she has unloaded there by the millions, by coughing and spitting, settle there for good; they slip into every fissure, into every nook and cranny, everywhere that dust piles up.[51]

How the *domestique* contracted the disease in the first place is not explained here, but Juillerat's point concerned the meaning of that initial outpouring of microbes for the future of the household. "From that day forward, every domestic that inhabits that kitchen, already anemic because of her lifestyle, . . . is almost fatally condemned to contract the merciless disease. These successive domestics constantly contaminate the entire apartment." It is not clear whether by "lifestyle" [*genre de vie*] he was referring to a servant's typical fifteen-hour workday or to questionable morals.

Less ambiguous, however, was the danger to the bourgeoisie, and Juillerat made sure no one misunderstood the need to watch over one's servants' health: "You see that, outside of the humane reasons that should prompt us to protect the life and health of those who serve us, our own self-interest demands that it be so." Apart from choosing an apartment with a spacious and sunny kitchen, Juillerat told his audience to disinfect both the kitchen and the *chambre de bonne* "each time you dismiss a domestic." [52]

At times, matters could get quite thorny for doctors and employers trying to guard against a "Tuberculosis Mary" contaminating the household. When the servant was a nanny, or had constant contact with children, the situation took on even greater urgency. If a doctor examined a domestic and found evidence of tuberculosis, how could he inform her employers of the danger to their family without violating the *secret médical*? This was the ethical question taken up by the Société de médecine légale in 1905, after participants at the International Tuberculosis Congress in Paris earlier that year had agreed that it warranted further study. Reporting the matter to the society's members, a Dr. Zuber sketched the background of a typical case.

> Here is how things usually happen. In one of the families that we treat, the parents have doubts about the health of the person who takes care of their children, because she coughs, feels tired, loses weight, etc.; the idea of tuberculosis and the dangers of contagion haunt them, and they ask us to examine the patient and to tell them the result. [53]

Zuber added that often the parents wished neither the reason for the examination nor its results to be revealed to the domestic. Such a demand, in his view, directly violated medical ethics and should not be entertained. Not only did the consent of the patient have to be obtained beforehand but she had to be fully informed of the reason for the examination, of its possible consequences for her, and of her right to prevent her employers from finding out its results. [54]

Nevertheless, Zuber noted, despite the various ethical protections afforded to the patient, there was a simple way for the doctor to ensure that the servant would "voluntarily" submit to the examination: "He will obtain from her a waiver of confidentiality by showing her that her refusal alone would be interpreted unfavorably." Obviously, the domestic was caught in a no-win situation: agree to the examination, and possibly lose her job, or refuse, and certainly lose it. If the procedure revealed an "open," or fully developed, case of tuberculosis, "the removal of the patient [from the household] is imperative." A compassionate explanation of the nature of the illness and the danger it creates for the children, Zuber wrote, should convince her of the necessity of leaving her employment and seeking treatment. More often than not, in his own experience, "the masters" proved to be "more or less generous" in helping to defray the costs of the fired servant's treatment.[55]

Dr. Zuber went on to relate by way of illustration some specific cases of consumptive domestics from his own medical practice. In one case, the domestic was fired after the diagnosis; several months later, the child she had been caring for came down with coxalgia (an ailment often tuberculous in nature). "We hesitate to see in this a simple coincidence." In another, the patient admitted that before taking the job, she had been released from the hospital with the recommendation that she not work around children. "She had taken no heed whatsoever of this recommendation, and this will often be the case, which justifies mothers' suspicions on the subject of their domestics' health."[56]

Finally, Zuber suggested a way to avoid the ethical dilemma in the first place and still protect the rights of all parties involved. Parents should require at least a lung examination for all prospective servants, after which the family physician could simply approve or disapprove of the hiring, without giving a specific diagnosis.[57] By not divulging any "medical" information, the doctor would be following the letter—if not the spirit—of the *secret médical*. Of course, the prospective domestic would be no better off, but the parents would be reassured. Rarely in any discussion of domestic servants and tuberculosis was there significant concern expressed for the actual health of the *domestique*, nor was she ever portrayed as a victim rather than a vehicle of tuberculosis, the endangered rather than the danger.

For the strategists of the War on Tuberculosis, both the wife and the *domestique* played the part of accessories to contagion, just as slum housing represented the incubator of microbes. Their role was an unwitting one at best, willful at worst, but in either case they needed to be watched. The ignorant wife could be educated, while the domestic could only be guarded against—or fired.

To the extent that its aim was the renovation of urban dwellings or the construction of cheap, sanitary housing on a large scale, the housing component of the War on Tuberculosis must be considered a failure.

All the improvements for which the casier sanitaire claimed credit, for example, were made voluntarily by the property owners. The state was unwilling to go beyond classification, surveillance, and cheerleading—to threaten the sanctity of private property—while it urged mutualists and philanthropists to put *their* money where the *administration's* mouth was. In this respect, housing policy was typical of the entire anti-tuberculosis campaign.

However, it would be a mistake to conclude that the considerable sound and fury of the battle against slums signified nothing. The need for physical improvements was only one of the driving forces behind the attack on unsanitary housing. In the War on Tuberculosis, seeing could often be more important than doing. The housing-tuberculosis connection provided a medicalized outlet for bourgeois disgust with and fear of the working class; in so doing, it also allowed old notions regarding the pathogenic role of filth and stench to survive in the new age of microbes. More important, the link between slums and tuberculosis gave rise to new ways of keeping track of the working class. Household education and didactic visits from upper-class ladies held out the promise of remaking working-class families in the image of the bourgeoisie. This subjective method of observation was complemented by the casier sanitaire, the objective eye of the administration inside the working-class home. With such means at its disposal, the state could contemplate, as Senator Volland had feared, "waging the war against microbes even into the privacy of our homes."[58]

CHAPTER FIVE

Morality and Mortality

*Alcoholism, Syphilis, and the "Rural
Exodus" in the War on Tuberculosis*

We must . . . seek out and incriminate . . . the two other
causes of death that cling to our society's flanks, syphilis and
alcoholism—those two Fates that join together with tuberculosis to form a trio far more terrifying than that of ancient
mythology.

—*Dr. Maurice Letulle, 1902*

Incriminating syphilis and alcoholism along with tuberculosis as a, in
Letulle's words, "terrifying trio" was the third major strand of the dominant etiology and a key strategic maneuver in the War on Tuberculosis.
It was through this trio that moral depravity came to be considered at
the turn of the century, along with slum housing and contact with microbes, a principal causal factor in the spread of tuberculosis. In 1905,
Louis Rénon, a professor at the Paris Faculté de médecine, published a
book entitled *The Diseases of the People: Venereal Disease, Alcoholism, Tuberculosis.*[1] This thorough investigation of both the medical and
social dimensions of the three great "scourges" of modern life left no
doubt that there was a connection among the three—a connection that
threatened the moral and physical well-being of France. At the center
of the problem, embodying the concerted assault of alcoholism, syphilis, and tuberculosis, lay the cabaret[2] and its associated evil, prostitution.

Letulle and Rénon were by no means alone in perceiving this triple
threat. From approximately the mid-1880s until World War I, medical
and governmental authorities in France proclaimed frequently and
forcefully certain interrelationships among alcoholism, syphilis, and tuberculosis and, in mobilizing against them, articulated a view of French
society in danger of biological and moral decline. The connections they
perceived among the three diseases illustrate not only certain currents
in French medical science at the time but also powerful tensions and

fears at work within French society as a whole. Moreover, like other aspects of the dominant etiology of tuberculosis around the turn of the century, the linkage of these three scourges appropriated and updated some much older ideas about the disease's causes. Vice and heredity in particular—like overcrowding and bourgeois disgust with working-class living conditions—were carried over from the pre-germ theory era into the social etiologies of the Belle Epoque but infused with slightly different meanings. Earlier vague formulations concerning "vice" or "excesses" developed into denunciations of specific transgressions (chiefly, alcoholism and prostitution) and were localized in dangerous spaces such as the cabaret. Meanwhile, age-old ideas about the heredity of tuberculosis that were primarily backward-looking (that is, explaining the origins of a given case) became, amid fears of degeneration, urgent and forward-looking, warning of dire consequences in future generations.

Examining the moral dimension of etiology, or of attitudes toward health and disease in general, means confronting the elusive boundaries of "morality" itself. The ever-shifting categories "moral" and "immoral" are neither absolute nor immutable, and take on the qualities of different societies in different times and places. One doctor's perspective on the connection between alcoholism and tuberculosis may offer a glimpse at what "morality" encompassed in France at the turn of the century. In the course of denouncing drunkenness and revolutionary politics among workers, Dr. Henri Triboulet told his audience at the International Tuberculosis Congress in Paris in 1905, "Let us add to our national motto these three terms, which will never disgrace it: *cleanliness, sobriety, prosperity* [*propreté, sobriété, prospérité*]." [3] This proposed revision of national identity (to supplement "liberty, equality, fraternity") arose out of a specific configuration of anxieties, notably including fears of revolution and demographic decline. In this context, "morality" seems to have denoted principally a combination of the following qualities: moderation (especially in alcohol consumption and sexual activity); a stable and clean household consisting of a monogamous husband and wife with children; and hard work. The absence of these qualities was blamed for various social pathologies, and tuberculosis was prominent among them.

In its most basic form, this segment of the dominant etiology took a triangular shape, contending that both alcoholism and syphilis caused (or contributed to the prevalence of) tuberculosis. In its individual manifestations, this argument was usually made with respect to the effect

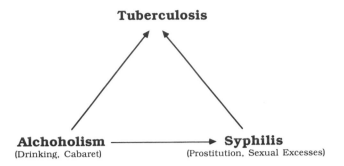

9. The moral etiology of tuberculosis (arrows indicate causal relations).

on tuberculosis of either alcoholism or syphilis—in effect, filling in one
or the other of two sides of the triangle, with tuberculosis as the
nexus—but occasionally all three scourges were linked in a single text
or intervention. Causal relationships—or "morbid associations," in the
words of one doctor—were most often expressed in terms of predisposition to tuberculosis, using metaphorical language concerning the quality of a "soil" or "terrain" and its receptivity to a "seed." Typically, the
full link expressed itself along the following lines: a certain number of
patients, previously alcoholic (or syphilitic), had developed tuberculosis; this evidence led to the conclusion that alcoholism (or syphilis) predisposed its victims to tuberculosis; therefore, the *medical* fight against
tuberculosis must begin with a *social* fight against alcoholism (or syphilis), specifically with a regulatory crackdown against cabarets (prostitution).

At issue here is not whether *in fact* alcoholism or syphilis had an
etiological effect on or an epidemiological correlation with tuberculosis.[4] Rather, it is the type of evidence in use at the time and how it was
used that are of interest. The perception of a connection, rather than
the medical "truth" of the connection, is the relevant fact here. The
ways in which the connection was perceived, expressed, and portrayed,
the conclusions that were drawn from the perceived association, and
the political and social implications contained in its expression offer
greater opportunities for meaningful analysis than would a truly "scientific" historical epidemiology.

Perceived connections among the three diseases certainly did not
(alone) cause perceptions of national decline. Rather, both the two-way
and three-way "morbid associations" served as avenues through which
anxiety was expressed and reinforced certain opinions about what con-

stituted immoral and dangerous behavior in society. The associations deserve special attention for two major reasons. First, they established a *moral* etiology of tuberculosis, France's leading killer, and thus persuasively linked behavior with disease, morality with mortality. Second, the connections consolidated seemingly separate phenomena into a generalized syndrome of national decline and constituted a means of expressing fear of such decline in medical—hence, objective and scientific—terms. Moreover, in doing so they justified surveillance of cabarets and prostitutes, useful targets for blame in their embodiment of certain types of antisocial behavior. Concern about prostitution and cabarets predated the alcoholism–syphilis–tuberculosis connections, but these connections both intensified the concern and integrated it into a broad diagnosis of French moral and physical decline.

The notion of "degeneration," as applied to societies' physical and moral well-being, was widespread throughout late nineteenth-century Europe.[5] In France, however, it fused with the continuing anxiety over low birth rates and demographic decline—particularly in relation to Germany and Great Britain—and fashioned a peculiarly French anxiety of national decline. The tuberculosis–alcoholism–syphilis triangle aptly expressed the degeneration paradigm; tuberculosis, the nation's leading cause of death, was the crucial link in connecting that paradigm to the French demographic decline.

PRELUDE TO MORAL DECAY: THE "RURAL EXODUS" AND ITS ROLE IN TUBERCULOSIS

In his two books on the population of Paris in the early nineteenth century, Chevalier painted a fearsome picture of a city under siege from its own poverty-ridden underbelly. Respectable Parisians recoiled in horror at the sight of the "dangerous classes," the ill-fed, ill-housed proletariat and *Lumpenproletariat* that spread crime and disease throughout the city. Chevalier emphasized the provincial origins of the desperate new Parisian poor and cited rural migration to the capital as the most salient factor—numerically and socially—in the city's nineteenth-century growth.[6]

But these migrants, Chevalier's early- and midcentury "dangerous classes," were dangerous (or perceived to be so) because of what they represented to individual bourgeois observers (crime, contagion) or to the city's public order (unrest). Theirs was a local menace. By 1900, the menace was a national one: less visceral perhaps, but on a much larger scale. The last half of the nineteenth century was certainly a period of substantial rural-urban migration. At the peak of the exodus in the late 1870s, up to 170,000 people per year left the French countryside for the city; in the late 1890s, the figure rose again as high as 130,000 per year. While the population of the Seine, the department that consisted of Paris and its suburbs, increased 87 percent between 1872 and 1911 (from 2.2 million to 4.2 million), many rural departments lost one-fifth of their inhabitants during that time, led by the Lot with a decline of 27 percent.[7]

But these statistics reveal less than do the contemporary *perceptions* of desertion and loss. In the minds of many observers, rural-urban migration threatened nothing less than France's demographic, sanitary, and moral survival. Concern over the "rural exodus" expressed several different strands of anxiety at once. It did not appear to help France's demographic emergency to have legions of young peasants forgo starting a family in favor of working in the city, where high death rates awaited them. As will be shown below, rural-urban migrants were thought to be more susceptible to deadly diseases such as tuberculosis and to play a key role in spreading them in both the city and the village back home. Furthermore, the morally pure and purely French lifestyle of the countryside, *la France profonde,* seemed to be dying out, abandoned by those whose duty it was to preserve it for the future. Similarly, the deserters from the farms and fields seemed to be swelling the ranks of customers in the cities' cabarets and brothels, hastening the nation's moral downfall.

Continual recapitulation of one particular narrative theme characterized discussion of the rural exodus from the 1890s on: a young man or woman, disillusioned with life on the farm and seeking wealth or opportunity, leaves the village for the big city; once there, the dreams turn to dust, and the dreamer sinks into poverty, immorality, crime or prostitution, and disease. It was a familiar literary motif, and its element of tragic inevitability lent it considerable evocative power. The key to the nationalist/political resonance of this theme was not only its familiarity but—particularly among the doctors, hygienists, and government officials addressing the tuberculosis problem—the extrapolation of the theme from the individual to nation. When the fate of France itself was at stake, the personal became political, the tragedy became a national one, and inaction seemed unthinkable.

A 1908 medical thesis offered a fairly typical view, through one of the classic core narratives,[8] of the rural exodus and its relation to tuberculosis.

> The young peasant, healthy and robust, dazzled by what he saw in the big city during his military service, deserts health, deserts home and family, and comes to enlarge the incalculable number of malcontents and have-nots who begin to see that life is not all roses and that health is not always in abundant supply. . . . Poverty, alcohol, and tuberculosis catch up with the stragglers and rip them apart without mercy.[9]

Other doctors joined in the chorus of despair and tried to warn those who had not yet left the countryside:

> If these words came to the attention of someone in the countryside, I would tell him: "You were born in the countryside, stay there." Stay there, [and] resist this absurd, reprehensible impulse, which these days drives rural people to desert the native village to seek fortune in the big city.

The great fortunes of the city, these doctors warned, were a mirage. "For every peasant who came to [Paris] covered with dirt and returned home as lord of the manor, how many—alas—have succumbed to the struggle[?]"[10] Many authorities accepted uncritically (and repeated) this notion of peasants seeking to strike it rich in the city. Few mentioned the devastating poverty of some rural regions, or indeed any other type of "push" motive, as possible factors in migration. Thus, even before the full sociomedical etiology of tuberculosis had been set forth, the soon-to-be-victim of the disease was depicted as at least partially at fault for choosing the conditions that would lead to his own downfall.

One exception to this rule provides a variation on the "fortune-seeker" theme, while avoiding to some extent the victim-blaming tendency. Louis Renault, in a medical thesis on tuberculosis among Bretons, recognized that the attraction of the city might have something to do with economic conditions at home.

> They fall under the irresistible spell of the big City, where wages are higher, without realizing that the cost of living is also higher than back home. Knowing a few rare examples of fellow villagers who left with nothing and found success, they hope to have the same experience and they abandon their native soil to seek adventure. . . . [T]o escape the threat of poverty, they head off to a worse fate: the poverty of large cities.[11]

As much as delusions of grandeur, Renault blamed France's mandatory military service for encouraging rural-urban migration. "Many young people," he explained, "after three years in a city, no longer want to go back to work in the fields." Moreover, their army comrades boasted of the advantages offered by urban life and ridiculed them for being mere peasants.

> Their envy is sparked: ambition and pride urge them on. When they return to their homes, the pastoral life seems hard and monotonous to them; at the first opportunity, they permanently desert their native land . . . [and] it will not be long before they know firsthand all the anguish of poverty, hunger, and disease.[12]

Greed, naïveté, suggestibility, and increased communication, particularly through railroad transportation and military service, were generally agreed to be responsible for the exodus of sixty thousand people per year (according to one estimate)[13] from the wholesome farms and villages to the diseased cities of France.

Once they got there, doctors and hygienists warned, the migrants' country background made them more susceptible than city natives to the many "morbid influences" awaiting them. Accustomed as they were to fresh air, regular work, and a well-ventilated house, they were ill-prepared for the effects of city air, overwork, and "revolting slums." Intending to return to their *coin de terre* with the money earned in the city, many migrants skimped on their diets and housing to increase their savings; this, too, made them "quite often the prey of tuberculosis, the 'city disease' . . . for *campagnards*."[14]

Yet in all of the rural exodus literature, the most commonly cited trap awaiting the new urban arrivals—and the most common gateway to tuberculosis—was debauchery. Establishing the inevitability of the descent into urban depravity and disease was crucial if rural-urban migration was to be integrated into the problematic of national moral-demographic decline.

Georges Bourgeois sought to explain the particular vulnerability of Breton migrants to tuberculosis by invoking "[their] poor hygiene, alcoholism, and [their] *lack of moral resistance*." This explanation, he added, was "unfortunately applicable to [most] immigrants, no matter where they come from."[15] This lack of moral resistance reinforced the sense of inevitability surrounding the slide into vice. Powerless to resist, the newcomer to the city was doomed; as all of the core narratives on this point make clear, opportunities and enticements to debauchery were everywhere.

His life disrupted, the transplant wastes little time becoming intoxicated by the pleasures of Paris. Often led on by friends, he soon learns the way to the *marchand de vins,* especially since his dark and dreary lodgings hold little appeal for him.

Not only did the cabaret satisfy the worker's need for sociability and relaxation but alcohol also provided a temporary relief from fatigue or poor nourishment.

Subjected to intensive labor or deprived of a sufficient diet, the worker hopes to find in alcoholic beverages the comfort . . . he needs. He drinks, soon becomes intemperate, and alcoholism leads to tuberculosis.[16]

Medical opinion seemed to be unanimous on this point: the progression from migration to tuberculosis passed through the cabaret.[17]

Several doctors also warned of a corollary to the rule of tuberculosis among rural-urban migrants. As many observers pointed out, the true dimensions of the problem could not be accurately understood through urban mortality statistics, because many tuberculosis victims returned to their home village or province, either to die among family or in the hope of a cure in the country air. The result of this reverse migration was the introduction of tuberculosis, the "city disease," into the countryside. The mere possibility of this contamination threatened the traditional and deep-seated image of rural France cherished by the urban bourgeoisie, and it prompted considerable anxiety in the medical community.

Louis Cruveilhier, the author of one study of this phenomenon, sought proof of its importance in his contention that tuberculosis mortality was highest in those departments out of which the most people emigrated. (Aside from numerous statistical anomalies in this argument,[18] Cruveilhier did not consider the possibility that both emigration and tuberculosis could result from poverty, and that the poorest departments tended to have the highest rates of emigration. However, it is less the factual accuracy of the argument than its place in the overall moral etiology of tuberculosis that is of importance in this context.) The urban-to-rural spread of tuberculosis typically occurred as follows, according to Cruveilhier. The peasant family lived in a humble dwelling that, while not exactly "very salubrious," was relatively free of germs and harmless to its occupants' health "as long as all members of the family stay[ed] home in the countryside."

This is no longer the case as soon as a son who had gone to the regiment, or to the city as a factory worker or as a mason—or a daughter who had been a wet nurse—comes back home with the germ of tuberculosis. How easy contagion will turn out to be in such a milieu, poorly ventilated, never exposed to the sun, humid and cold, where tubercle bacilli maintain their full virulence.

The previously harmless features of the rustic house became deadly once the tubercle bacillus was introduced from the city. As soon as any family member experienced any kind of physiological stress, "contagion is then unavoidable." The likelihood of contagion was further enhanced by the fact that quite often in these households, the contaminating son/ brother shared not just a bedroom but also a bed with other family members.[19] Such core narratives, and the problem of rural tuberculosis as a whole, served to universalize the syndrome of rural exodus and its effect on the national health. Under such conditions, it was impossible to approach the problem as a local one, or as one limited to certain social milieus.

Among the measures recommended to deal with the rural exodus and its role in tuberculosis, some aimed at neutralizing the "contagious" return of tuberculous migrants to the countryside. Cruveilhier, for example, urged that both urban and rural authorities be warned of "the dangers posed by the return of *tuberculeux* to their native land unless severe and effective measures are taken concurrently to isolate them as much as possible, in order to protect those who offer them hospitality."[20] Other doctors proposed focusing such isolation policies on the city itself, so that susceptible migrants would not come into contact with tuberculosis in the first place.[21]

However, there was widespread accord on the most urgent measure of all: halting, even reversing, the depopulation of the countryside. Only policies striking at the root causes of the rural-urban migration, observers agreed, could have any lasting effect. Certain contributory factors such as military service could be mitigated, some felt, and they applauded the government's decision in 1905 to reduce mandatory service from three years to two.[22] Yet several observers stressed that an overhaul of the French system of education was necessary if rural children were to be cured of the impulse to leave the countryside. The current system, wrote one doctor, "orients all children toward tuberculosis and toward bureaucracy." "The education of farmers' children . . . must not make them aspire to careers in banking or commerce. On the contrary, we must . . . keep them on the paternal land and prepare them to become . . . educated farmers." With an education appropriate and relevant to their lifestyle and surroundings, peasant children would be able to "develop from an early age their penchant for agriculture." There would be no reason for them to want to desert their rural roots.[23]

A few doctors even dreamed of reversing the fundamental trends of the Industrial Revolution and repopulating the countryside through rural factories and the revival of small-scale home industries. Two versions of this vision in particular depict a new industrial order in such a way as to constitute a sort of "counter-core narrative," substituting optimism and renewal for the gloomy fatalism of the standard rural-exodus narratives. Charles Fauchon, in his 1903 pamphlet, *Tuberculosis, A Social Question,* mentioned the recent construction of a tobacco factory in a large city and mused,

> Suppose, on the contrary, that this factory . . . were built along a railway line, in the countryside[;] workers could live there cheaply, far from the unhealthy stimulations of cities, in hygienic houses . . . isolated from one another and surrounded by spacious gardens. There they would find excellent living conditions from every point of view, and tuberculosis could not find any victims in these milieus.

This vision of a remoralized workforce, isolated from urban depravity and ensconced in a clean, sober domestic atmosphere, reconciles modern industry with the demands of public order and health;[24] it represents a kind of turn-of-the-century hygienists' utopia and reveals by opposition many of the anxieties that found voice in the mainstream War on Tuberculosis.

Lucien Graux, also writing in 1903, went so far as to claim that the new Industrial Revolution was already under way and already refashioning the moribund working-class family.

> Already it seems that an economic revolution is in the works. The consequences of hydroelectric power are incalculable. Factories are springing up at the base of mountains, on sunny and windswept plateaus, far from unhealthy cities. Electric power . . . in every home will once again make domestic industry run, and the laborer will be able to work in his reconstituted household.[25]

While Graux's vision emphasized the return of the working-class woman to the home and the resulting reconstitution of the family, he shared with Fauchon a preoccupation with recapturing the rural essence of Frenchness that had been vitiated by modern urban life and that manifested itself in the modern, urban, industrial disease, tuberculosis.

Against the background of rural depopulation and the influx of up-rooted peasants into urban factories and cabarets, hygienists and public officials set their sights on the triangular association of alcoholism, syphilis, and tuberculosis. In doing so, they intensified the tendency to ascribe moral value to the disease that claimed more lives than any other.

ALCOHOLISM AND TUBERCULOSIS: TARGETING THE CABARET

In a recent essay, Nourrisson emphasizes the contingent and shifting nature of the alcoholism–tuberculosis link between the mid-nineteenth and mid-twentieth century. Harmless and even therapeutic until the last third of the nineteenth century, alcohol became enemy number one of the War on Tuberculosis by the turn of the century. The fledgling anti-tuberculosis campaign borrowed from and built on the strength and membership of the established antialcoholism movement. After World War I, Nourrisson argues, huge wine production surpluses necessitated a medical "rehabilitation" of alcoholic beverages in general, and the link with tuberculosis declined (even though wine itself had never been specifically implicated). Not until after 1945 did alcoholism regain its privileged place in the generally accepted etiology of tuberculosis.[26] Nourrisson's argument is provocative, and the broad outlines of his chronology are instructive. His essay should serve as a cautionary tale to anyone tempted to portray the evolution of medical or etiological science in a linear fashion. A more detailed investigation here of the development of the alcoholism–tuberculosis connection before World War I, breaking it down into its constituent elements and exploring its ramifications, will help establish the immediate social meaning of the connection, if not the ultimate reasons for its rise and fall.

Pre-germ theory medical texts in the early nineteenth century focused on the role of alcohol abuse in such sudden and exotic afflictions as apoplexy and even spontaneous combustion. Around the time of the Bourbon Restoration, medical dictionaries, while attributing revivifying powers to alcohol in small quantities, warned of these two risks as well as "imbecility," pupil dilation, coma, convulsions, "insensibility," paralysis, "and even death" in cases of abuse.[27] It should be noted that nineteenth-century medical references to "alcohol" meant primarily distilled spirits; fermented drinks such as wine, beer, and cider were often referred to as "hygienic beverages."

A more extensive and detailed enumeration of the pathological effects of alcohol appeared in 1838 in the *Annales d'hygiène publique,* the nation's first public health journal (founded in 1829). In the empirical and public policy-oriented style characteristic of that journal, Dr. Charles Roesch mentioned a multitude of illnesses under the heading "Drunkards' Illnesses and the Types of Death to Which They Succumb." From "melancholia" to cholera, including obesity, gangrene, "bilious fever," and softening of the bones, the list covered much ground and notably included "pulmonary phthisis," albeit without comment or elaboration. The bulk of the article considered in detail the medicolegal aspects of only a few of the conditions to which drunkards were said to be predisposed: apoplexy, spontaneous combustion, impotence, sterility, and epilepsy.[28]

Perhaps the most interesting feature of the Roesch study is its practical recommendations, aimed (like much of the material in the *Annales d'hygiène publique*) at eliciting action from governmental authorities. The recommendations were remarkable in that unlike the legions of later proposals, they did not focus on the cabaret or the *débit de boisson*. Roesch urged strict punishment of public drunkenness and related disorders, an end to the practice by household heads of giving drinks to their domestic servants (to revive their energies), and fabrication only of expensive, high-quality eau-de-vie, in order to put its purchase beyond the economic reach of poor families. Further, he fiercely denounced the *colportage* (ambulant sale) of spirits, precisely because the amount and pace of drinking was greater at home than at the cabaret or the *marchand de vin*. Roesch's only regulatory measure involving débits per se proposed that none be licensed to sell only eaux-de-vie.[29] As will become clear below, this failure to indict the cabaret as fundamental to the sociomedical problem of drink and disease provides a striking contrast to the dominant opinion of the Belle Epoque. Just as striking is the absence in these early texts of tuberculosis as a major alcohol-related problem.

By the late Second Empire (at which time the concept of "alcoholism" had been more or less established), the connection of alcohol and tuberculosis seems to have become a more pressing medical issue, but opinion was far from unified. "You understand how important it would be for this question to be resolved," wrote Dr. A. Fabre in the medical journal *Gazette des hôpitaux* in 1868. However, from Fabre's point of view, the resolution was important not because of any action the public authorities might need to take with regard to alcoholism but because many doctors at the time actually *used* alcohol in their treatment of pulmonary tuberculosis.[30]

Fabre summarized the contemporary debate as follows:

> We find ourselves here in the presence of two contradictory opinions: on the one hand, some doctors consider alcohol the least bad remedy for phthisis . . . ; on the other hand, Bell, of New York, Kraus, of Liège, and Launay, of Le Havre, maintain that alcohol produces phthisis and in particular the galloping form of this illness.[31]

He went on to explain that Magnus Huss had found, during autopsies of "drinkers," dried tubercles in the lungs, suggesting that alcohol had arrested or cured incipient phthisis. Other researchers had claimed, on the contrary, that alcoholism brought about and accelerated the progress of the disease.

Fabre proposed to resolve the question by examining the history of one of his patients with consumptive symptoms, an *ivrogne* who admitted drinking a liter of absinthe per day. The doctor cast doubt on the diagnosis of other cases usually cited to support the pathogenic link of alcoholism with consumption: perhaps these robust young people, alcoholic but with no family history of consumption, died in fact of various forms of pulmonary "inflammation" rather than of consumption itself. In the case at hand, the young man's lungs at autopsy showed grayish, compact masses quite distinct from actual tubercles. Alcohol was indeed the source of the patient's illness, in Fabre's opinion, but the illness was not tuberculosis; rather, it was "a variety of caseous pneumonia probably developed under the influence of alcoholism." The sequence went as follows: "First exaltation, then sedation, produced by the same agent, alcohol; exaltation, then dulling of the nutritive system, successively determined by the same illness, inflammation."[32]

The successive, opposite effects of alcohol and alcohol-determined inflammation led Fabre to his paradoxical conclusion: "Knowing that alcohol can have precisely opposite effects, depending on the manner in which it is used, you will understand that the most effective treatment of accidents produced by alcohol consists of the use of alcohol itself." If alcohol had caused any morbid effects in the body at all, matters would only be worsened by the complete withdrawal of alcohol from the system, for the body had become "habituated to a stimulant." The doctor, then, needed to administer a stimulant, "and the best one, in this respect, is precisely alcohol." With moderate doses, the doctor could regulate the patient's gradual withdrawal from alcohol, although

Fabre expressed pessimism over the prospects of successfully combating the social problem of alcoholism in this way. "Deadly poison or precious remedy, depending on whether it is abused or used wisely, you understand that alcohol occupies an important place in both pathology and therapeutics and that it has necessarily aroused strong contradictions until we realized the opposite effects it can determine."[33] In this analysis, the doctor becomes a kind of artist, walking the tightrope between poison and remedy only by virtue of a subtle, professionally informed manipulation of substances. Fabre gave no dogmatic conclusion regarding tuberculosis, but the case studies he cited implied that despite some appearances, alcoholism caused only nontuberculous pulmonary inflammations.

If Fabre's study did not resolve (or even address head-on) the question of alcoholism and tuberculosis, it did express the confusion and difference of opinion that continued to reign over the issue for several decades. In Louis Landouzy's 1881 lecture series, "How and Why One Gets Tuberculosis," which covered an exhaustive list of causes and manifestations of tuberculosis, there was only a single oblique mention of alcohol or alcoholism as a contributory cause of the disease: a reference to "excesses of all sorts." Landouzy discussed alcoholism only as a unique terrain or soil on which tuberculous infection evolved in a particular fashion.[34]

Even after Koch's discovery in 1882, uncertainty persisted. An 1887 medical encyclopedia, under the entry "Phthisis," reviewed the debate just as Fabre had done, and took the middle ground.

> We will take another point of view. Alcoholism ends in the decay [dé-chéance] of the organism; the fact is undeniable, but the causes of this dé-chéance are organic lesions. It is by altering tissues and apparatuses that alcoholism deteriorates the individual. Now, if alcohol provokes lesions which impede the diet, such as chronic gastritis, . . . tuberculosis may appear, as it appears in cases of undernourishment.

Thus, alcoholism led to tuberculosis only when it produced lesions in the body's gastrointestinal system. When alcohol affected primarily the nervous system or circulatory system, however, "it does not seem that it especially favors the development of tubercles."[35] While this passage shows little certainty in the causal linkage of alcoholism with tuberculosis, the article does presage later work in its use of the word déchéance (fall or decay) to describe the effects of alcohol on the body. From the "déchéance" of the individual body to the "déchéance" of society as a whole was a step that later observers would not hesitate to take.

A similar encyclopedia article appeared the next year, in 1888, in which Dr. Victor Hanot took a somewhat stronger stand in linking alcoholism to tuberculosis. He took pains, however, to cite the arguments of both sides in the debate: on the one hand, alcohol has no relation, an inverse relation, or even curative properties with regard to tuberculosis; on the other, alcoholism predisposes to the disease. Researchers cited in the article as denying the pathogenic link had found, among other things, that drunkards and cabaret proprietors rarely suffered from tuberculosis and that the disease progressed more slowly in habitual drinkers than in nondrinkers. One of these researchers, Dr. Emile Leudet, found only 20 tuberculosis victims out of 121 alcoholics under his care. Leudet called alcohol an *aliment respiratoire* that slowed the loss of nutritive elements and conserved energy in the body, thereby exercising a *favorable* influence on health.[36]

Hanot ended by rejecting Leudet's thesis, siding instead with another recent study, in which patients had "very manifestly" contracted their illness after "immoderate usage of alcoholic beverages." Furthermore, tuberculosis developed quite rapidly in these patients, as it had in its "galloping" form observed by other authors in alcoholic patients. "We must therefore admit . . . that the abuse of alcoholic [beverages], supplemented by other excesses and by poverty, which ordinarily accompany drunkenness, predisposes to phthisis, or causes it to break out."[37] A consensus among doctors appeared to be in the making, according to which alcoholism was a major predisposing factor to tuberculosis. Hanot's qualification "supplemented by other excesses" is also curious, and typical of later writings on the issue. This implies a connection with sexual excess and venereal disease, and it would not take long before this link became explicit.

Medical opinion gradually crystallized during the 1890s around the belief that alcoholism was a major—if not the single most significant—social cause of tuberculosis. By 1898, when Dr. Constantin Thiron spoke to the fourth French Congress for the Study of Tuberculosis in Man and in Animals, the alcoholism–tuberculosis connection seems to have achieved the status of dogma that it would retain until World War I. Thiron's paper, despite its somewhat unwieldy title, "Alcoholism, Considered as One of the Major Predisposing Causes, by Heredity or Acquired Individually, of Tuberculosis," pithily expressed the social and political tensions underlying the connection. Thiron first asserted

that "nobody at any time" had contested the proposition that alcoholism predisposes to tuberculosis (a manifestly false assertion, as the documents quoted above show) and went on to debunk the popular wisdom that alcohol had hygienic or therapeutic value.[38]

"Hereditary alcoholism" preoccupied Thiron: the children of alcoholics were "feeble, anemic, . . . scrofulous, irritable, disobedient and
vicious, . . . sickly [tarés], . . . turbulent and restless." Alcoholics were
also prone to "excesses of all kinds"—not only immoral but propagat-
ing pathology into future generations. Among the consequences of their
immorality was, inevitably, poverty: "poverty appears as a result of alcoholic vice and passion."[39]

Having accounted for poverty, Thiron confronted the *politics* of
drinking directly—and in a surprisingly polemical manner.

> As for the question of pauperism, of *socialism,* and of the struggle for life,
> the worker could be happier if he eliminated the cabaret and alcohol from
> his ordinary habits, substituting for them sobriety, thrift, good nourishment
> and refreshing sleep; poverty is in part nothing but the result of the loss of
> time, money and health through alcoholism.[40]

Socialism would seemingly disappear with the eradication of alcoholism. In this passage, bourgeois moralizing and the dark political associations of the cabaret fused to give the fight against alcoholism and its
link with tuberculosis added strength. That Thiron's argument was
firmly grounded in a particular social and political position scarcely
needs to be belabored. When Thiron finished by denouncing alcoholism
and tuberculosis as "the principal causes of the depopulation of almost
every country,"[41] the association of the two scourges can be said to
have achieved its mature form.

Just two years later, in 1900 (the same year that the medical journal
La Tribune médicale ran a year-long series of articles on "the crusade
against tuberculosis and alcoholism," pointing out the danger posed by
the "alcoholic peril" to France's "virility, and even [to] its existence"),
the first French government commission on tuberculosis performed its
work and presented its conclusions. The portion of the commission's
report devoted to the effects of alcoholism on tuberculosis expressed
many of the same anxieties that underlay the medical studies noted
above. The report used the term *dégénérescence* (degeneracy or degeneration) to evoke the joint ramifications of alcoholism and tuberculosis
on French health and society.[42] The author of this section of the commission's report, Dr. Edouard de Lavarenne, claimed that the depart-

ments with the highest per capita consumption of alcohol also had the highest percentage of military conscripts rejected for physical deficiencies—and therefore "the most candidates for tuberculosis." "This is because alcoholism has a direct action on the race, and by debasing it . . . it dooms children more and more to the déchéance of which tuberculosis is one of the most habitual outcomes."[43] It is significant that de Lavarenne used not only the army as the index (and guarantor) of national vitality but also tuberculosis as a measure of France's déchéance. Clinical observation and experimental research had already shown, de Lavarenne argued elsewhere in the report, "the stigmata of physical and intellectual degeneration borne by the descendants of alcoholics." These "hereditary defects" predisposed them to tuberculosis.[44] This was not the same heredity that caused tuberculosis in the essentialist era. In the Belle Epoque, heredity went hand in hand with contagion as a cause of disease, predisposing the soil to be fertile when the seed fell upon it. The confluence of these indicators—military strength, debased heredity, and tuberculosis—pointed to continued decline for the nation. Tuberculosis assembled various threads of anxiety into one coherent package of alarm.

Racial degeneration and depopulation also preoccupied Rénon. Alcoholic heredity, he warned, threatened to perpetuate substandard human specimens, subject to a multitude of biological and moral disorders, into future generations and to result in "the physical degeneration of the species."[45] Rénon's *Maladies populaires* did not, of course, pertain principally to the entire human "species" but rather to what was commonly called the "French race." Such terminology underscores the extent to which, even at a time of truly international medical knowledge, when scientific literature and congresses crossed borders routinely, tuberculosis was perceived in France as a *French* problem above all.

As far as depopulation was concerned, however, alcoholism was not directly a culprit; in fact, alcoholics tended to have many children, Rénon contended. "Unfortunately, society gains nothing from it, because they are bad children. This is not a selection of the race, it is on the contrary a destruction of the race." In effect, France had turned natural selection on its head, procreating particularly the unfittest. "It is nonetheless indisputable that alcoholism does not cause declining natality; what causes it is something else, the progress of neo-Malthusianism."[46] This late-nineteenth-century movement, appropriating Thomas Malthus's ideas about the relationship between population and means of subsistence, urged working-class families to restrict births voluntarily to improve their standard of living.[47] Pronatalists, in turn, accused the neo-Malthusians of complicity in France's depopulation and decline. Alcoholism, Rénon and other mainstream doctors lamented, only compounded the problem by tainting what little human legacy *was* being left behind.

In most cases, empirical proof of the causal role of alcoholism in tuberculosis involved four types of evidence: anecdotes from clinical practice and the apparent distribution of tuberculosis along sexual, geographic, and occupational lines. The anecdotal evidence consisted of case histories from a doctor's private or hospital practice, or simply impressions and observations from daily life. For example, in his medical thesis entitled *How Parisian Working-Class Families Are Disappearing from Tuberculosis,* Isidore-Paul-Alphonse Ladevèze profiled the patients in the hospital ward where he practiced.

> Among our 26 male patients, we found 19 that were manifestly alcoholic, or 72 percent. And we should note that some of them were robust workers that one would never have suspected of [having] tuberculosis, and in whom we found only alcoholism as a predisposing cause. Among women, only 3 of 18 were manifestly alcoholic, but we know that women do not easily admit their bad habits.[48]

There were no rules governing such evidence; each doctor gave free rein to his impressions and judgment (including who might be "suspected" of tuberculosis and that women were unwilling to admit their bad habits). Yet the "results" were generally accepted as statistically precise and were often cited by other authors. For example, Ladevèze referred to the clinical observations of Dr. Jules Lancereaux regarding the causes of tuberculosis:

> In a recent communication to the Academy of Medicine, M. Lancereaux ... attributes [cases of] tuberculosis—from the perspective of circumstances that could prepare the terrain and make it favorable to [the disease's] development—as follows:

Tuberculosis and alcoholism	1,229
Insufficient ventilation, Sedentariness, Overcrowding	651
Poverty and deprivation [*Misère et privations*]	82
Poverty and pregnancy	91
Tuberculosis in the family (probably heredity)	93
Contagion	46
Total	2,192

> We see in this table the preponderant influence of alcoholism.

Ladevèze accepted these results as statistically valid even while con-
fessing, "[I] do not fully understand the forty-six cases under the rubric
Contagion."[49] His puzzlement actually highlights the curious nature of
such "proofs." They testify to the impulse in the medical community,
especially where social etiology was concerned, to sanctify through
quantification and systematization what were essentially anecdotal,
subjective interpretations. Lancereaux's table was characteristic of
much of the work in this field in its attempt to ascribe to every case of
tuberculosis a single, exclusive social "cause."

In any case, such evidence was generally accepted as proof of the
alcoholism–tuberculosis connection. Ladevèze also referred in his thesis
to the sexual distribution of tuberculosis, in which the greater mortality
from the disease among men than among women was used to indicate
alcoholism as a causal factor. The gender differential had been exactly
the reverse in the early nineteenth century, Ladevèze pointed out; to
explain the shift, "one can only think of alcoholism, [which is] more
developed among [men]."[50] Jacques Bertillon took this evidence a step
further in a 1910 article, "Alcohol and Phthisis," claiming that tuberculosis mortality rates were roughly equal for boys and girls until age
fifteen. This corresponded, he noted, with the time when "the two sexes
are equally sober." "Afterward, the vulnerability of the bearded sex [*du
sexe barbu*], which is also the drinking sex, manifests itself." Moreover,
Bertillon maintained, the gender differential in mortality did not manifest itself in the countryside—further proof that "alcohol makes the bed
for tuberculosis" (*l'alcool fait le lit de la tuberculose*).[51]

The geographic line of reasoning typically held that the departments
in France with the highest per capita consumption of alcohol suffered
the highest mortality from tuberculosis. (Occasionally, it extended to
the comparison of nations and ascribed France's high rank in mortality
among European nations to its high alcohol consumption.) Maps were
commonly reproduced with departments shaded according to their alcohol consumption and tuberculosis mortality. They were not unequivocal—often showing little more than vague concentrations in both categories around Normandy, Brittany, and the Ile de France—but they
were interpreted as quite clear evidence of the link. Bertillon, a doctor
devoted to the use of statistics in public health, once again took the
reasoning one step further. On the map showing alcohol consumption
by department, he drew a line representing the northernmost limit of
wine growing. With the exception of the East, the areas south of the
line showed significantly lower rates of alcohol consumption. Similarly,

the wine-growing regions seemed to have generally lower tuberculosis mortality. Distilled spirits, Bertillon concluded, were responsible for the difference.

> Thus, it seems to be eau-de-vie that regulates the distribution of phthisis throughout France; that is, of all causes that can prepare us to receive the terrible tubercle bacillus, there is none more effective than alcohol. The other causes (more numerous and very complex) pale before it like the stars before the sun. It is the master![52]

Alone among those who denounced the role of alcoholism in causing tuberculosis, Bertillon opposed the idea of a regulatory crackdown designed to shut down débits de boissons. Because the real culprit was eau-de-vie, he advocated measures that would encourage *débitants* to sell, "instead of eau-de-vie or absinthe, good French wine. This will make the Midi happy, and at the same time it will diminish tuberculosis in the North."[53]

Always statistically minded, Bertillon went so far as to claim that if the departments of the North and East drank wine instead of eau-de-vie, their tuberculosis mortality would fall to the level of the wine-growing Midi (that is, to 25,500 deaths per year from 42,190), thus saving 16,500 lives per year. ("What sanatorium could even hope for such a result?")[54] Such a conclusion typifies two tendencies in the dominant sociomedical methodology of the period: first, the extrapolation from (sometimes shaky) statistical evidence to unrestrained speculation sanctioned by numerical precision; second, the reference to a statistical "norm" or minimum attainable rate of tuberculosis (that of the Midi), which implicitly represented a social or cultural ideal—the robust, wine-drinking, truly French regions untainted by alcoholism and its attendant vices. This "southern norm" is analogous to the rural ideal depicted by the critics of the rural exodus; in both cases, the corresponding policy goal was somehow to get "back" to the truly French and healthy (imagined) past.

The last type of evidence commonly used to bolster the alcoholism–tuberculosis connection was occupational mortality. Bertillon, for example, compared the material situation of innkeepers, or *cabaretiers,* with that of other store owners, and found them roughly equivalent: "generally poorly housed, leading an enclosed life, and also subject to the emotions that often go along with commerce." The only difference, Bertillon wrote, was that cabaretiers were forced to spend long hours every day in an "alcoholized atmosphere": "even when they try to stay sober, they absorb alcohol through their lungs and through every pore, so to speak." This atmosphere explained the much higher mortality from tuberculosis among innkeepers in England than among other shopkeepers.[55] While other hygienists generally limited themselves to commenting on the drinking habits of cabaretiers when citing these same statistics—failing to echo Bertillon's assertion about absorption of alcohol through lungs and pores—the lesson was clear: workers in occupations prone to heavy drinking suffered a higher incidence of tuberculosis than did other workers.

Although innkeepers served as the prime exemplars of the occupational connection between alcoholism and tuberculosis, other workers occasionally provided variations on the same theme. The hygienist Robert Romme, for example, wrote in 1901 that postmen suffered disproportionately from tuberculosis, because they engaged "unconsciously" in "intense alcoholization."

> The postman has a registered letter, a parcel to deliver, an invoice to collect, information to gather? Then it's a chance to have a drink at the grocery store, the bar, the dairy, the butcher's shop, and in this way postmen end up drinking ten or fifteen small or large glasses of wine, beer, absinthe, vermouth, etc., every day. It's a rare postman who, after ten years' service, doesn't show some signs of alcoholic saturation. And once the soil is prepared for the specific seed to be sown, the Koch bacillus . . . does the rest.[56]

Whether it was conscious or unconscious, alcoholism did its damage. The combined effect of the various forms of evidence was to project utter medical certainty between the 1890s and 1914 on that which had earlier been debated and uncertain: alcoholism was a prominent—to many, the most prominent—cause of tuberculosis.

The central role of the cabaret in anxiety over the alcoholism–tuberculosis connection has already been suggested. Indeed, the seeming impossibility during the War on Tuberculosis of discussing this etiological issue (that is, the role of alcohol in tuberculosis) without focusing on the cabaret can be seen through a closer look at some representative texts. The slide from "problem" to "place" in nearly every medical discussion of this topic is remarkable and suggests levels of meaning beneath the ostensible aims of the texts.

Louis Landouzy, elegant orator and tireless leader of the struggle against tuberculosis in France, presided over the French delegation to the 1912 International Tuberculosis Congress in Rome. His report to the congress, "The Role of Social Factors in the Etiology of Tuberculosis," made it clear that his failure in the 1881 lectures specifically to mention alcoholism among the causes of tuberculosis no longer represented his opinion on the matter. Leaving to other speakers the details of the alcoholism–tuberculosis connection, Landouzy wished to emphasize one particular aspect of the problem:

> I shall only mention here the cabaret . . . as a public space where for hours, *in an atmosphere already deleterious in and of itself,* consumptives cough in people's faces and spit on the ground, infecting those around them—who are easy to contaminate, since chronic alcoholism has already put them in a certain state of déchéance.[57]

Its atmosphere "already deleterious in and of itself," the cabaret was also a prime locus of contagion for a particularly susceptible clientele. It was shown in chapter 4 that one of the ways slum housing contributed to the spread of tuberculosis was via the cabaret (to which the working-class husband/father resorted to escape his unpleasant home). Here (and in other texts), as a *lieu de collectivité,* the cabaret provides a setting for contagion as well, thereby representing by itself all three strands of the dominant etiology—contagion, slum housing, and immorality.

It is not surprising that when Raoul Brunon, a doctor in Rouen who spent most of his career in the forefront of the antialcoholism movement in France, wrote a textbook on tuberculosis, alcoholism figured prominently in it. Brunon's attention, too, seemed to slide toward the cabaret when he attempted to prove the connection between alcoholism and tuberculosis. He offered two case studies from his own practice to support his contention.

> Forty-eight-year-old man. He began coughing six months ago. . . . Since childhood, he has smoked, drunk coffee and eau-de-vie. Habitually [drinks] two coffees per day, and often absinthe as well. . . . For eight years, he has worked as a weaver in a large urban establishment. *He is actively involved in politics and admits that, because of this, opportunities to go to the cabaret are more frequent than before.* He is of strong Norman stock, a real colossus. He nonetheless has a rapidly developing form of tuberculosis.

The second patient, "also . . . a colossus," had been a débitant for fifteen years:

> He took over a failing business and, "to boost business, [he] raised quite a few glasses with his customers." . . . Starting two years ago, he no longer drinks. It is too late. His life is in grave danger.[58]

That the cabaret appeared in the two case studies cited to prove that drinking caused tuberculosis is no coincidence. In particular, Brunon's reference to the worker's political activity (and his "admission" that he went to the cabaret) strongly suggests that the doctor was concerned as much with the débit per se as with the pathogenic effects of alcohol.

Nor was Brunon's clinical evidence unusual in evoking the political role of the cabaret.[59] The most forthright statement of the political anxiety over the cabaret—or perhaps the most extreme political agenda— came from Henri Triboulet at the 1905 International Tuberculosis Congress in Paris. At one point in his speech entitled "Alcohol–Tuberculosis," referring to "our adversaries," Triboulet paraphrased working-class demands for higher wages, shorter hours, and better housing. Triboulet then ridiculed these demands, claiming that workers would merely squander their extra hours and wages drinking at the cabaret. He proposed abstinence instead.

> The doctor knows ... that, for rest and proper nourishment, one needs money. And, to get this money, instead of proposing political and social upheavals, which are discussed all the more willingly the less probable they are known to be, the doctor contents himself with recommending a simple method, as hygienic as it is economical: abstention from alcohol.[60]

Pursuing the political argument even further, Triboulet clarified his point: squandered money was not the only connection between the cabaret and left-wing demands. Revolutionary politics—the politics of the cabaret—was in fact a politics of *drunkenness*.

> With the habituation of the nervous system to alcohol comes the miscomprehension of social laws: the politics of the cabaret, full of hatred, makes a great deal of noise and accomplishes nothing. With hygiene, let us substitute the politics of sobriety: with healthy organs, comprehension of all things is just and sound. ... Thanks to hygiene, let us add to our national motto these three terms, which will never disgrace it: *cleanliness, sobriety, prosperity* [*propreté, sobriété, prospérité*].[61]

While it would be rash to attribute Triboulet's political views to all of the doctors and hygienists who made the connection between alcoholism and tuberculosis (after all, even leftist agitators acknowledged some kind of connection), his outburst was undeniably significant as a look behind the "science" of the dominant etiology. Not only was the cabaret indicted as politically (as well as morally and physically) pathological but reform involved nothing less than a reformulation of national identity (and the triad of the French Revolution) along moral and hygienic lines, with "prosperity" its ultimate end.

The medical literature's focus on the cabaret and the intense anxiety it seems to have provoked were also apparent in the policy measures proposed to fight the alcoholism–tuberculosis relationship; most of them dealt strictly with the cabaret. As Brunon put it, "Prevention is in part contained in these few words: RESTRICTION OF THE NUMBER OF CABARETS." The public health community was in overwhelming agreement that local authorities' right to license new débits should be curtailed and many existing alcohol outlets closed down. Equally popular was the proposed elimination of the home distillery privilege (*privilège des bouilleurs de cru*), which allowed the extensive production of distilled spirits. The first governmental commission on tuberculosis in 1900 went further than some by suggesting "administrative regulations in the aim of hindering the *frequenting* of cafés and cabarets." Others called for cutting taxes on "hygienic" fermented beverages (wine, beer, and cider); for antialcohol education programs in the schools and army; and for cooperative restaurants that would amply and cheaply nourish workers without serving alcohol.[62] In parliament, representatives of the antialcoholism movement repeatedly introduced bills restricting cabaret licenses or limiting the privilège des bouilleurs de cru. None of these legislative measures came to fruition before World War I.[63]

In the late twentieth century, after the triumph of the "disease model" of alcoholism, there may be less blame or moral stigma visited upon the alcoholic for his condition than in earlier times. The extent to which alcoholism served to fix blame for tuberculosis around the turn of the century in France is suggested by some revealing passages in the vast body of medical literature on the link between the two phenomena. Dr. Fauchon's pamphlet *La Tuberculose, question sociale* addressed the hypothetical parents of a child lost to tuberculosis: "This seed of tuberculosis, it is neither you nor your domestics that gave it to your unfortunate child, it is your neighbors the alcoholics . . . and you are justified in saying: 'Without those miserable alcohol drinkers who infected my child, he would still be with us.' "[64] Another doctor writing in *La Tribune médicale* in 1901 was scarcely more charitable, declaring that the association of alcoholism and tuberculosis "is no longer a matter . . . of microbes but of an adversary perhaps even more formidable, because it is man himself who, by his lack of will, his bad instincts, his passions, becomes his own enemy." In a similar vein, a participant in a 1903 conference on alcoholism and tuberculosis spoke of "a cowardice of character, which leads to . . . a willful illness."[65] In other pronounce-

ments, the moral judgment was more subtle, but it is clear that blame
was strongly attached to alcoholism—and through it, to tuberculosis—
at the time of their association.

From the early nineteenth century to World War I, the medical attribution of tuberculosis to alcoholism progressed from debate and uncertainty to unanimity, and eventually allowed wide-ranging policy recommendations and moral pronouncements to be made. In contrast, the
syphilis–tuberculosis connection followed no such course but continued
to be expressed, despite a notable lack of scientific evidence indicating
a direct causal link.

SYPHILIS AND TUBERCULOSIS: TARGETING THE PROSTITUTE

The prostitute, immorality incarnate and an object of social anxiety in
France comparable to the cabaret, became associated with tuberculosis
through the study of venereal disease (especially syphilis) as a matter of
public health warranting the attention and surveillance of the authorities. Because prostitution was universally considered to be the primary
means of transmission of venereal disease, the incidence of syphilis in
France became a kind of index of national morality. The history of the
syphilis–tuberculosis link, when compared with that of alcoholism and
tuberculosis, reveals at the same time less medical certainty and precision regarding pathogenesis and a similar underlying sociopolitical
agenda.

Before germ theory and Koch, there was some precedent for considering syphilis a predisposing influence on the development of tuberculosis. At least one of the early-nineteenth-century medical encyclopedias
listed syphilis (and antisyphilis therapy) among twenty-eight causes of
pulmonary phthisis—including cancer, hysteria, and hypochondria—
mentioned in medical literature.[66]

But by the time the syphilis–tuberculosis link became the object of
more frequent study, beginning in the 1880s, discussion of syphilis was
permeated with social and political issues such as prostitution and depopulation. Under the entry "Syphilis," an 1883 medical dictionary
prominently featured a discussion of the control of prostitution and
complained about the disease's role in national decline. "It is undeniable
that syphilis, by the harmful influence it exercises on natality and on the
vigor of the younger generations, is an important factor in the depopulation and bastardization [*l'abâtardissement*] of the race."[67] Both low na-

tality and vitiated heredity—two components of racial decline and social "counter-Darwinism"—were ascribed in part to syphilis.

A Dr. Granier gave a paper in 1885 before the Société de thérapeutique of Paris that connected syphilis with tuberculosis in an intriguing way. Granier's paper can be situated within a strange sort of medical debate over the connection, a debate without overt disagreement but full of ambiguity and uncertainty. Granier began by referring to previous research on the question, which seemed to show that syphilis (by generally debilitating the body) favored the development of tuberculosis and accelerated its pace in subjects already predisposed to the latter disease. One authority had called syphilis "an undisputed source of the degeneration of the species and a no less indisputable source of consumption." Granier's summary of the state of medical opinion on this issue nevertheless equivocated on the exact nature of the pathogenic influence. "Perfect agreement, on the one hand, in admitting a determinant influence of syphilis on the development of tuberculosis in predisposed subjects; on the other hand, in denying a direct, special influence of syphilis on tuberculosis." [68]

Granier went on to claim, seemingly in opposition to this conventional wisdom, that syphilitic infection *itself,* in a predisposed subject, could evolve into tuberculosis, "with no penetration whatsoever by an external germ." [69] This contention of "morbid spontaneity," of course, flew in the face of Koch's discoveries of 1882, according to which only the entry of the tubercle bacillus into the body could cause tuberculosis. Although presented as little more than a hypothesis, Granier's contention testifies to the increasingly close association between vice and tuberculosis that had begun to develop in the French medical community. Two medical encyclopedias published soon after Granier's findings tended to downplay (albeit ambiguously) the direct influence of syphilis on tuberculosis, while highlighting the generally degenerative effects of syphilis on the species as a whole. It predisposed to tuberculosis only "as any debilitating cause" did, not in a particular or uniquely pernicious manner. [70]

"Morbid Associations: Syphilis and Tuberculosis; Soils and Seed" was the title of Landouzy's presentation at an 1891 tuberculosis conference in Paris. The most curious of all texts linking syphilis with tuberculosis, the piece is all the more significant in that it represented the opinion of France's leading "phthisiologist." In a comment of only two and one-half pages, Landouzy presented differing, even apparently conflicting, views of the link. While his title suggested a predisposing relationship (direct or merely "debilitating") of syphilis to tuberculosis, Landouzy did not address the issue of predisposition per se. Instead, he posited a "sclerogenetic" effect of syphilis, which resulted in a slowly evolving, "torpid" tuberculosis; he even suggested that such a *sclérolate de tuberculose*" brought about the improvement of certain symptoms.[71]

Why, then, did Landouzy also lament, "[What a] bad, very bad morbid association [is] that of tuberculosis and syphilis proceeding in tandem"? (*Mauvaise, très mauvaise association morbide que celle de la tuberculose et de la syphilis marchant de pair!*) Its context suggests that this particular exclamation referred to cases in which an already tuberculous patient acquired syphilis. This sequence, according to Landouzy, gave the tuberculosis renewed severity and *hastened* its development.[72]

This brief article leaves many questions unanswered. In justifying the subject of his paper, Landouzy pointed to "the frequency of syphilis" and "the nonrarity of the association of syphilis and tuberculosis." What he meant by the latter is less clear; he defined neither "association" nor "nonrarity." Nor did Landouzy suggest whether the frequency of the association had a causal basis or was coincidental. The reference to "soil and seed" in the article's title is equally unclear, since cases of tuberculosis aggravated by the presence of syphilis are mentioned only in passing. On the surface, at least, Landouzy seems to have concluded that prior syphilis somehow impeded the development of tuberculosis: it constituted an "acquired terrain" on which the tubercle bacillus produced "a very particular harvest." He went on to urge researchers to study the evolution of tuberculosis on "terrains rendered pathologically improper" to the "easy development" of the bacillus.[73]

An 1894 report in a medical journal set forth a contrasting view of syphilitic "soil." Professor Carl Potain, teaching at the Hôpital de la Charité in Paris, examined a twenty-nine-year-old syphilitic who had begun to show symptoms of pulmonary tuberculosis. The combination, in Potain's experience, was common, "and in the large majority of cases, it is syphilis that opens the scene, tuberculosis only developing later." The issue was quite clear, leaving no room for equivocation or ambiguity: "Syphilis calls forth tuberculosis [and] furnishes it with a good soil on which to grow."[74]

René Jacquinet, one of Landouzy's students at the Paris Faculté de médecine, published his thesis on syphilis and tuberculosis (as well as a related study in *La Presse médicale*) in 1895. Far from describing the torpid *tuberculose sclérosante* of Landouzy, however, Jacquinet presented observations of a quite different nature. Most of Jacquinet's case studies, in fact, all of whose subjects were syphilitic prior to tuberculous infection, exhibited a severe, rapid tuberculosis—fatal in a very short period of time.[75]

Jacquinet admitted that it was difficult to establish statistics on the coexistence of syphilis and tuberculosis and on the temporal or causal sequence of the diseases. Nevertheless, nearly all of the authors he quoted on the subject portrayed the predisposing or "provocative" effect of syphilis on tuberculosis as frequent. To conclude his section concerning the etiological role of syphilis, Jacquinet quoted the venereal disease authority Alfred Fournier, who also characterized the progress of syphilis-caused tuberculosis as rapid and quickly fatal. "According to my own experience," Fournier said, "as well as what has been said by . . . the most authorized observers, I would not hesitate to inscribe syphilis in the etiological chapter of pulmonary tuberculosis."[76]

Jacquinet did cite his mentor Landouzy, indeed quoted him at length, on the sclerogenetic effect of syphilis. This apparent internal contradiction, not characterized as such by Jacquinet, can perhaps be explained by the timing of the syphilitic infection involved. Jacquinet presented Landouzy's findings as bearing only on infections that were already many years old when the tuberculosis began; in contrast, Jacquinet devoted most of his own attention to still-active, virulent syphilis.[77] This distinction (made more clearly in Jacquinet's thesis than in *La Presse médicale*) offers a possible explanation for syphilis producing both torpid and rapid tuberculosis, but it does not explain the conclusion of Jacquinet's thesis, attributed to Landouzy: "Among infectious associations, there is none worse, none more formidable, than the combination of a syphilis and a tuberculosis."[78] It is difficult to understand why a *retarding* effect would be likened to an *intensifying* effect and called the worst infectious "association" possible.

Despite the ambiguity of the syphilis–tuberculosis link, some sort of association certainly existed, if only as a result of the frequency of references in the literature; and if syphilis were associated with tuberculosis, it was inevitable that prostitution would enter into the association. It did so in various ways, and not always with direct reference to venereal disease. It should be borne in mind, however, that all discussion of syphilis (including its relationship to other threats and "scourges") contained, implicitly or explicitly, a discussion of prostitution.[79]

An interesting example of the way in which prostitution insinuated itself into discussions of tuberculosis arose in the proceedings of the

French government's first tuberculosis commission in 1900. Professor Charles Bouchard, calling the commission's attention to "the frequency of tuberculous contamination by prostitutes," proposed that tuberculosis be added to the list of venereal diseases for which prostitutes were periodically examined by the authorities. Bouchard's resolution justified this measure as follows:

> The extended and prolonged contact of the oral mucous membrane of a tuberculous person with the same mucous membrane of a healthy person, *as often happens during the genital act,* is a very favorable condition for the transmission of tuberculosis.[80]

This passage apparently indicates that *kissing*—which "often happens" during sexual intercourse—can transmit tubercle bacilli. The resolution continued,

> This circumstance, even more than alcoholism, is the cause of the extreme frequency of tuberculosis in prostitutes;
> ... [T]his same cause makes the prostitute a frequent source of tuberculosis.[81]

His striking conclusion followed logically: "Transmitted under the conditions indicated above, tuberculosis acquires the character of a veritable venereal disease."[82]

Several features of this proposition deserve further comment. First, the association of the prostitute with alcoholism was presupposed and needed no proof. Second, the prostitute with tuberculosis was seen not as a victim or potential patient but as a potential "source" of contagion. Finally, while Bouchard's actual etiological contention was simply that kissing could spread germs, the displacement of the issue to that of prostitution was seemingly instantaneous and unselfconscious. Blame was placed on a safe target (and not, for example, on just *anyone* who engaged in kissing), and further surveillance of prostitutes was rationalized. The second, "permanent" government commission on tuberculosis does not appear to have investigated the question in depth, but it also received evidence according to which prostitutes were among "the most serious agents of the propagation of tuberculosis."[83]

Both prostitution and syphilis reappeared in connection with tuberculosis in Rénon's 1905 textbook, *Les Maladies populaires*. While Rénon classified syphilis as one of several illnesses (along with typhoid fever, influenza, measles, and smallpox) that predisposed to tuberculosis, he did not draw as direct a causal tie in this direction as he did from alcoholism to tuberculosis. The association was no less strong, however, for lacking a physiological pedigree, as will be shown below in a discussion of the ultimate triangular link.

Three other similarities between the syphilis problem and the alcoholism problem are illustrated in Rénon's book: racial degeneration, the threat to the social fabric, and the association with the cabaret. The first has been touched on at length above, and Rénon simply reiterated similar concerns about degeneration in his book.[84] As for the social fabric, its most fundamental underpinning was the family, and syphilis had a ruinous impact on the family.

> It means the end of the marriage, discussions, separation, divorce. It also means the contamination of the wet nurse and its results: unlimited blackmail or a scandalous trial for damages. It means, finally, the material ruin of the family, and after the illness, the incapacity [and] the death of the family head, [and] destitution.[85]

In Rénon's view, symptoms and scandal went hand in hand; the clinical entity could not be conceived of apart from its social ramifications. The physical and moral dimensions of syphilis were inseparably intertwined, and each had dire consequences.

The cabaret, subtextually omnipresent in Rénon's book, was explicitly implicated on several occasions in the genesis of the three associated scourges. As far as syphilis was concerned, sailors from the French navy and merchant marine were among the groups subject to the cabaret's deleterious influence. The frequency of syphilis among the sailors was understandable, wrote Rénon,

> if one thinks of the evil that can be done by all the shady cabarets in port cities [tous les cabarets interlopes des ports], frequented by sailors who go there after long periods of continence. Alcoholism and venereal diseases reign there in tandem.[86]

Also reigning at the cabaret, of course, though not mentioned by name, were the prostitute and the end result of all these pathologies, tuberculosis.

COMPLETING THE TRIANGLE: IMMORAL PLACES, IMMORAL BEHAVIOR

The confluence of alcoholism, syphilis, and tuberculosis—the complete triangular association—operated in a subtler way than did the two-part connections discussed above. Above all, the triangular link demonstrated the force and frequency of the specter of the cabaret (and, to a

lesser extent, the prostitute) in turn-of-the-century fears of French decline and degeneration.

Before considering the triangular link in its full three-part form, it is
worth mentioning that on occasion during this same period, medical literature explicitly linked alcoholism and venereal disease without the
nexus of tuberculosis. For example, the 1901 International Congress on
Alcoholism heard a paper in which it was argued that while alcohol had
an undeniable influence on venereal disease by encouraging sexual excesses, it was "tipsiness" rather than drunkenness or chronic alcoholism
that correlated most closely to the contraction of venereal infection.[87]

Another of the rare medical expositions of the alcoholism–syphilis
connection was more provocative in its social implications. This study,
by Dr. Barthélemy of the clinical staff of the Paris medical faculty, appeared in the *Annales d'hygiène publique* in 1883 (before the other links
described above had coalesced). As a follow-up to one of his earlier
studies, which had posited an aggravating effect of alcoholism on syphilitic chancres, Barthélemy looked into the surprising frequency in the
initial study of serious cutaneous infection among women. He found
that all of the women so affected were "*femmes de brasserie*," pub wait-
resses known to offer additional services to their customers, and that
all of them were forced by their employers to drink excessively.[88]

On further study of the situation of femmes de brasserie in general,
Barthélemy found that most were syphilitic; indeed, they were the principal source of venereal disease among "the young men of the *Ecoles*."
In the interest of public health and better surveillance of "clandestine
prostitution," the doctor recommended that these "establishments
served by women" be suppressed in their current form as "insalubrious
establishments of the first degree." Barthélemy justified such a regulatory measure (at first sight incongruous in an article entitled "Influence
of Alcoholism on Syphilis") by "the frightening proportion in which
[syphilis] contributes to the depopulation of the species . . . and at the
very least to the degeneration of the race."[89] This is one of the first
instances of the cabaret *and* the prostitute being medically implicated
in depopulation and degeneration. It would not be the last.

It is impossible to pin down chronologically the origins of the three-
way alcoholism–syphilis–tuberculosis connection. In a paper presented
at a 1891 tuberculosis conference that may represent the first explicit
reference, Dr. E. Tison included a case study of an alcoholic and syphilitic patient who died of tuberculosis. Tison concluded that the progress

of the tuberculosis was more rapid than normal in this case (not *scléro-sant*) and that "pulmonary [tuberculosis] followed organic weakening by syphilis and alcoholism."[90] Somewhat indirect references to this triangular connection can be found in writings on tuberculosis around the turn of the century as well. For example, Romme maintained in 1901 that the "seed" of tuberculosis found "a particularly propitious soil" in unsanitary lodgings, whose inhabitants were "ravaged by syphilis and alcohol."[91] In most cases, references to the three-way connection were oblique, or remained at the level of allusion.

Rénon went beyond allusion in 1905 when he confronted the triangular link explicitly and in detail. Both in his lecture at the international tuberculosis congress of that year and in his book *Les Maladies populaires,* Rénon clearly targeted alcoholism, syphilis, and tuberculosis— and the behavior they represented—as dangerous threats to French society. First, he laid the medical groundwork for the connections: both alcoholism and syphilis seem to favor the development of tuberculosis; in addition, the déchéance that predisposes to tuberculosis can be inherited, and the children of alcoholics and syphilitics (as well as the children of tuberculous parents) are likely future victims of tuberculosis.[92] Rénon then proceeded, in his lecture, to sketch the outlines of the "social defense against tuberculosis" that he had in mind. In this fight, the cabaret was a formidable adversary. "I regret that we cannot diminish the strength of this *enemy of the people,* the cabaret." However, action against the threat was both possible and necessary. "The fight against syphilis and other intoxications, in solidarity with the fight against tuberculosis, will find serious support in . . . [a] union of all efforts to defend the *physical and moral* interests of the community."[93] Rénon not only turned the language of revolution on its head with the epithet "enemy of the people" but also demonstrated how inseparable were the physical health and the moral health of France in the diagnosis of social pathology.

The crucial role of the cabaret in uniting all three scourges was never more succinctly expressed, however, than in *Les Maladies populaires.*

Alcoholism is the great purveyor of tuberculosis. "*La phtisie se prend sur le zinc,*" said M. Hayem, and this is true. It is the associate of syphilis, in those shady cabarets [*cabarets interlopes*] found in abundance around barracks [and] factories, bars where one gets alcoholism on one side of the counter and syphilis on the other [*débits où l'on s'alcoolise d'un côté du comptoir et où l'on se syphilise de l'autre*].[94]

Once again, the word *associate* was used to define the connection among the scourges. The cabarets (and, by adroit implication, prostitution) were all the more dangerous in that they were "spread out" around factories and garrisons, where they turned vital workers and soldiers into degenerates and sapped France's economic and military strength. The triangle was completed not through tuberculosis this time but rather via the nexus of the cabaret's zinc countertop: "You get phthisis at the *zinc*"; on one side of it, you get alcoholism and, on the other side, syphilis.

Mortality in general (and its leading cause, tuberculosis, in particular) posed a vexing problem to a demographically stagnant nation that perceived itself as in danger of decline. The problem was even more worrisome, however, when it appeared that physical or numerical decline was inextricable from—indeed, both evidence and a result of—vice, political subversion, productive incapacity, moral "déchéance." Through vice and heredity, it was feared, a kind of subspecies was being propagated in France, a lower race of "candidates" for tuberculosis and other afflictions, morally and physically degenerate. Resulting mortality kept population from increasing, so lower quality was matched by lower quantity.

General fears of national decline, combined with a specific and acute Germanophobia in the aftermath of the Franco-Prussian War of 1870, allowed the appropriation of ostensibly medical issues for the expression of political concerns, or at least the evocation of such concerns in medical discourse. For example, at the Toulouse conference on alcoholism and tuberculosis in 1903, one speaker recalled the words of Gambetta after the Prussian capture of Metz in 1870.

> In the presence of so many evils and the prodigious effort they require, the country should once again hear the great voice which rose up in the somber days of 1870, after the capitulation of Metz, and which kindled hope in our hearts: "Frenchmen, lift up your souls and your resolution to the level of the terrible perils which weigh on the *Patrie*.
>
> "It still depends on us to leave behind ill fortune and to show the universe what a great people is made of, [a people] which does not wish to perish and whose courage is aroused even in the midst of catastrophe." [95]

In this instance, alcoholism and tuberculosis not only were compared metaphorically to national military defeat and *la patrie en danger* but also served as a reminder of the need to preserve the greatness of the French nation and to prove that greatness in response to the threat of decline.

Furthermore, perceived moral and physical degeneration fed political fears of domestic as well as foreign threats. In addition to Triboulet's diatribe against the politics of the cabaret, the characterization of the Paris Commune of 1871 as the work of alcoholics was quite common. Barrows has shown that "the terrible year of 1870–71 triggered an immediate and dramatic shift in the perception of drink."[96] The entire experience of that year, the *"année terrible,"* had ingrained a lasting fear of French decline that could take (and in many minds had taken) biological as well as political form. Nevertheless, the medical form of this fear seems to have intensified during and after the 1890s, particularly during the decade 1895–1905. Other historians of France have also pinpointed this period as one of heightened medical attention to preventive social and hygienic policy and have attributed this attention in part to the demographic anxiety of the time.[97] Degeneration symbolized many perceived trends and threats, from loss of productive economic capacity (through lost man-hours due to illness and an unreliable workforce) to declining national vitality and virility (through a declining birthrate) and loss of national stature in the world arena.

The structure and evolution of the three-way association exemplify the peculiar interactions of scientific medicine with society as a whole. In the case of the alcoholism–tuberculosis connection, debate among doctors and scientists gave way in the last decade of the nineteenth century to near-unanimity and an abundance of physiological evidence supporting the etiology. In contrast, the syphilis–tuberculosis "association" was never actually a debate, even though ambiguous and seemingly conflicting data were presented in connection with it. Moreover, the type of scientific proof of a causal or predisposing relation common in the literature on alcoholism was comparatively meager in the work on syphilis, apart from statements concerning the effects of debilitating diseases in general. Yet overriding social and moral factors seem to have imposed a strong triangular association, regardless of the clinical evidence.

The concept of heredity clearly played a major role in the diagnosis of degeneration, and its use marked a significant change in medical thought in France.[98] As was the case with overcrowding and filth, an element of pre-germ theory etiologies persisted into the time of the War on Tuberculosis but in somewhat altered form. In the essentialist era of the early and mid-nineteenth century, before Villemin and Koch, tuberculosis had been understood as an inherited disease—that is, acquired principally and directly by heredity. Heredity was thus essentially a *backward-looking* concept, used to explain why people were afflicted with tuberculosis at that time. By the turn of the century, heredity had given way to contagion and behavior as a direct cause of tuberculosis; however, it remained an indirect cause through the concept of inherited predisposition. In this usage, amid concerns over national demographic decline, heredity was a largely *forward-looking* concept that explained why the future consequences of all three scourges were so grave.

Both alcoholism and syphilis served to bring a moral and behavioral element into the etiology of tuberculosis, a rampant—and for years inexplicable—killer. Moral judgments have often characterized societies' responses to disease throughout history—the example of AIDS, among others, shows this to be no less true in the late twentieth century—and have rendered mysterious threats comprehensible and less threatening to many members of those societies. In this respect, the role of syphilis in France at the turn of the century is crucial, for it did not enter the dominant etiology with as much accumulated "science" behind it as did alcoholism. Judged by the standards of the time, that is, fewer studies and more tenuous types of evidence linked syphilis to tuberculosis than linked alcoholism to tuberculosis.

If syphilis was thought to affect the body's resistance to tuberculosis only in the same manner as many other diseases, why did it become closely connected to tuberculosis? Several answers can be conjectured. First, syphilis was closely associated with infertility and birth defects, and the connection thus spoke to fears of depopulation. Second, it reinforced the moral/behavioral etiology of tuberculosis; in so doing, it may also have strengthened the repressive power of the reigning bourgeois ethos of family and monogamy. Third, syphilis introduced the prostitute as a mortal danger; she was already the consummate symbol of degeneracy and social pathology in France. In the words of Alain Corbin, "the prostitute figures at the center of the tragedy of this time because she contains and symbolizes at once the venereal evil, alcoholism, tuberculosis and *dégénérescence.*"[99]

Alcoholism, syphilis, and prostitution all focused attention on that other potent symbol of social fear, the cabaret. The continual intrusion of the cabaret into medical investigations and explanations is one of the most salient and striking features of the alcoholism–syphilis–tuberculosis connection. Inherently "shady," the cabaret lay at the confluence of several social pathologies: economic unproductiveness, immoderation, sexual promiscuity, prostitution, and left-wing politics. The central role of the cabaret in the moral etiology of tuberculosis also allowed it to fit relatively seamlessly with the other two strands of the dominant etiology as a whole, those involving contagion and housing. For example, the cabaret became a breeding ground for bacilli and a locus of contagion; meanwhile, the lamentable conditions of the worker's slum lodgings further encouraged him to spend his time at the cabaret.

The doctors who were in the forefront of the evolving triangular association did not simply use the problems of tuberculosis, syphilis, and alcoholism as a front or a sham hiding their true social and political agenda. Neither, however, was the connection a straightforward, ideologically neutral medical attempt to improve public health. Rather, there was a subtle slide from the ostensibly empirical scientific observation of pathological correlations to a broader social diagnosis. This diagnosis captured, channeled, and expressed a wide range of anxieties, which included but were not limited to concern over the health of Frenchmen. It did so in a manner that seems to have been compelling, and it was also politically expedient.

The connection of alcoholism and of syphilis with tuberculosis—and, later, the mutual association of all three scourges—indicted certain *social* pathologies in the *biological* decline of France (and, by extension, its political and economic downfall) at the turn of the century. The focus on the cabaret and on prostitution added potency to the moral etiology of disease, and embodied in familiar targets manifold threats to the nation.

CHAPTER SIX

Le Havre, Tuberculosis Capital
of the Nineteenth Century

Le Havre . . . occupies the first rank among the most
unhealthy French cities. . . . Phthisis is, in Le Havre,
perpetually endemic.
> —*Joseph Richard, medical thesis, 1901*

The city of Le Havre has never been unhealthy.
> —*Théodule Marais, mayor, 1903*

Mayor Marais's sanguine claim that his city had never been unhealthy
was belied not only by all available statistics but also even by the actions
of the local government and civic leaders from the 1880s on. Year after
year, from the time such figures were kept, Le Havre ranked highest
in per capita tuberculosis mortality of all major French cities. It was
consistently at or near the top in overall mortality as well. Social investigators, hygienists, and public officials regularly decried the lamentable
state of Le Havre's housing stock and its notorious degree of alcohol
consumption. Moreover, to an extent unmatched in any other French
city, local elites attempted to respond to the challenges of ill health and
urban pathology with a strategy of public and private action aimed at
the material and moral improvement of the working class. This chapter
tells the story of these efforts: their origins, their vicissitudes, the directions in which they were oriented, the controversies to which they gave
rise, and their impact.

How did the War on Tuberculosis actually work at street level? Some
answers have already been suggested. The experience of Le Havre more
than any other city, with its exceedingly high incidence of tuberculosis
and its vigorous reform efforts, can serve as a window on the everyday
ramifications of medical knowledge. Le Havre is in no way typical as a
case study of tuberculosis in nineteenth-century France; it is an extreme
example. But for this very reason, the tensions, anxieties, and responses
aroused by tuberculosis are exaggerated there and exposed to view.

They appear in dramatic relief, and seen in relief the local meanings of tuberculosis become clearer.

One hundred years ago, wealthy Havrais notables literally looked down on the poor. Le Havre occupied a strip of land bounded by the Seine on the south and on the north by the hills that stretch from the coastal town of Sainte-Adresse to Graville northeast of the city. Working-class families occupied the flat quarters near the port, the workplace of many of the city's residents. The merchants and bankers who made their fortunes from Le Havre's growing commercial role in the nineteenth century moved upward, building elegant hillside mansions on the edge of town, overlooking the overcrowded slums below. This sharp difference in geographic elevation expressed in spatial terms the vast extremes of wealth and poverty generated by the city's rapid commercial and industrial growth.[1]

In the nineteenth century, Le Havre was the primary seaport of Paris and France's gateway to the world across the Atlantic. Its location near the capital at the mouth of the Seine and the gradual improvement of its port facilities since its founding by King François I in 1517 made Le Havre a premier point of transit for passengers, raw materials, and manufactured goods entering and leaving France. On the eve of the First World War, Le Havre was the second largest seaport in France (after Marseille) and the largest transatlantic port; between one-fourth and one-fifth of French maritime commerce passed through the Havrais docks each year. Le Havre's importance as a port shaped every aspect of the city's life: its major industries, including shipbuilding and metallurgy; the mercantile and financial elite, with commercial interests as far-flung as the sugar and cotton plantations of the New World, that dominated the city's economy and politics throughout the nineteenth century; and its working population of sailors, dockworkers, and laborers, whose employment was not only grueling but unreliable, dependent on the caprices of weather and international markets.[2]

Like Paris, Le Havre experienced rapid and dramatic population growth during the mid-nineteenth century. A city of fewer than 27,000 inhabitants in 1823, it doubled in size by 1846; in 1881, Le Havre had grown to a population of 106,000; and in 1901, it exceeded 130,000— the ninth-largest city in France. Over the entire nineteenth century, only Roubaix and St.-Etienne among major French cities grew at a faster rate.[3] As in Paris, the sudden pressure exerted by this growth on the city's physical and social structures caused considerable anxiety among political leaders. The concentration of so many people in the close

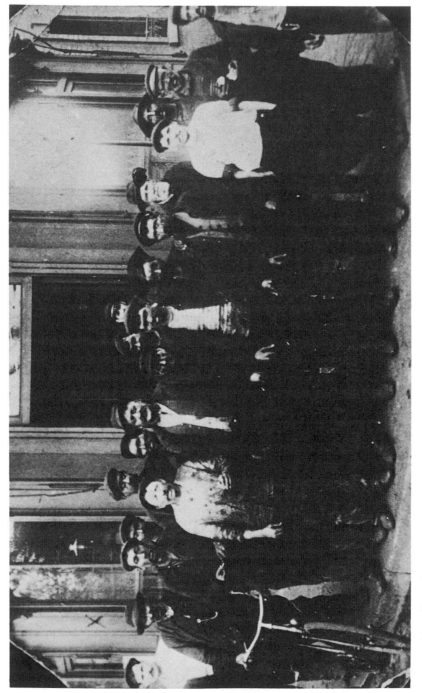

10. Coal handlers of Le Havre's waterfront, ca. 1910. Photo courtesy of Jean Legoy, Le Havre.

quarters of the central city—especially working people confronting the contradictions of dire poverty in the midst of great mercantile and industrial wealth—gave a troubling immediacy to the prospect of disease and unrest; on the heels of two cholera epidemics and two revolutions in France during the 1830s and 1840s, few could ignore the threat posed by the nation's increasingly pathological cities. A perceived penchant for drink and depravity among the "dangerous classes" only exacerbated the fears of local and national elites.

In the case of Le Havre, a cadre of philanthropically minded public figures led by Jules Siegfried spearheaded a wave of reform initiatives in the city during the early Third Republic. Siegfried, who achieved a national reputation as a centrist republican legislator and cabinet minister, dominated politics in Le Havre during his tenure as mayor (1878–1886) and throughout his thirty-six years in parliament as deputy and senator (1886–1922). Personally or through his disciples and allies, Siegfried made his influence felt at City Hall, and in no domain was this influence stronger than in health policy and sanitary reform. The first municipal board of health in France[4]—Le Havre's Bureau d'hygiène—was his creation in 1879, and he also became known nationally as a champion of colonialism and working-class housing.[5]

As early as the Second Empire, however, there were signs that a new awareness of hygienic matters in general, and the problem of tuberculosis in particular, was emerging in Le Havre. In the 1850s, Dr. Adolphe Lecadre began issuing periodic reports on the city's "sanitary situation"; most of them were published in the bulletin of the Société havraise d'études diverses, the local *société savante*. In an 1868 report—just after Villemin's efforts to prove the transmissibility of tuberculosis but well before both the establishment of the Bureau d'hygiène and Koch's pivotal discovery of the tubercle bacillus—Lecadre foreshadowed several aspects of the later dominant etiology and War on Tuberculosis. Chief among these was the *localizing* impulse. Lecadre proposed to explain much of Le Havre's mortality by breaking down death rates from certain causes street by street, according to the residence of the victims. First among the killers he included in the category of "local" or housing-related diseases was tuberculosis. Writing during the not-quite-contagionist interim between Villemin's and Koch's experiments, as the tide was beginning to turn against the likes of Pidoux and Peter, Lecadre asserted that tuberculosis was "transmitted by the effluvia inherent in housing."[6] On its face, such a declaration seems straightforwardly miasmatist, but its use of the word *transmitted* and its focus on housing (rather than, for example, swamps or soil drainage) prefigure to some extent the key role played by unsanitary slums in the later, contagionist etiology of the disease.

It was neither obvious nor at random that Lecadre chose to analyze tuberculosis and other diseases locally, by ascribing them to certain buildings, streets, and neighborhoods. Several revealing phrases in his report show that this strategy was both conscious and clearly delineated. Certain causes of death were to be excluded from the analysis by *quartier*.

> Some illnesses . . . are specific to certain ages. . . . Other diseases, such as those of the heart, are frequently caused by the exaltation of the passions, overwork, the depletion of physical strength, a dissolute lifestyle, etc., [and] cannot affect certain streets [differently].[7]

In other words, those diseases for which no known social or behavioral cause existed—Lecadre noted tuberculosis, infantile diarrhea, typhoid fever, and the measles as four that accounted for a significant number of deaths—would be broken down by street and neighborhood to find specifically local correlations. Other possible causal factors (such as work or diet, for example) failed to appear in the statistics, because Lecadre's method excluded nongeographic variables. This predetermination of the conclusions in the approach was not uncommon in mid-nineteenth-century epidemiological studies. Unlike other aspects of social relations, housing was perceived as subject to—and in need of—remedial action.

There were other hints as well in Lecadre's early reports of what would later be the dominant etiology of tuberculosis. For example, in that same 1868 report, he noted that the disease frequently struck unmarried residents of lodging houses, who fit a certain social profile:

> We see among these consumptives . . . a goodly number of sailors, [including] many outsiders[;] and at the top of this list must be placed the Bretons, who came to Le Havre seeking the work that their native land refused them[;] among the women [are] a large quantity of servants, mostly young girls, [who] left the countryside, where they were often quite healthy, to come lose their health in the insalubrity and laxness—and for some of them dissoluteness—of the city.[8]

Here, in addition to housing, the rural exodus, domestic servants, and immorality are all associated with urban mortality from tuberculosis—much as they would be forty years later. Lecadre's analysis was hardly as sustained or emphatic on these points as the dominant etiology would later be, but it shows that much of the official bourgeois reaction to tuberculosis, on the local as well as the national level, predated germ theory and derived more from social change than from strictly scientific developments.

In later reports throughout the 1870s, Lecadre continued to emphasize the pathogenic role of unsanitary housing, while at the same time elaborating on other causes of tuberculosis. By and large, these were the classic elements of pre-germ theory etiologies. Masturbation, sexual excesses, sedentary lifestyles and occupations, the exposure of wet or sweaty skin to sudden temperature changes, and various other environmental influences took their places alongside heredity in Lecadre's catalog of predisposing factors. He equivocated on the contagion question (acknowledging spousal transmission in cramped domestic situations) and quibbled with those who accused alcoholism alone of causing tuberculosis, to the exclusion of other factors.[9] For the most part, however, in his steady stream of reports on Le Havre's demographic and sanitary condition, Lecadre reinforced his contention that nothing was more continually and evidently associated with tuberculosis than poor housing.

> Where do we see phthisis principally appearing? [I]n narrow streets, in cramped lodgings, in buildings where many large families are crowded together. The primary and principal cause of the frequency of phthisis is poverty[;] not the poverty that *lacks bread* but the kind that lingers in unsanitary lodgings, deprived of suitable air, ill-clothed, often wallowing in uncleanliness, suffering the terrible effects of overcrowding.[10]

This attitude exemplifies what Cottereau has called the "glissement écologique," or ecological slide, which transfigures social relations into spatial relations.[11] Lecadre in effect attributes tuberculosis to "poverty," but interprets poverty as a spatial or environmental rather than economic problem.

More of a chronicler than an advocate, Lecadre offered in his reports few proposals—either individual or social—for remedying the deteriorating health situation in Le Havre. One especially revealing passage in an 1877 report highlights his view of the proper role of medicine and public health in society. Writing specifically about possible responses to the city's growing tuberculosis problem, Lecadre uncharacteristically set forth an agenda.

Because civilization, whose progress is so beneficial, has its excesses which
often do real harm to society, let us react against these excesses, not only by
example, but also by incessant observation and by constant studies of public
and private hygiene.[12]

Rather than urge strong governmental or philanthropic initiatives to
"react against these excesses," the doctor proposed a battle without
intervention. The phrase "incessant observation" encapsulates Lecadre's personal mission as well as his prescription for improving society.
It was a prescription that would soon go a long way toward fulfillment
with the establishment of the Bureau municipal d'hygiène in 1879.

REMAKING THE WORKING CLASS:
HOUSING, HEALTH, AND MORALIZATION

Before examining the history of France's first municipal board of health,
in large part the creation of Jules Siegfried, it is worth considering some
of Siegfried's other reform efforts—in particular, the workers' social
club and sanitary low-cost housing—as part of his wider vision of a
more orderly and healthier society. Historians have portrayed the Protestant legislator as the quintessential Third Republic *notable,* with his
mercantile wealth, his power base in a local fief, and his political agenda
of class rapprochement. An avatar of late-nineteenth-century liberalism,
a "professional paternalist" in the words of Sanford Elwitt, Siegfried
built his career on two axes: the expansion of French markets and influence through free trade and colonialism, and social harmony through
the moralization and *embourgeoisement* of the poor. "To reconcile the
working class through the union of capital and labor, without endangering the established social order, this was the task Jules Siegfried set
for himself," wrote the historian of Le Havre, Jean Legoy.[13]

In the France of the 1870s, the task was hardly a simple one. In the
aftermath of the Paris Commune, the gulf separating the classes seemed
to many an abyss. Mutual fear and contempt characterized each group's
perceptions of the other. In such a state of affairs, true reconciliation
was unthinkable. All the items on Siegfried's social agenda shared one
basic aim: to remake the working class in the image of the bourgeoisie.
Perhaps the archetypal reform in this spirit initiated by Siegfried was
the workers' social club, the Cercle Franklin.

The crux of the social question, Siegfried felt, was hard work. The
harder one worked, the more money one made. If workers could be

encouraged to grasp this basic truth, he insisted, all concerned would
be better off, and the social question would peacefully disappear.

> With orderly and economic habits, through regular work and rising wages,
> workers can satisfy their needs and those of their families. Unfortunately,
> while some cannot find regular work, others—more numerous— . . . lose
> themselves in the life of the cabaret; whereas, in order to achieve the welfare
> they desire, they should be applying themselves courageously to their
> work.[14]

Such misguided souls played right into the hands of "vulgar agitators"
with "subversive theories," who "exploit[ed]" honest workers for their
own purposes. The consummate liberal, Siegfried believed that only the
free play of market forces could determine fair wage levels or the proper
relationship between labor and capital. However, something could be
done about the lifestyle and "habits" that caused workers to fall prey
to subversion: in particular, *la vie du cabaret,* which robbed the poor
of their money, their health, and their faculties of judgment and moderation. (Although it would not reach its apogee until the turn of the
century, the "moral etiology" that implicated cabarets and alcoholism
as causes of tuberculosis was already in evidence in Le Havre in the
1870s.) Siegfried agreed with most hygienists and moralists that the
demoralizing and unhealthful life of the cabaret was only able to exercise its allure because of the dreary and insalubrious home life of the
poor. Drinking and debauchery claimed so many disgruntled workers
because after a long and tiring day of sometimes back-breaking labor,
they simply could not bring themselves to face the filthy and *"bien
triste"* quarters awaiting them at home. "Can we be astonished that,
lacking the comfort that the wealthy can afford, they go out to find
some distraction?" "Sirs," Siegfried told a lecture audience in Le Havre
in 1874, "the cabaret is the worker's worst enemy."[15]
    The antidote could only be one that addressed the root cause luring
customers to the cabaret. Siegfried called his strategy *"moralization
through distraction."*[16] He proposed a *"cercle d'ouvriers,"* modeled
after the Workingmen's Club of Manchester and an analogue in Mul-
house: a gathering place for workers of all occupations, where they
could be entertained and enlightened while relaxing among their peers
in a leisurely atmosphere. In Le Havre, the workers' social club would
be named after Benjamin Franklin, whom Siegfried admired as "a great
American citizen, a friend of order and liberty as well as a partisan of

hard work and education."[17] In this, as in all of his writings and speeches, Siegfried's Protestant background is very much in evidence; indeed, his entire social reform program cannot be understood without taking into account the crusading religious zeal that animated it. The bywords "order" and "work" are never far away in these texts from their companions "liberty," "morality," and "well-being." Throughout the early Third Republic, Protestants were disproportionately represented among the ranks of French social reformers and philanthropic leaders.[18]

Le Havre's bourgeoisie, of course, could afford the home life and diversions that preserved the individual from destructive and subversive ideas; the working class, much more vitally in need of such off-the-job distractions, could not. Siegfried set out to fight the paradox that only those least needful of this particular service could afford it. He argued that, in fact, not only was a cercle d'ouvriers in the workers' best interests but it was also in the self-interest of the wealthy and powerful. In pleading with the latter to finance the establishment of the Cercle Franklin, Siegfried planted barely veiled hints in their minds about the consequences of shortsighted conservation of wealth.

> It is right and legitimate to work to acquire a fortune; but . . . the error . . . is in believing that it can only benefit oneself. An error, sirs, which does not go unpunished; à père avare, fils prodigue, and slowly accumulated money, selfishly guarded, can disappear . . . with a rapidity that we all know.[19]

All classes of society were joined together, Siegfried maintained, by ties of social solidarity. Bourgeois philanthropy, when directed toward projects such as the Cercle Franklin, amounted to self-preservation, particularly when one considered the alternative.

> To do good for others is not only an act of charity but also an act of intelligence, because it does good for oneself. To understand this . . . is the real way to hold at bay that great cause of ruin for our country, that peril that constantly threatens us[:] Revolution.[20]

Idle (working-class) hands were the devil's playground, and idle (bourgeois) money was an invitation to disaster. Simmering class resentment, which had erupted three years earlier in the Paris Commune, could be contained only through a farsighted program of charity, a remoralization of workers that transformed them into respectable, if low-income, facsimiles of the bourgeoisie. Here again, Protestant reforming zeal and moralism infuse Siegfried's politics, along with class-based pragmatism. Attributing the absence of revolution in England to mutual respect among the classes and the prudent philanthropy of the wealthy, he cannot have left his audience in doubt as to the import of his warning.[21]

Such frank pleas for contributions show Siegfried to have been remarkably open about his political and philanthropic strategy; he also seems to have been adept at selling his plan. The Cercle Franklin was built in 1875 and officially opened its doors in January 1876. The new facility offered lectures, concerts, and a library for its members, along with recreational activities such as gymnastics, fencing, and billiards. The initial response was enthusiastic: more than two thousand Havrais joined the club in its first year of operation. However, its popularity soon waned—no doubt thanks, in part, to the annual membership fee of five francs, more than a day's wages for some workers—and less than ten years later, in 1885, the Cercle Franklin was all but defunct.[22]

If Siegfried and his fellow reformers in Le Havre were discouraged by occasional setbacks and signs of failure, they showed no signs of it. The workers' social club was neither the only nor even the most ambitious of their projects during the early Third Republic aimed at improving the health and morals of the city's poor. The possibility of building sanitary, low-cost workers' housing on a large scale preoccupied Siegfried throughout his career, and he saw in it a chance both to root out the material causes of disease and to remove the crucial first step on the slippery slope that led workers to the cabaret, depravity, and death.

The history of official concern over the deplorable state of working-class housing in Le Havre begins in earnest as far back as the 1840s and 1850s, when the city's population first showed signs of imploding. When thousands of poor migrants from Normandy and Brittany came to the port city seeking work and lodgings, even the demolition of the fortifications surrounding the old city and the annexation of several adjacent communes could not accommodate the new arrivals. Merchants such as Siegfried, reaping vast profits from the rapidly growing commerce of the port, built mansions on the hillsides overlooking the old town, and even the less opulent houses being constructed in outlying neighborhoods were far beyond the means of most Havrais workers. As a result, the decrepit apartments and boardinghouses of the center city—in particular, the Notre-Dame and Saint-François quarters adjoining the old port—simply became more and more crowded.[23]

Following the national law of 1850 on housing sanitation (Le Havre was, after all, not the only city experiencing such problems), the Commission on Unsanitary Housing (Commission des logements insalubres) convened in the city in 1851. The commission investigated complaints and reports of particularly egregious sanitary negligence on the part of landlords; it requested compliance when it found repairs or improvements needed, and it had the power to refer cases of recalcitrant *propriétaires* to the city council and to the courts. Most often, the commission compiled exhaustive and detailed reports but preferred a strategy of coaxing landlords into repairs (however piecemeal) to pursuing legal action against them.[24]

Nevertheless, the commission's reports provide unique access to official perceptions of the laboring poor and their daily lives. The dominant tone of this narrative genre—little changed around the turn of the century from what it had been forty years before—is one of shocked disgust. For example, in a typical report from an 1893 visit to a building on the rue du Grand-Croissant in the Saint-François quarter, the commission's members found a house "unfit to house even animals." On the ground floor, a partially enclosed toilet opened onto the open door of a butcher's shop; a side of meat hung above the entrance "as if to receive the emanating scents of the facilities." On the fourth floor, they found a courteous woman in a quite clean apartment, who showed them the steady trickles of urine that ran down the wall next to her bed, filling the apartment with "a persistently acrid odor." They came from an overflowing toilet one story above, and when the commissioners investigated those units, under the rafters, they were overcome. "Here, we must give up trying to depict the appearance of these sordid places" (*Ici, nous renonçons à dépeindre l'aspect de ces lieux sordides*).[25] Such rhetorically dramatic expressions of outraged reticence were commonplace in nineteenth-century hygienic and moralistic reform literature; often, as in this case, they were belied by the detailed descriptions of the offending circumstances that followed. Although such protestations most often alluded to sexual improprieties or to the proximity of near-naked bodies,[26] here the locution seems to have referred principally to excretory functions, as it was surrounded by descriptions of filthy latrines and other more makeshift evacuation systems.

In this example as elsewhere, the housing commission's reports struggle to make sense of a kind of subspecies living in their midst, a mystifying and somewhat threatening "Other," wallowing in quarters not fit for animals and yet seemingly indifferent to their plight. Both the threat and the indifference are highlighted in another report from the same year, after a visit to a building on the rue d'Albanie in the Notre-Dame quarter. Again the commissioners' attention was drawn to the toilet facilities, or lack thereof. They burst out laughing when they opened the door of the water closet on the fourth floor, exclaiming "Oh, how necessity is the mother of invention!" There on the floor, in the place of a latrine, was a common metal household storage box, "voluminously full!" A commission member asked one of the tenants why there was no seat and no proper latrine.

> "A seat?" She seemed not to understand, as if we were speaking of a luxury unknown to her. There had never been one. As for the latrine, she told us, it had been taken away, a few days earlier, because it was full, and had never been returned.[27]

They asked her if the rent was expensive. "Oh yes, sir," she answered, "very expensive: 160 francs per year." When they asked if all of the tenants paid the rent regularly, the woman's tone turned incredulous. "Oh, of course not, we would have to be stupid to pay rents like those. The landlady comes around demanding her money, but everyone tells her the same thing. She goes ahead and tells us to leave, but nobody moves." The commission's response to this colloquy is extremely instructive.

> With this answer, we left, taking with us the following moral: the people that live in these hovels . . . belong to a race apart: Like all others, they avidly desire material comforts, as long as they can enjoy them for free. They are told to leave, because they don't pay; but they prefer to stay. Therefore, they must be happy there.
> However, here we have a question of public health and the public interest. We cannot tolerate in the middle of the city such hotbeds of infection.[28]

It is jarring to find the commissioners, at times so compassionate and solicitous of the needs of Le Havre's poor, pronouncing such a harsh judgment on the buildings' inhabitants: that they lived in squalor because they wanted to, that they should be willing to pay if they wanted anything better. These comments make sense only if one takes at face value the qualification of the residents as "a race apart." In and of themselves, such creatures may not have been worthy of official concern or even pity; but given the threat of contagion—the possibility that the unspeakable pathologies bred in such conditions could spread outward, threatening even respectable citizens—remedial action was imperative.

Many reformers, including Siegfried, were not content to let the Commission des logements insalubres investigate cases of reported negligence or insalubrity. Only an entirely new environment could remake the material and moral life of the worker.[29] Vital to Siegfried's efforts to build hygienic *cités ouvrières* was working-class ownership of the new homes.

> The worker who hopes to become a homeowner devotes all of his attention to his house; he develops an interest in his domestic life, . . . abandons the cabaret, and becomes a veritable conservative. . . . Do we want to combat poverty and the errors of socialism at the same time? Do we want to augment the guarantees of order, of morality, and of political and social moderation? Then let us create cités ouvrières![30]

The enemy again was revolution; along with a bourgeois morality, property ownership—an economic interest, however slight, in the status quo—was seen as a means to the desired end. Built simply but attractively according to the laws of hygiene, the cités ouvrières would marry aesthetic and sanitary virtues with this economic interest, creating a pleasant place to spend one's leisure hours and eliminating the deadly temptation of the cabaret.

In light of later reformers' preoccupation with fighting socialism, it is ironic that in the early days of the Second Empire, the first initiative toward the construction of a cité ouvrière in Le Havre was itself socialist in inspiration. Several local followers of the utopian socialist Charles Fourier, eager to apply some aspects of the philosopher's hypothetical "phalanstery" (a community whose residents live and work together in harmony according to their individual and collective desires), brought forth a detailed proposal in 1852. The plan, for which land had already been set aside in the Leure quarter on the eastern edge of the port, would have provided fifty-two new housing units in five two-story buildings, with spacious gardens, ample sunlight, and sanitary facilities that would have satisfied even the most fastidious housing commissioner. However, despite the repeated urgings of Louis-Napoleon Bonaparte (both as president and later as emperor) for the realization of just such housing projects, the prefect of the Seine-Inférieure rejected the proposal on the grounds that its authors had not provided enough information on how the project would be financed.[31]

After the abortive Fourierist plan, it was not until 1870 that another working-class housing project was launched in Le Havre; this time, it had the backing of Siegfried and other prominent members of the city's merchant elite. Together, they contributed 200,000 francs as start-up capital for the Société havraise des cités ouvrières, which in late 1870 began construction of its first group of seventy-seven houses, collectively known as the Cité havraise, in a relatively sparsely populated area in the northeastern part of the city. In 1884, the society added another group of forty houses, the Cité Desmallières, several blocks to the east, near the city limits separating Le Havre from the commune of Graville. All these units, though small, were actual houses in the "pavillion style," separated from each other, with courtyards and gardens. In contrast, the eighty-two housing units provided between 1899 and 1906 by the Société havraise des logements économiques (a group unaffiliated with Siegfried's society) consisted of six separate *pavillons* and one four-story building containing seventy apartments. Little is known about this second organization or the housing it provided; in any case, it did not meet the strict definition of a cité ouvrière, because its units were for rental only, with no possibility of eventual ownership by the tenants.[32]

This idea, of course, lay at the core of Siegfried's vision for workers' housing: ownership. Residents paid a monthly *redevance*—considerably higher than rents for similar lodgings elsewhere in the city—that was credited toward the ultimate purchase of the house. The entire sum would have to be amortized within a period of twenty years; as it turned out, few made it that far. In both the Cité havraise and the Cité Desmallières, the tenancy of at least half the units turned over within the first ten years of operation. Fewer than a third of the would-be home owners made it to twenty years and actual ownership. Moreover, there is no indication that tenants earned any kind of equity with their payments, equity that they might have been able to apply to the purchase of another house if they left the cité before the twenty-year amortization.[33]

In that respect as well as others, the reality of the cités fell short of the reformers' aspirations. Despite the seeming urgency of public health considerations in the workers' housing enterprise, there were no provisions in the Cité havraise for either water supply or for waste disposal (it was not connected to the city's still-limited network of sewers), and the sand used in the construction materials retained moisture and kept the houses somewhat dank. The first residents of the cité were forced to use the woodsheds in back of their houses for toilets. Such glaring oversights, coupled with the units' high turnover, can only have thwarted to a great extent the lofty goals of Siegfried's meliorist paternalism.[34]

This is not to say, however, that extravagant claims were not made on behalf of the cités ouvrières, particularly where health was concerned. During the key years when the long-term and large-scale success or failure of the concept was at stake, its proponents mustered impres-

sive statistics in its defense. An 1884 report to the Société havraise d'é-
tudes diverses enthusiastically touted the benefits of workers' housing
projects, based on fifty years' experience in London. There, overall mortality in the philanthropic housing projects amounted to less than a
third of the rate for the city as a whole. Tuberculosis mortality in the
London projects was reported to be about half as high as the citywide
level.[35] Similarly, in 1885, a prominent physician in Le Havre proclaimed the 117 houses in the Cité havraise and the Cité Desmallières
"almost entirely free" of tuberculosis, thanks to "the excellent hygienic
conditions" of the homes. Six years later, the same doctor gave more
precise figures in a newspaper report, attributing to the cités just 1 tuberculosis death per thousand inhabitants per year, compared to 6.3 in
the Notre-Dame quarter. The newspaper concluded, in a ringing endorsement of the workers' housing strategy, that the number of deaths
from tuberculosis in Le Havre annually could be cut almost in half if
the city had proportionally as many cités ouvrières as London.[36] For a
city with the highest tuberculosis mortality per capita in all of France
(and likely in all of Europe), a 50 percent reduction would have been a
monumental achievement. Even allowing for hyperbole and statistical
exaggeration, such enthusiasm in the press and in the medical community suggests at the very least that (1) improved housing was widely
seen as an effective remedy against the scourge of tuberculosis, and (2)
the cités ouvrières enjoyed significant public support.

That support was not unanimous, however, and expressions of skepticism occasionally clouded the otherwise rosy light in which the workers' housing projects were publicly portrayed. In the first place, many
taxpayers objected to the original investors in the projects being guaran-
teed a certain rate of return on their investment. This appears to have
been a fairly common feature of such societies' charters, a concession
by the city to those who put up the capital for construction—much like
a tax break to encourage certain investments deemed socially useful.
However, it did not sit well with some observers, who wondered what
right the wealthiest négociants in Le Havre had to an automatic claim
on the public treasury, particularly if their motives were strictly charitable.[37] In these matters, the line between "philanthropist" and "inves-
tor" was a thin one.

The lengths to which reformers urged the state to go in making cités
ouvrières financially attractive to prospective tenant/owners also raised
some hackles. A letter to the editor in the newspaper Le Courrier du
Havre in 1893 denounced the bloated bureaucracy and unfair favorit-

ism that would likely result from Siegfried's low-cost housing bill, then under consideration by parliament in Paris. The angry correspondent painted the proposed law as positively unpatriotic.

> Let us take from the well-off class of workers—because the bill applies only to this group—let us take two young men returning from their military service, having just acquitted an equal debt to their *patrie*. Are they not entitled to be treated by their country on an equal footing? They should be; but if the Siegfried law passes, they will not be.[38]

Suppose they both wanted to settle down with their families and become home owners, the letter continued. One chose a "Siegfried house"; the other, "more independent," built his own house. Under the new bill, the first would be exempt from all taxes for twelve years and would enjoy other benefits as well. "For him, the cité in question will mean the easy life, a chicken in the pot just like under Henry IV." The other home owner would have to pay not only his own share of taxes but enough to make up for his "privileged" counterpart's exemption on top of it. "No! no!" the author fulminated, "[s]uch a law is impossible in a country like ours."[39] While it is conceivable that this letter to the editor was simply the work of a disgruntled landlord fearing subsidized competition, it nonetheless shows the extent to which the cités ouvrières were seen as intended only for a select stratum of the working class and sanitary housing in general as a "privilege" rather than a right or a social necessity.

Others attacked the shortsightedness of housing improvements per se, for failing to take into account the fate of those displaced who could not afford the "improved" lodgings. (Although this criticism does not apply to all cités ouvrières, as they were not always built on the sites of older housing units, it does highlight the perceived tendency in social reform to provide for workers of relatively greater means while ignoring the most needy.) In 1884, residents of the notoriously unsanitary Saint-François quarter demanded that a square then being cleared in front of the Saint-François church be extended through the entire facing block of houses, to bring needed light and air to their neighborhood. A journalist named Lécureur with the newspaper *Le Havre* reported the residents' demand but asked what would happen to those who lived, however miserably, in those buildings. "Nothing is more laudable," Lécureur allowed, "than to rescue people from death [by] remov[ing] them from the harmful influence of a milieu where disease, especially the horrible *phthisie* . . . , has taken up permanent residence." Strictly speaking, there was not a shortage of housing in Le Havre, he argued, but the displaced could not afford the sanitary lodgings that were available. He told of receiving complaints from former residents of several streets in the old neighborhoods of the center city, whose modest apartments were demolished when the streets were widened for hygienic purposes.

> Unable to come up with the money needed [to stay in the area], they were forced to take refuge in [the] Le Perrey [quarter], in appalling little nooks a thousand times more insalubrious even than the poor apartments from which they had been expelled. . . . [O]ne has the right to ask if this is real progress, and for whom[?][40]

Lécureur acknowledged that the question was a "delicate" one, but he maintained that if such "improvements" continued, without regard to the "*expulsés*," there were only three possible outcomes, all of which would be "absolutely disastrous" for Le Havre: the displaced workers and their families would have to either move outside the city limits, take up residence in the newly constructed buildings with no intention of paying the higher rents, or leave the area entirely because it had become "uninhabitable."[41] Once again, other interests may have been at stake in this critique, but it at least raised the question of whether such measures constituted true "progress," a question that had no place in the unshakably positivist worldview of Siegfried and his fellow reformers.

Philosophical doubts aside, perhaps the most damning criticism of the low-cost housing movement held that its claims of success in fighting disease and depravity were skewed by a rigorous screening process. An anonymous letter to the editor of Le Havre's *Petit Républicain* in 1891 leveled that charge in a searing, cynical diatribe against the cités ouvrières. Amid the familiar litany of complaints about heavy tax burdens and "the shackles of bureaucracy," the author questioned whether housing actually played as great a role in public health as was generally believed. "Housing is not everything," he wrote. Meager diets and overwork contributed heavily to the poor health of the working class, a fact that was hidden by the statistics coming out of the new housing projects.

> In the cités ouvrières, they tell us, mortality rates are extremely low! But of course; they are just like the mutual aid societies: not everyone who wants in is allowed in! A serious investigation always takes place first.[42]

The society demanded of all prospective tenants, the author alleged, "guarantees of order, morality, good health, etc." Such demands, he added, would have been viewed as preposterous coming from an individual private landlord.

> A serious selection process, a careful triage, appropriate means of collecting information: what better way of keeping out the disease-ridden poor! What better way of obtaining statistical results proving that so few people die in the philanthropic cités! *Parbleu!*[43]

The same triage kept out anyone of questionable "moral condition," he further contended, thereby preserving the image of the cités ouvrières as wholesome communities of happy families.[44] While it is impossible to either verify or disprove these allegations, the mere fact that they were made publicly, in the pages of a newspaper—even allowing for exaggerations—suggests that the glowing reports of the projects' success should be taken at less than face value. Even if the selection process did not work in this elaborate manner, with its hints of espionage, the steep *redevances* required of residents acted as a de facto triage, excluding the majority of Havrais workers who could scarcely pay their rent, much less a considerably higher monthly mortgage payment.

In its response to the perceived role of slum housing in the spread of disease, Le Havre was different from Paris and other French cities in one crucial respect: its civic leaders attempted from a very early date and in a sustained manner to create a new and better housing stock. In contrast to a strategy of administrative surveillance and record keeping, there was an effort in Le Havre to alter the situation on the ground. The city, behind the impetus of Siegfried, was a national pioneer in this domain. However, the new housing never materialized on as large a scale as its leaders had hoped. Even double the 117 houses built by Siegfried's society could not have made more than a small dent in the public health crisis of a city of 130,000 people. Furthermore, it is clear that moral concerns played as great a role in the city's housing reform programs as sanitary ones, although the social reformers of the time might not have recognized any difference between the two. The strategy of surveillance was also very much in evidence—yet another area in which Le Havre was a trailblazing city.

KNOWING THE CITY: THE BUREAU D'HYGÌENE

Perhaps the most long-lasting and widely imitated of Siegfried's social reforms was the Bureau d'hygiène, France's first municipal health department, created in 1879. After 1902, every French city of more than

twenty thousand inhabitants was required by law to establish a health
bureau modeled on that of Le Havre; its pathbreaking work earned
it national and international acclaim among doctors, hygienists, and
politicians. As a precursor and, later, outpost of the War on Tuberculosis, the Bureau d'hygiène attempted to translate the medical and hygienic knowledge of the dominant etiology into *local* knowledge and
to track the disease administratively through the city and through the
years.

Along with Siegfried, the person most responsible for the establishment of the Bureau d'hygiène was Joseph Gibert, a Swiss-born physician who settled in Le Havre after attending medical school in Paris.
Gibert is known to some historians of France as a principled convert to
the cause of revisionism in the Dreyfus case; the doctor interceded with
his friend and fellow Havrais Félix Faure, president of the republic, and
was shocked and dismayed when Faure admitted that Dreyfus had been
convicted based on secret "evidence" but invoked *raison d'état* in refus-
ing to reopen the case.[45] But Gibert spent most of his career, outside
of his private practice, seeking ways to improve the desperate sanitary
situation of his adopted city. In 1878, the first year of Siegfried's tenure
as mayor of Le Havre, the two friends first put the idea of a municipal
health department before the city council, on which Gibert also served.
The doctor spoke eloquently about the need to preserve the country's
human resources, a need that was especially acute in light of the country's demographic and political decline as a world power. "If we are
not first [among nations] in the production of human life"—a reference
to the country's falling birthrate—"let us strive to be first in the saving
and husbanding of this incomparable treasure, and preserve it, through
a practical and serious organization of public hygiene, from the
scourges that constantly threaten it." Gibert told the council members
that the nation would applaud Le Havre's initiative "if every year more
healthy and robust defenders are saved for its battalions, more hands
are saved for its workshops, [and] more young girls are prepared by a
salutary education for their role as mothers."[46] From the very beginning, then, concerns over national decline, military might, productivity,
and parenthood conditioned the fight against tuberculosis and other
causes of death, on the local as well as the national level.

Although several members of the city council suggested modifications to Gibert's and Siegfried's proposal to reduce its cost, the only real
opposition to the plan came from Louis Brindeau. (Twenty-four years
later, as mayor, Brindeau would praise the bureau and its work in glow-

ing terms.) The councilman objected that the creation of a new city department would entail excessive expenses. Mayor Siegfried intervened to suggest to the council some specific benefits the bureau would bring. It would monitor, he said, the day-to-day sanitary topography of the city. "Thanks to the reports of the Bureau d'hygiène, it will be possible to compile a synoptic map of the progress and intensity of diseases in [our] neighborhoods." Gibert concurred that only through detailed knowledge, by mapping the incidence of diseases such as tuberculosis in the city's streets and neighborhoods, could science determine their true causes. Brindeau insisted that "to create a special office of hygiene is to spend a great deal [of money] . . . for statistical information." He suggested instead that the same amount of money be spent on sewers, public baths, and other material sanitary improvements, while existing commissions and departments could compile all necessary statistics without the additional expense.[47]

Brindeau could not stem the positivist tide, however, and the reformers' arguments regarding the need to collect more comprehensive and systematic information won the day. Le Havre inaugurated its new Bureau d'hygiène in 1879 and began an era of exactly what Lecadre had called for: "incessant observation." The bureau was given authority and responsibility over all health-related matters, and its day-to-day functions included maintaining France's first casier sanitaire, a record of the place, time, and cause of every death in the city, as well as keeping track of births; disinfecting the lodgings and personal effects of victims of contagious diseases (including tuberculosis); inspecting samples of foods and beverages for quality; administering smallpox vaccinations; following up complaints concerning various causes of insalubrity; inspecting schools, other public facilities, and industrial establishments; and surveillance of registered prostitutes for venereal diseases.[48]

Right from the start, the bureau was forced to come to grips with tuberculosis, the city's leading killer. During the 1880s, its periodic reports gradually elaborated all three elements of what would later become the dominant etiology of the disease (contagion, housing, and immorality), while at the same time the major French medical journals and the professors at the Paris *faculté* were only taking the first tentative steps toward the same ultimate conclusion. The bureau's very first report, on its operations in the first three months of 1880, placed great emphasis on tuberculosis, pointing out that no epidemic or any other cause ever approached it in the number of deaths it accounted for. This early report, marking a sober realization of the difficult tasks facing the bureau, singled out two particularly pernicious causes of tuberculosis. Though it mentioned heredity, contagion (two years before Koch), poor nutrition, and lack of ventilation as contributory factors, the report denounced above all "venereal excesses among adolescents and alcoholic excesses," often found doing their damage together in the same person. Four years later, in 1884, the bureau's director, Dr. A. Launay, lamented in a brief passage on tuberculosis that "alcoholism continues its ravages" and otherwise shed no new light on the matter.[49] In Le Havre, one of the most "alcoholic" cities in France,[50] the moral etiology of tuberculosis took hold quite early.

By 1887, five years after Koch's discovery of the tubercle bacillus, as most of the medical profession was slowly being won over to the contagionist perspective on tuberculosis, the view from Le Havre had further evolved in the direction of what would become the dominant etiology. Doctor Gibert, in summarizing the epidemiological evidence gathered by the Bureau d'hygiène, cast the decades-old concern over slums and overcrowding in the new light of contagion. "There is a constant relationship," he wrote, "between . . . population density and pulmonary phthisis." To illustrate his point, he compared the figure of 1 tuberculosis death per thousand population in the cités ouvrières to 5 per thousand in Notre-Dame and Saint-François. (Reformers preferred this particular comparison to strict neighborhood-to-neighborhood ratios, because it purported to encompass socially identical populations in different environments.) While allowing that "we must admit the influence of contagion," which had been scientifically proven, Gibert could not yet bring himself to abandon completely some older miasmatist notions, as in this equivocal statement: "Overcrowding, whose importance is so great in Le Havre, acts no doubt through the vitiation of the air, but also . . . through contagion." The moral etiology, too, had progressed in terms of sophistication and statistical certainty; here Gibert contended that "alcoholism, by weakening the individual who indulges in it, prepares the way for contagion, and this can explain the enormous number of consumptives in Le Havre." It was not until roughly ten years later that this formulation became the widely accepted dogma of official French medicine. Interestingly, this 1887 report is one of the extremely rare official documents from Le Havre to actually make reference to the city's standing as tuberculosis capital of France and probably all of Europe. In partial explanation of that status, Gibert also claimed that Le Havre "appears to be the European city where the most alcoholic beverages are consumed." For the most part, local officials preferred not to call attention to the city's unenviable standing, while still insisting on the need for public health reform.[51]

Ten years after the bureau's creation, the new etiology of tuberculosis had taken hold in Le Havre, and the local manifestations of contact with bacilli, substandard housing, and immoderation assumed preeminent importance in the bureau's reports. The degree of emphasis accorded to any individual factor varied with local circumstances; for example, in 1890, the bureau's advisory committee made the bold claim that the true causes of tuberculosis were only known (and knowable) thanks to the establishment of the bureau itself. "Nobody knew, before the creation of the bureau, what its topographical distribution was. To-day . . . it is easy to know the true causes of its propagation." The meticulous mapping of every death from tuberculosis revealed that its primary cause was overcrowding (which facilitated contagion), since mortality was highest in the most densely populated districts of the city. When commenting on the sexual distribution of the disease, the bureau invoked alcoholism to explain the significantly higher incidence among men than among women.[52]

Several points that went unacknowledged throughout the history of the bureau's work on tuberculosis should be addressed here. The advisory committee's assertion notwithstanding, observers such as Lecadre had linked the disease to overcrowding and housing conditions long before the creation of the Bureau d'hygiène, although without framing the issue in the language of contagion. Moreover, by deciding to investigate tuberculosis geographically, that is, by using the casier sanitaire data to represent its incidence spatially through the streets and neighborhoods of the city, the bureau predetermined the outcome of its inquiries. Had similar records been kept regarding differential tuberculosis mortality by occupation, wage level, place of birth, or any other variable, different conclusions certainly would have been reached. However, given the novelty of Le Havre's Bureau d'hygiène, even in 1890 the advisory committee may have felt the need to justify its continued existence and rightful place in the municipal administration. It had to claim that important progress was being made, if not in material changes at street level, then in the realm of local knowledge.

Similar claims of progress continued into the 1890s and beyond, despite occasional administrative difficulties and Le Havre's persistently high death rate from tuberculosis. A shortage of office staff forced the bureau to suspend the maintenance of the casier sanitaire in 1893; it was not until mid-1901 that temporary outside assistance brought the records fully up to date, whereupon they lapsed again for at least nine more years.[53] "Little by little, we are making progress," Gibert reported in 1897, "but it is still not enough." Other officials shared his optimism but not his caution; shortly after taking office in 1908, with Le Havre still ranking consistently at or near the top among French cities in both tuberculosis mortality and overall mortality, Mayor Henri Genestal confidently proclaimed, "The state of public health in our city is *excellent*."[54]

Throughout its early years, the Bureau d'hygiène attempted to preach the antituberculosis gospel of prudence and cleanliness to the population of Le Havre. Its functions included supervising the municipal disinfection service, a service for which the bureau constantly strove to incite demand. Gibert was "pleased to report" to the advisory committee in 1896 that "the population is taking up the habit of having their lodgings disinfected after deaths from pulmonary tuberculosis." He urged his fellow doctors to encourage this practice further, until the time when all tuberculosis deaths would be followed by disinfection as a matter of course. At the same meeting, other members of the committee pursued Gibert's line of reasoning and called for mandatory declaration of all diagnosed cases of tuberculosis. Declaration to local authorities was already required by law for several other contagious diseases and would have facilitated universal disinfection. While one doctor called for mandatory declaration along with the isolation of tuberculosis cases within hospitals and the distribution of spittoons and anticontagion instructions to all those afflicted with the disease, another committee member demurred. Any measure that singled out tuberculosis victims, he argued, would rob them of hope. Many patients who showed signs of the disease had been carefully shielded from that fact by their physicians, and so strong was the popular association of tuberculosis with despair and death that to reveal the truth would shatter their illusions of possible recovery and a normal life.[55] These were precisely the same dilemmas and controversies that the entire French medical profession was facing—although the critical mass of activist doctors and social reformers in Le Havre seems to have caused the issues to appear there several years earlier than elsewhere in France—and despite the energy and money spent, the Havrais came up with no unique or original practical solutions to the problem of tuberculosis. In the domains of administrative surveillance and statistical knowledge of the disease, however, as in mortality, Le Havre far outdistanced all other French cities and the central government as well.

The health department's crowning achievements in this regard were its two published decennial reports, the first covering the 1880s (published in 1893) and the second the 1890s (published in 1903). Prosaically entitled *Relevé général de la statistique démographique et médicale,* each was a prodigious accomplishment, an encyclopedic monument to the statistical *quadrillage* of a city and its population. For example, each volume contained detailed foldout maps of Le Havre; each map was marked with a pattern of dots, each dot representing a death from tuberculosis, for the years covered in that volume. (See fig. 11.) Together, the maps testify not only to the bureau's thoroughness in collecting data but also to its leaders' passionate commitment to medical topography as a means of fighting disease. Such maps of disease incidence, also known as "spot maps" or "dot maps," were not new in the 1880s. Epidemics of yellow fever and cholera had previously given rise to case mapping in various British and American cities. But Le Havre's tuberculosis maps of the late nineteenth century signaled a shift in the object of mapping from the exotic, exogenous, and epidemic to the familiar and endemic.[56]

Mayor Brindeau wrote the preface to the first decennial report in 1893. As a city councilman fourteen years before, Brindeau had been the lone voice in opposition to the establishment of the Bureau d'hygiène. In his lengthy preface, he recalled that the proposal had "encountered a fairly intense opposition." "Some keen minds contested the usefulness of an institution whose organization, costly as it was, would only produce . . . statistics which were quite interesting from a scientific point of view, to be sure, but would bring no practical result." Without ever admitting that these were precisely his own objections (or that he was the *only* member of the city council to voice them at the time), Brindeau suggested that the experience of fourteen years had shown them to be well intentioned but unjustified. The wisdom and diplomacy of the bureau's collaborators, he wrote, had succeeded in convincing private interests—here he was presumably referring to the proprietors of factories and plants classified as unsanitary establishments—to conform their practices to the principles of public hygiene, even though the bureau lacked the legal authority to enforce its policies. Brindeau further pointed to a two-thirds decline in diphtheria deaths since the bureau began its disinfection service in 1885 as evidence that the office had had a positive practical impact. Yet notwithstanding his earlier skepticism regarding the utility of statistics, even Brindeau had to admit that the bureau's statistical work, as summarized in the decennial

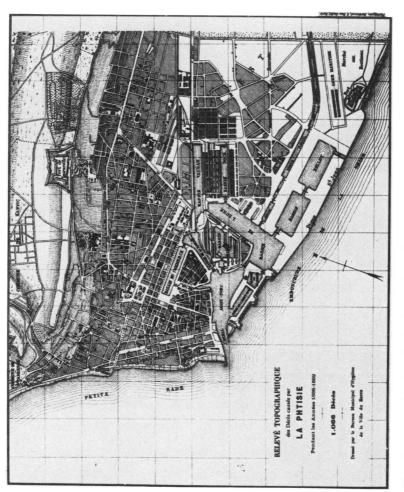

RELEVÉ TOPOGRAPHIQUE
des Décès causés par
LA PHTISIE
Pendant les Années 1888-1889

1.066 Décès

Dressé par le Bureau Municipal d'Hygiène
de la Ville du Havre

11. Spot map showing deaths from tuberculosis in Le Havre, 1888–1889. From *Relevé général de la statistique démographique et médicale, 1880–1889.*

volume, was the pride of its brief history. In approving the publication of the volume, he pointed out, the city council had agreed to use it as the basis for considering sanitary improvements. "We can therefore say that the cleaning up of Le Havre will be the practical conclusion, so to speak," of the bureau's massive statistical compilations.[57] This was the great and largely unfulfilled promise of the Bureau d'hygiène. In the end, even the most sophisticated statistics could not raise money, expropriate a slumlord, or house and feed a day laborer and his family.

As far as tuberculosis was concerned, the body of the two decennial reports was concerned with elaborating the street-by-street, house-by-house understanding of the disease, in which all components of the dominant etiology took their place. In the chapter of the 1880–1889 volume entitled *Mortality by Street,* recognizing that poverty, poor housing, and disease often went hand in hand, Doctor A. Lausiès questioned the true role of poverty in determining mortality. "If poverty [*la misère*] means a shortage of the material things in life and entails a lowered resistance to causes of death, it is difficult to appreciate the part played by those too-often concomitant phenomena, ignorance and vice." To untangle the web of factors, Lausiès called attention to the seven streets at the top of the mortality list.

> Without a doubt, poverty is extreme in all of them, but they suggest some quite different [nuances]. The rue de la Vallée is full of Bretons, poor for the most part, whose passion for alcohol is well known; the rue d'Albanie has never evoked images of a comfortable life; as for the rue des Boucheries, it brings together all the causes of insalubrity. The social milieu is perhaps poorer there than anywhere else, and ignorance plays a role there along with alcohol.[58]

The tragedy of poverty seems to have been altered in its moral status, in the view of Lausiès, when ignorance and vice were also present, as in the rue des Boucheries. "More than anywhere, it seems that the residents, deprived of air, sunlight, and cleanliness in this narrow street, wallow in their misery and abandon themselves with a kind of fatalism to the inability of ever getting out."[59] In other words, Lausiès hinted, economic poverty is one thing; but the moral defects of the rue des Boucheries population made them truly different, much as the unsanitary housing commission perceived some slum dwellers as a race apart.

Elsewhere in the 1880–1889 report, Doctor Gibert stressed a different theme within the dominant etiology, momentarily downplaying specifically local factors. "What dominates the entire question of phthisis, in Le Havre as in London and Paris and in all human agglomerations, is

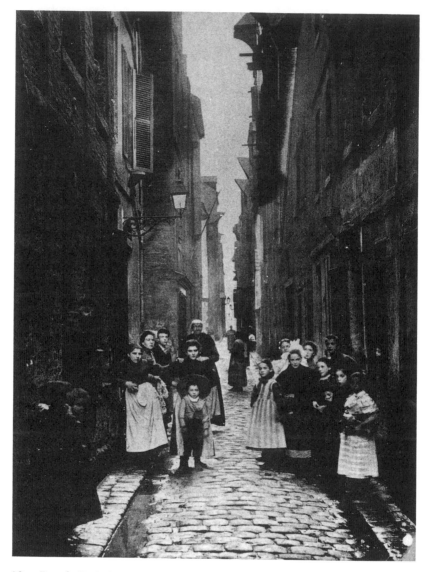

12. Rue du Petit Croissant, a street that perennially accounted for many tuberculosis deaths in Le Havre, ca. 1900. Photo courtesy of Jean Legoy, Le Havre.

contagion and nothing but contagion." Gibert called for a single "social remedy" to combat contagion and eliminate tuberculosis: housing reform. The cités ouvrières should be multiplied, he wrote, and spacious, well-built workers' apartments should be constructed on the outskirts of the city, so that "air could circulate freely, and so that contagion from house to house could be avoided." [60] In this one volume, then, in 1893, a fully elaborated version of the dominant etiology was put forward in Le Havre, well before its diverse elements were assembled in coherent form elsewhere.

By the time the second decennial report (covering the years 1890–1899) was published in 1903, there appears to have been a subtle shift in the attitudes of the city government and the Bureau d'hygiène toward health and mortality. In his preface, Mayor Marais struck a defensive posture from the start. "The city of Le Havre has never been unhealthy [and] is making progress in terms of salubrity, [while] new improvements must be pursued and will be obtained." Marais obviously felt the need to contradict a certain perception of his city, whether through specific criticisms from the outside or simply a general image of Le Havre as diseased and unclean. In his discussion of the bureau's statistics, he proudly noted a decline in overall mortality from the 1880s to the 1890s of 30.9 to 29.7 per thousand per year.

> A proportion still too great, certainly, whose significance must be attenuated to some extent by the contribution of the transient population [*le contingent fourni par la population flottante*], but which justifies in any case our continuous search for improvement.[61]

The claim that Le Havre's high mortality was due in large part to nonresidents who transited through the port or otherwise found themselves in the city when they died (of illnesses contracted elsewhere) dates back at least as far as the reports of Adolphe Lecadre; however, it came to be asserted with greater frequency and insistence in the first decade of the twentieth century.

Later in the same volume, the bureau's director, Dr. Henri Pottevin, sought further explanations for Le Havre's death rate—from tuberculosis in particular—that might absolve the city's health policy of blame, or at least mitigate its responsibility. Other cities such as Paris "exported" their tuberculosis patients, Pottevin contended, either to the suburbs or to family members in the provinces. Because these former Parisians died outside the city limits, their deaths were not included in the capital's statistics, thereby artificially depressing its mortality figures. In contrast, "Le Havre keeps all of its *tuberculeux*," Pottevin explained, "and therein lies one of the primary causes of our [high] tuberculosis mortality." He pointed to "the predominance of the poor element" in the city's population as an additional reason for the misleadingly high statistics, along with the fact that most Havrais were of Norman or Breton origin. Since nationwide, these were "the French races most heavily afflicted" with tuberculosis, Le Havre's high rate was understandable.[62]

All of these protestations seem intended to explain away or make excuses for the city's continually high mortality figures. They are also part of a broader pattern that goes beyond the interpretation of statistics. Local officials consistently downplayed both the role of material well-being in the incidence of tuberculosis and the need for remedial material action to fight it. In the same report, Pottevin reviewed a wide array of strategies recommended by various medical authorities—from sanatoriums to wage increases for workers—only to conclude that "the essential part of the antituberculosis program, and perhaps the only one in which our immediate action can be effective, is the work of social education." Teaching the poor not to spit on the ground, to have their lodgings disinfected, and in general to avoid infecting those around them when they became sick—this was the bureau's crucial duty in the War on Tuberculosis.[63] If the welter of social factors that contributed to the spread of disease could be distilled for the most part into a matter of personal negligence, the failure of the state or private philanthropy to commit substantial resources to the battle would be to some extent justified.

The hypersensitivity of Havrais officials to their city's death rate continued through the years preceding World War I. In 1911, for example, Dr. Adrien Loir (then director of the Bureau d'hygiène) went to great lengths to explain away the overall mortality figure from the previous year. In the bureau's annual report, Loir explained that several circumstances beyond the administration's control inflated the numbers for Le Havre, especially in comparison to other cities. "Our mortality statistics in Le Havre are augmented by three important causes": (1) counting residents of suburban towns who died in the city's hospitals as part of Le Havre's total deaths; (2) a peculiarity of major ports, the influx into the city of would-be emigrants from the "interior," who took up temporary residence in Le Havre pending departure only to fall ill and die in its hospitals; and (3) assigning to Le Havre the deaths of foreigners who drowned in the port area, who disembarked from ships already ill, or who died aboard ship less than two days before arrival in Le Havre.[64]

Although many cities made similar claims about being unfairly burdened in official statistics with deaths that rightly belonged to other jurisdictions, there may well have been some truth to Loir's contentions. Nevertheless, the insistence of city officials in pressing these claims and the variety of excuses invoked suggest that other factors were at work in these years. For one thing, a national public health law passed in 1902 not only required all cities to establish health offices modeled on that of Le Havre but also mandated special inquiries and remedial measures for those cities that exceeded the national average in mortality for three years in a row.[65] Furthermore, health statistics (including overall mortality and tuberculosis mortality) for all major French cities had been compiled and published by the Ministry of the Interior only since the late 1880s; this *Statistique sanitaire des villes de France* for the first time allowed cities to be compared in matters of health and disease. In Le Havre, the defensive attitude surfaced especially in the decennial report covering the 1890s. The compilation of the report coincided with a period of intense public discussion and debate concerning public health—and tuberculosis in particular—with governmental commissions investigating various problems and possible reforms and with parliament debating at great length the public health law finally passed in 1902. If ever Le Havre's status as tuberculosis capital of France were exposed to public view, this was the time.

In fact, the fate of the 1902 public health law parallels the course of antituberculosis efforts in Le Havre and of the French War on Tuberculosis as a whole. The law seemed to pursue an aggressive strategy in the area of information gathering and surveillance alongside a cautious approach to material intervention. Its principal provisions included the establishment of bureaux d'hygiène, the mandatory declaration by physicians to local authorities of all cases of certain contagious diseases (tuberculosis was not among them), and requiring special investigations whenever a city's mortality rate consistently exceeded the national average.[66] In a circular to departmental prefects in 1907 concerning the application of the law, Prime Minister Georges Clémenceau insisted that one of the chief roles of government in public health matters was as "propagandist" and "apostle," educating the population to ease the acceptance of hygienic ideas and practices.[67] Moreover, several years after its passage, the nation's public health authorities agreed that the law was rarely enforced and that without enforcement, it could have little effect. Even the new bureaux d'hygiène created by the 1902 law remained nothing more than "phantom boards" and accomplished very little, some hygienists complained.[68] In Le Havre, where the health board was much more than a mere phantom, the enforcement of public health regulations was still no sure thing, ranging from vigorous to half-hearted.

ENFORCEMENT, CONTROVERSY, AND PROTEST

The enforcement of sanitary regulations in two separate incidents, thirty years apart, perhaps best evokes the unfulfilled promise and unsustained energy of the War on Tuberculosis in Le Havre. They also illustrate the extent to which (and in what form) mainstream medical knowledge concerning tuberculosis reached the general population. In the early 1880s, when boundless energy and optimism animated the hygienic campaigns of Siegfried and his circle, city officials were willing to use the tools of public health expertise to combat insalubrity, even when the sanctity of private property was at stake. In contrast, three decades later, with no such property interest involved, not even citizens' demands could rouse the administration to action. The first case involved a pair of buildings on the rue Saint-Thibaut in Le Havre, built between 1865 and 1871 for low-income housing, with the mayor's authorization to bypass local building standards. In August 1881, the city's Commission des logements insalubres inspected the buildings and found them unsanitary. The commission's report called the houses "a receptacle of intolerable odors and miasmas [and] a hotbed of infection, dangerous for [their] occupants and neighbors." Following this report, the city council in October 1881 declared the buildings unfit for habitation. The buildings' owners, the Bénard brothers, appealed the city council's decision to the Conseil de préfecture at the departmental level. They admitted that the structures were less than solidly built, "in order to be rented to workers," but maintained that the courtyards were large enough and the ventilation sufficient to meet hygienic standards.[69]

The Seine-Inférieure prefect's office sent two members of the departmental Conseil central d'hygiène to inspect the Bénards' properties. The buildings' occupants welcomed them courteously and made no complaints about their living conditions. The inspectors found neither illness nor "*déchéance physique*" among the inhabitants; furthermore, they claimed to have investigated the buildings' mortality figures from the previous two years and found them below the city average. The Commission des logements insalubres report, they insisted, was "forced, exaggerated." "The filth and poverty . . . of the tenants, source of an unpleasant and noxious stench," should not be confused with unsanitary features of the buildings themselves, the inspectors maintained. If the same inhabitants were moved to more "comfortable" lodgings, their "carelessness, laziness, disorder, and poor conduct would reproduce the same state of affairs in very short order."[70] Blaming the ill health of the poor on their own habits and morals, of course, was to become a standard feature of the French response to tuberculosis.

The prefect's inspectors concluded that to uphold the city council's decision would be unjust, inasmuch as "the salubrity of housing has its degrees"; an overly strict enforcement of sanitary regulations would entail a loss of so many housing units that "social necessity" demanded a hands-off approach. After all, they reasoned, "these are the lodgings of poor workers," who could not afford to pay higher rents elsewhere. "Where would these 132 unfortunates go" if their buildings were condemned? They recommended a pragmatic response, in which such buildings would be improved by limited remedial construction but not ruled off-limits for housing entirely.[71]

The most significant aspect of the Bénard case may be the way in which Le Havre city officials and the Bureau d'hygiène responded to the departmental report. In July 1882, four months after the prefect received his inspectors' conclusions, the city's lawyer asked his staff to check the bureau's files for the actual mortality statistics in the Bénards' buildings. The bureau had of course been keeping the casier sanitaire—records of causes of death in every building in Le Havre—since its establishment in 1879. The city's figures told a story very different from that of the departmental inspectors' report. Although it is unclear whether the casier sanitaire data applied to all or only some of the housing units at 40 and 42 rue Saint-Thibaut, they showed more than double the number of deaths reported by the prefect's inspectors, including four from pulmonary tuberculosis and five from infantile enteritis since late 1879. As mayor of Le Havre at the time, Siegfried cited the casier sanitaire statistics in a letter to the Conseil de préfecture of the Seine-Inférieure. "No demonstration could be more conclusive," he wrote, "nor justify more amply the protective measure taken by the city council"—namely, the complete condemnation of the buildings for human habitation.[72] In essence, Le Havre officials were attempting to use a new administrative tool, the casier sanitaire, to force action by private interests in the name of public health.

Le Havre's municipal archives show that the city continued to press its efforts to condemn the buildings, though they do not reveal the affair's ultimate outcome. In August 1882, the Conseil de préfecture overturned the city council's *interdiction d'habitation* but ordered repair work done within two months. The following April, the work was still not even close to completion, and Mayor Siegfried instigated further legal proceedings against the Bénards. In late June 1883, the city engineer reported that the repairs had either not been done or had been done improperly; thereafter the available evidence falls silent.[73] Whatever the final dispensation of the Bénard case, it provides a snapshot of official Le Havre's attitude toward tuberculosis and public health around the time of Koch's discovery of the disease's microbial agent. Before contagionism had fully penetrated the public sphere in France, the municipal government had not only developed a sophisticated administrative tool (the casier sanitaire) to monitor the sanitary status of the city's housing but also shown a willingness to use it to bring about material change. Just as important, perhaps, is the fact that the Le Havre administration never went to such lengths again, though it maintained the casier sanitaire for many years thereafter.

In fact, the city's approach could scarcely have been more different thirty years later, when another "affair" related to unsanitary housing came before Le Havre's Bureau d'hygiène. In September 1912, Mayor Henri Génestal received a letter from Auguste Clouet, a concerned constituent who had approached him in person a few weeks before. Clouet was anxious about the health of his young nephew, Robert Lefebvre, who since the death of his mother had been living with his grandparents at 66 rue du Perrey in Le Havre. Clouet's concern stemmed from the fact that the child's mother had died of tuberculosis and from the filthy state in which the grandparents kept their house. Clouet sought to gain custody of the child—promising to send him to live in the countryside—and asked for the mayor's help.[74]

The mayor asked Adrien Loir, director of the Bureau d'hygiène, to have a member of the bureau's staff look into the situation at 66 rue du Perrey. The staffer, M. Legangneur, reported back within ten days, taking the view that the Lefebvre boy and his grandparents lived quite healthy and contented lives amid considerable poverty and squalor.

> The walls are uniformly dirty and one has to wonder if the floor even exists. The beds are sordid pallets, and yet one senses in these people an air of satisfaction (they have always lived this way), and the old couple seems to give all their affection to this child.

Legangneur observed the household twice a day for a week and felt confident that "in the middle of this poverty, the child is happy; in any case, despite his dirty face and his tousled hair, he seems full of health." The grandparents, he felt, were too set in their ways to learn even elementary hygiene, but they, too, had always enjoyed fine health. Legangneur could find no reason to strip the elderly couple of custody.[75] His report is extraordinary in its implicit mockery of the housing etiology of tuberculosis and its departure from the positivist social engineering usually advocated in public health literature at the time. Its paternalistic tone toward the poor is more representative of the genre. But most interesting of all is what it says about the evolution of antituberculosis policy in Le Havre during the early Third Republic.

There are several possible explanations for the apparent change in the city's health enforcement policy over these three decades. One is that the change was more apparent than real: the handling of the Robert Lefebvre matter could be attributable to the idiosyncrasies of Legangneur, the health board's inspector, or to other factors affecting the board's operations in 1912. A sense of ambivalence about the problem of unsanitary housing or the perceived lack of a clear mandate to deal vigorously with health matters in the private sphere could also explain the quite different handling of the two cases. However, both the substance and the style of official documents concerning these affairs point to another interpretation: a gradual waning of the urgency and priority that tuberculosis, public health, and the housing question had commanded from the 1880s through the first years of the twentieth century in Le Havre. By 1912, the fusion of anxieties that animated the War on Tuberculosis had passed its peak, and other issues assumed priority on local and national agendas.

Dispute and controversy over tuberculosis in Le Havre were not limited to matters of individual negligence or unsanitary housing. Establishment of an antituberculosis dispensary in the city aroused a storm of protest and anxiety among various groups of residents; its story, more than any other, reveals how and how much medical knowledge about tuberculosis had filtered through to the general population, and the extent to which Le Havre's social fault lines—like those of the nation as a whole—structured and shaped official responses to the disease.

Plans to establish a dispensary in the city were fraught with conflict from the very start. In 1902, two separate groups submitted proposals to the mayor and city council. The first, led by two doctors from Le Havre's Pasteur Hospital, advocated a public institution run by the municipality and built as an annex to the hospital on hospital grounds. The second group, calling itself the Ligue havraise contre la tuberculose, consisted of a cross-section of the city's medical, philanthropic, commercial, and political elite: Jules Siegfried and his brother, Ernest, along with former mayor Génestal and future mayor Brindeau, were among its members. This influential group proposed a privately run dispensary, partially supported by public subsidy, unconnected physically or administratively with the hospital. It would be a "Calmette-type" antituberculosis dispensary, providing free medical consultation, material aid in the form of linens and in some cases rent assistance, and most of all "education and propaganda" on how to avoid transmitting the disease to others. The sponsors first suggested a site on the cours de la République—the former Dollfuss dispensary (apparently a venereal disease control facility for prostitutes), which had the advantage of already being under city management.[76]

But so did the hospital, and the doctors behind the competing plan objected to the Dollfuss site. Recognizing the potential for contagion hysteria, they told the city council that such an installation would "contaminate" the building and environs on the cours de la République, particularly through the handling and washing of patients' laundry. Laundry machines would need to be purchased or built, Doctors Courbet and Laurent continued, for it would be "a veritable crime" to subject employees to the danger of washing clothes and linens by hand. They went on to cite the cost of hiring an experienced bacteriologist and procuring other equipment, as well as the lack of public control over a publicly subsidized facility, in opposing the Ligue havraise plan. In contrast, the hospital already had the personnel and equipment needed, and it was located in the hills on the outskirts of town; locating the new dispensary on the hospital grounds would therefore minimize both danger and cost.[77]

Nevertheless, the city council rejected the Courbet and Laurent plan and sided with the prominent city fathers—at least in part. In July 1903, the council approved a subsidy to the Ligue havraise contre la tuberculose, but it attached some strings. Its tight budget forced it to scale down the amount of the subsidy from what the league had requested (16,000 francs for start-up costs and 12,500 francs per year for operations) to a mere 6,000 francs per year. (The dispensary eventually made up for this shortfall with 20,000 francs per year out of the national pari-mutuel revenues from horse-race betting.) Moreover, in an apparent concession to neighborhood complaints, the city council vetoed the Dollfuss site, calling it "absolutely incompatible with the proposed usage."[78]

The Ligue havraise responded with an alternative proposal, this one strikingly similar to that of their opponents, although it kept the dispensary under private control. The league had its eye on a site adjacent to the Pasteur Hospital, outside of the grounds proper on the rue de Tourneville; this adjoining property had been acquired by the hospital for a planned expansion, but the hospital administration was willing to lease it to the antituberculosis league on very favorable terms. The site's main advantage, however, its location on the outskirts of Le Havre, in a less densely populated and healthier hillside neighborhood, soon turned into the very bane of the proposal.[79]

The well-to-do population of the rue de Tourneville, unaccustomed to disease in their neighborhood, did not take kindly to the prospect of a dispensary on their street. In early August 1903, thirty-eight residents sent a petition of protest to the mayor and city council. Their street was already too narrow for the traffic that used it, they wrote. Without sidewalks, pedestrians were forced to press themselves against the walls running alongside the street when vehicles passed. In their petition, the residents raised the specter of long lines of tuberculosis patients on this street every day during consultation hours. "These patients, whose greatest relief is expectoration, will strew the surface of the street with their sputum, and passersby will have no choice but to carry along with them these agents of propagation . . . of the Koch bacillus!!!" If the city went ahead with this measure of "reverse hygiene," the petitioners contended, it would actually be helping to "propagate the terrible disease rather than eradicate it." They gravely warned that the municipal authorities would bear full responsibility if the plan went ahead and tuberculosis became "epidemic" in the neighborhood. The petition concluded by urging that a "more appropriate site" for the dispensary be found, either inside the hospital grounds or outside of the city entirely.[80]

But the residents of the rue de Tourneville did not stop there. In August and September 1903, they sought to marshal authoritative medical evidence to back their dire claims about the danger of a dispensary on their street. After citing Emile Duclaux of the Institut Pasteur in support of their argument, they contacted two prominent Havrais physicians and solicited their expert opinion on the matter. Both were unequivocal. "Numerous patients will loiter about in this small space and create a permanent source of contamination," wrote Dr. Lausiès. Dr. Bernardbeig called the dispensary "a danger of permanent contagion for the neighboring houses" and lamented that so many tuberculosis victims—heedless of the hazards of spitting—refused to use spittoons, even when given their own portable "hygienic" models. Despite the petition's complaints about the dangerously narrow streets and unsanitary gutters, both doctors agreed that the neighborhood was a healthy one, theretofore all but free of tuberculosis. Both cited this fact as a further argument *against* locating the dispensary there, implying that those who suffered from the disease should be sent to an unsanitary part of the city for consultation or that tuberculosis could be physically walled off in poorer neighborhoods, where it posed little threat to the bourgeoisie.[81]

The Public Assistance Committee of the city council met to consider the issue, and in November 1903, it voted against the league's proposal. The committee's report quoted at length from the rue de Tourneville petition and cited several other reasons for opposing the site adjacent to the hospital. However, the Le Havre authorities neither rejected the dispensary entirely nor relegated it to a remote area outside of the city, as the petitioners and their medical experts had urged. Instead, they allowed the Ligue havraise contre la tuberculose to suggest another site, and the league obliged, paradoxically settling on an inner-city location. However, unlike the cours de la République and the rue de Tourneville, the new site on the rue Haudry was in a working-class neighborhood, a fact that might help explain the apparent deviation from the experts' advice.[82]

When the population of the rue Haudry learned of the new plan in fall 1904, it, too, reacted strongly and resolved to fight it. No fewer than 229 residents signed a petition sent to Mayor Théodore Maillart— an overwhelming response, particularly when compared with the 38 signatures on the Tourneville petition. The "laboring" people of the rue Haudry (as they called themselves in their cover letter to the mayor) sarcastically questioned the reasons behind the choice of their street for the antituberculosis dispensary, pointing out that the first two proposed sites had been rejected after neighbors made public their concerns about contagion.

> The arguments given by the residents of the cours de la République and the rue de Tourneville appeared to make the difference for the authorities involved. By what miracle could these arguments have lost their strength? And must we be contented, in order to impose a source of infection on a *poor* neighborhood, with the reasoning that *the rich didn't want it?*

The angry petitioners went on to explain that the rue Haudry was not served by a sewer line; that liquid wastes stagnated in the relatively flat street's gutters, rather than draining off; and that their children, unlike those of the rue de Tourneville, did not have gardens or yards in which to play and had to use the street as a playground. They would therefore be "in daily contact with morbid germs" in the dirty water from the dispensary's laundry and in the patients' sputum. The residents pleaded with the mayor to "defend [their] right to life" and veto the site. Their plea was to no avail, however. A year later, on October 29, 1905, soon after the close of the International Tuberculosis Congress in Paris, the Ligue havraise inaugurated the Brouardel Dispensary at 16 rue Haudry. The eminent hygienist Dr. Paul Brouardel himself, after whom the dispensary was named and whom Maillart called "the most illustrious enemy of tuberculosis," attended the ceremony; the mayor called his presence "a guarantee of success." [83]

The degree of that success is unclear; the impact of the dispensary on tuberculosis mortality in Le Havre cannot be ascertained with any certainty. The number of Havrais who actually came into contact with the institution seems to have fluctuated widely. For example, there were 746 initial medical consultations at the dispensary in 1912; in the following year, which saw a sharp increase in deaths from tuberculosis, there were 2,859 consultations. Each year, roughly 120 families borrowed linens from the dispensary, and several hundred had their homes disinfected. Other services included "*secours de loyers*" (the league paid out between two and three thousand francs one year in rent assistance, although there is no record of how many households were helped in this way), bacteriological tests for the presence of the tubercle bacillus, laundry service, residential painting and cleaning, and, of course, free portable spittoons. Greater frequentation of the dispensary, however, could accompany both higher and lower incidence of tuberculosis. It was the hygienists' hope that more visitors receiving consultations would cause a decline in the disease. Conversely, however, an increase in tuberculosis would naturally create greater demand for the dispensary's services and cause the number of consultations to rise. There does not appear to have been an appreciable decline in Le Havre's tuberculosis mortality after the 1905 opening of the Brouardel Dispensary; most of the city's gradual pre-World War I decline had already occurred by that time. In fact, in six of the next eight years, tuberculosis mortality was higher than it was in 1905.

The story of the establishment of Le Havre's dispensary does, however, teach two relatively clear lessons. Wealth played an instrumental role in municipal health policy. It is not difficult to see the abandonment of the rue de Tourneville site for the rue Haudry as a concession to an influential constituency at the expense of a powerless one. Perhaps the most important lesson of this episode, however, is that by the very first years of the twentieth century, germ theory had become common knowledge. By whatever means and whatever the distortions in the transmission, the bacillocentric thrust of the dominant etiology and of the official War on Tuberculosis had penetrated the popular consciousness. The streets were full of contagionism.

It can safely be said that Le Havre did more to fight tuberculosis than any other city in France. It also had more of it to fight. Tuberculosis mortality *did* decline in Le Havre during the late nineteenth century and until the First World War, according to the available evidence—slowly and unevenly, but noticeably. However, the same was true for other large cities in France at the same time, where the decline was more even and at a slightly syncopated rhythm compared to Le Havre (see fig. 3 above, p. 8). It is extremely difficult to discern any connection between the various components of Le Havre's battle plan (low-cost housing, the Bureau d'hygiène, disinfection, the dispensary, etc.) and the incidence of tuberculosis; it is nearly impossible to draw any specific conclusions from the difference between the gradual decline in Le Havre and the gradual decline in cities that mounted little or no organized, sustained opposition to the disease in these years.

At every turn in Le Havre's struggle against the disease, moralization, administrative surveillance, and bacillophobic education assumed paramount importance; alteration of the material circumstances in which the victims of tuberculosis lived and died was relegated to the background. When material action was undertaken, as with the low-cost housing projects, financial and other concerns ensured that its impact was limited.

Le Havre's experience was as far from typical in France as is imaginable. However, its extremes—of both incidence and response—throw into especially sharp relief some of the key transformations of the nineteenth century and the ambivalent, often contradictory ways in which

France came to terms with the social aspects of health and disease. The city's experience also exemplifies what other authors have called the "ecological slide" and the "dispensary gaze." As noted above, Cottereau has described the "glissement écologique" as the expression of social relations in terms of relations with the environment.[84] While Cottereau's distinction between the "true" domain of the social and the mediated, suspect domain of the environmental is open to question, it is true that throughout most of the nineteenth century, any health problem that seemed to have a "social" existence or incidence was analyzed in *spatial* terms. Tuberculosis was no exception, even before germ theory gave its spatial distribution a contagionist significance.

In *The Birth of the Clinic,* Foucault described in his chapter titles two themes in the development of the "clinical gaze": "To See and to Know" and "Open Up a Few Corpses."[85] The health reformers of Le Havre essentially extended the clinical gaze from the individual body to the spaces between bodies in the city. To do so involved seeing and knowing the streets of the city and opening up those streets and their slums to the bright light of science and governmental surveillance. Taking his cue from Foucault, David Armstrong has identified the "dispensary gaze" as a strategy of controlling space within the city by mapping the movement of pathology within it. "The Dispensary represented the Panopticon writ large," he contends, "a whole community 'traversed throughout by hierarchy, surveillance, observation, writing.' "[86] That which Armstrong associates with the dispensary and the twentieth century, however, was in many ways a nineteenth-century phenomenon and predated the modern form of the dispensary. What might more properly be called the "hygienic gaze," in the nineteenth century, did indeed represent a strategy of controlling pathology through surveillance, knowledge, and writing; ideally, the influence of the Bureau d'hygiène (with dispensaries as its outposts) would radiate outward throughout the city, bringing in data and sending forth education. In its consummate form, it was a realization of the strategy that Lecadre had advocated against tuberculosis in the 1870s: "incessant observation."

Despite the best administrative efforts of the Bureau d'hygiène and the apparent success of contagionism in spreading bacillophobia, there are signs that the War on Tuberculosis did not define the limits of the disease's popular meanings in Le Havre. In the early years of the twentieth century, certain voices outside of mainstream medicine and the city government even expressed a defiant opposition to the dominant etiology of tuberculosis. For example, local trade union activists attributed

Le Havre's high mortality to a chain of factors inherent in the capitalist system. Alcoholism, in the view of a workers' temperance organization, was the principal cause of "the frightening progress of tuberculosis" in the city. However, the trade unionists distanced themselves from bourgeois doctors by attributing alcoholism to overwork and fatigue, which led workers to seek energy and sustenance in drink. Overwork, they charged, was built into industrial capitalism.[87] The argument implied that tuberculosis would be overcome only with the end of the capitalist regime. Meanwhile, the same group of activists opened a clinic and dispensary where union members and their families could seek treatment and assistance for injuries and illness.[88] Workers, it was believed, could not depend on mainstream doctors and official dispensaries to protect them. Only by agitating politically and taking charge of their own care within the workers' movement could they hope for better health.

Evidence of the strength and degree of acceptance achieved by this political perspective on tuberculosis in Le Havre is scattered and uneven. However, there was a sustained effort on the national level to create a left-wing alternative to the official understanding of tuberculosis. The origins and development of this effort are the subject of the next chapter.

CHAPTER SEVEN

Dissenting Voices

Left-Wing Perspectives on Tuberculosis
in the Belle Epoque

To find views of tuberculosis that directly conflicted with the dominant etiology, one must look for evidence outside the mainstream of medical literature. Popular genres such as political cartoons can provide some important clues in this regard. Two intriguing cartoons, side by side, suggest that in Belle Epoque France, the popular meaning of tuberculosis—especially its political meaning—at times eluded the control of the doctors and public officials leading the War on Tuberculosis. *La Voix du peuple,* the weekly news and propaganda organ of the Confédération générale du travail (CGT), came out with a special edition on May Day 1906. Two years earlier, at its Bourges congress, the CGT had decided to focus its energies on a single issue, the eight-hour workday, and to culminate its agitation with a wave of strikes on May 1, 1906. "As of May 1, we will stop work after eight hours," their slogan claimed. The May Day issue included a conspicuous indication that the extreme Left in France had claimed tuberculosis as a prominent issue in its agitation. In fact, the period leading up to May Day 1906 marked an important step in the creation of an alternative—and defiantly oppositional—body of medical knowledge.

The special issue of *La Voix du peuple* mixed propaganda urging workers to support the campaign for the eight-hour day with reports of ongoing labor unrest and police repression around the country. Two eye-catching cartoons (fig. 13) occupied the bottom left- and right-hand corners of page three. On the left, a sullen, sickly figure of indeterminate

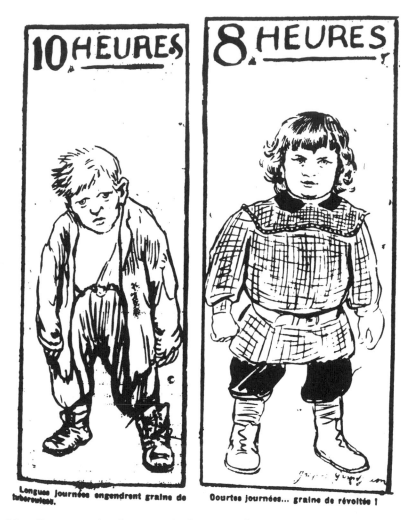

13.   Cartoons printed on page 3 of *La Voix du peuple*, May 1, 1906.

age—seemingly equal parts old man and scrofulous young boy—stares
wanly out from beneath the headline "10 HOURS," his workman's
clothes hanging loosely from his body. The caption reads, "Long days
breed the seed of tuberculosis." Across the page, under the headline "8
HOURS," a robust, smartly dressed youth, one hand clenched in a fist
and eyes fixed on some distant target, exudes strength and determination. His caption: "Short days . . . seed of revolt!"[1] In this journalistic
context, the opposition of these two simple images clearly identified
tuberculosis as two things: the result of long workdays, and a major

obstacle in the realization of the workers' true interests (through revolution). That a political cartoon could represent the disease in this manner testifies to the power of tuberculosis as a social signifier at the time.

La Voix du peuple was not just the newspaper of a major trade union federation. It was the official voice of revolutionary syndicalism, the internal threat most feared at the time by representatives of the established order in France. To be integrated into the CGT's eight-hour-day propaganda in such a way, tuberculosis must have achieved by that time a certain degree of recognition—at least in the syndicalist milieu and among most observers of the workers' movement—as a potent political issue, a key component of the "social question."

The story of how tuberculosis came to be seen as a side effect of industrial capitalism in general, and of overwork in particular, involves both the maturation of revolutionary syndicalism in France and the development of deep ideological cleavages within the medical profession itself. It also highlights the place of medicine and other specialized forms of knowledge in oppositional ideologies. Rather than attacking bourgeois power only in the domain of political economy, syndicalists broadened their assault to include fields such as medicine and public health, which by means of expert knowledge allowed society to be organized, normalized, and disciplined. The historiography of medicine in general and of tuberculosis in particular has tended to ignore such issues. Especially for the period after the rise of germ theory, conflict and opposition within medical science regarding the etiology and prophylaxis of disease recede from the historiographical picture. In fact, this period was alive with controversy, debate, and political division within French medicine.

Although its roots can be traced back beyond the era of germ theory to the early-nineteenth-century hygienists' work on inequality before death, the syndicalist view of tuberculosis reached maturity and gained currency during the two decades preceding World War I. Even within this period, its peak period of vitality as a weapon in syndicalist polemics lasted only from approximately 1900 to 1908. It is no coincidence that the heyday of revolutionary syndicalism in France converged chronologically with the peak years of both the mainstream War on Tuberculosis and the syndicalist, oppositional version. These were years of tremendous turmoil and strife, when the workers' movement sought to consolidate its status as a threat to the existing power structure and when many bourgeois observers feared the disgruntled French worker as both a political and a biological danger, a threat to public order and public health alike. When both the official War on Tuberculosis and the syndicalist critique achieved their greatest public expression in the period 1904–1906, the specter of revolution was more haunting than ever to the propertied classes, and workers struggled with ever greater force and determination against what they saw as social inequality and injustice. The sparks generated when revolutionary syndicalism converged with increased public attention to tuberculosis portray both syndicalism and public health in a new light.

THE ORIGINS OF THE OPPOSITIONAL CRITIQUE AND THE CONTOURS OF THE SOCIALIST CURRENT

On a fundamental level, the turn-of-the-century oppositional critique of tuberculosis had its roots in the work of the early hygienists during the July Monarchy. The studies of Louis-René Villermé, most notably, showed a direct correlation between poverty and mortality—the basis of later left-wing agitation. Yet Villermé left open both the extent and the exact nature of the causal connection between the various conditions that constituted poverty and specific causes of death. Moreover, he shunned even the slightest implication in his work that socialism or any socialist remedies would be an appropriate response to the deplorable conditions he uncovered.[2] Nevertheless, Villermé's work stood as a pioneering exploration of poverty as a public health problem, and it laid a foundation for future work by others who did not share his aversion to socialism.

Left-wing denunciations of the disproportionate incidence of tuberculosis among the working classes surfaced long before the official view had coalesced—and even before Robert Koch's identification of the tubercle bacillus. For the most part, the earliest expressions of discontent fall into two categories: quasi-romantic, paternalistic laments about the workingman's lot;[3] and analyses in the tradition of Marx, Engels, and scientific socialism, which tied overall mortality rates, for example, to the price of wheat and invoked tuberculosis only peripherally.[4]

Throughout the 1880s and early 1890s, left-wing critiques of official medicine in general and tuberculosis in particular were all but absent from both medical and socialist literature. During this period, as Koch's 1882 discovery penetrated through the profession and became medical dogma, the dominant etiology of tuberculosis began to take shape. Tuberculosis became firmly established as a "social disease," whose three determinant social causes were exposure to the tubercle bacillus, unsanitary housing, and immoral behavior. It was only by the late 1890s that theories of bodily exploitation had evolved sufficiently—and that the French workers' movement had regained enough strength—for the reformist and revolutionary strains to diverge. At the same time, the French trade union movement was gradually organizing workers and gaining strength; the formation of the CGT in 1895 marked a key step in this process. Socialist political parties were also growing during this time, although they did not achieve unity until 1905.

The consolidation of the dominant etiology and the strengthening of the workers' movement set the stage for the development of an alternative understanding of tuberculosis. Eventually, this oppositional critique split into two more or less distinct currents. The far Left, revolutionary syndicalist perspective rejected the dominant etiology altogether and saw tuberculosis as inherent in the logic of capitalism. The syndicalists focused their antituberculosis efforts on the fight for shorter workdays and higher wages in the short run and for the complete overthrow of the capitalist system in the long run.

In contrast, the "socialist" or "reformist" opposition accepted the fundamental tenets of mainstream Pasteurian medicine and of the official antituberculosis campaign. In particular, this socialist current emphasized two of the three main components of the dominant etiology of tuberculosis, the pathogenic role of unsanitary housing and of any exposure whatsoever to the bacillus, while downplaying the third component, alcoholism and other immoral behavior. Within this dominant etiology, the socialist critics sought to represent the workers' viewpoint by demanding that government attenuate those aspects of capitalism that they felt most directly threatened workers' health.

Several peculiarities of the socialist current make it difficult on occasion to distinguish it from the mainstream or "official" view of tuberculosis. The socialists aimed at changing laws and policies from within the economic and political power structure. They generally accepted the terms of debate set by the medical establishment and adopted the rhetoric of government officials and prominent doctors. Conspicuously absent from their polemics was the language of class conflict. This socialist current fought to represent the worker's voice within the official debate, to focus that debate on pathogenic factors imposed on workers by their economic condition, and to absolve workers of some of the blame directed at them in the dominant etiology of tuberculosis.

A debate in the pages of *Le Mouvement socialiste* in 1901 exposed the tensions inherent in the socialists' stance. Two doctors, Jules Thiercelin and Octave Tabary, disputed what contributions could best be made by socialists to address the prevalence of tuberculosis in the working class. Thiercelin urged the working class not to fall into the trap of the official War on Tuberculosis, lest it be diverted from the real struggle.

> I do not believe at all . . . that it is necessary, nor would it be effective, to undertake a specific war on tuberculosis; the working class, which is most afflicted with the Koch bacillus, could end up wasting a great deal of time in the war against various microbes: the latter are too numerous (even though unanimous public opinion is against them . . .).[5]

Microbes were not the enemy, nor were they even the effective cause of tuberculosis. To devote tremendous amounts of time and money to destroying bacilli, without changing the fundamental causes of working-class disease, would be futile.

> It is quite obvious, in effect, that the scourge is not the Koch bacillus, which has no doubt existed for a long time and will survive for a number of years hence, but the physiological poverty of the working class; thanks to machines and competition, the exploitation of one's fellow man no longer knows any limits, except one: the limit of the human organism's resistance, and today that limit is called tuberculosis.

Thiercelin used the example of England, where lower mortality from tuberculosis accompanied wage increases and reductions in work hours, to bolster his contention that only overall physical well-being and enhanced resistance to infection could vanquish the disease.[6]

Just as he would not be taken in by official slogans, however, neither could Thiercelin accept the conclusion of some anarchosyndicalists that any governmental action at all was a sellout of the working class. "We must not . . . get too accustomed to that simplistic solution . . . of waiting for a new society to resolve all of our current problems." Those who did so were nothing but "lazy and ignorant dreamers."[7] In fact, Thiercelin obliquely lumped together his opponents on the Left and Right with this curious characterization: "Against the governmental anarchy of today, we must oppose organization and regulation, to the benefit of all. It is we who are the party of order." Normally, "the party of order" (traditionally used in France to refer to the forces opposing revolution) would not be an epithet coveted by a socialist; Thiercelin appears to have been using this rhetorical device to advocate a sensible middle ground—a policy including income taxes and strict labor laws—between illogical alternatives.[8]

Dr. Tabary, in contrast, refused to sit back and criticize while there was urgent work to be done. To abstain from the War on Tuberculosis, he replied to Thiercelin, would be "a crime." "The socialist party . . . does not have the right to let its members die without protesting against the negligence of the propertied classes." Tabary lashed out at the "doctrinaires" who would wait for a maximum of suffering among the working class to bring about "the realization of their ideal of justice and solidarity." Isolated in their "ivory tower," they advocated an "all or nothing" approach to social reform, fearing that any improvement in the workers' condition would delay the ultimate emancipation.[9]

Fed up with the extremist revolutionaries, Tabary held in equal contempt the inaction that had characterized the official response to tuberculosis. The government had taken refuge behind grave pronouncements and encouraged the private sector to shoulder the economic burden of tuberculosis prevention and care. Tabary deemed the private sector's response laughable, given the scale of the problem. "The remedies brought about by bourgeois philanthropy have so far been ridiculously impotent and stingy." Instead of depending on the generosity of the rich, Tabary maintained, socialists should incorporate the necessary "radical measures" into their political program. Among those measures, he stressed national insurance against tuberculosis for all workers as a crucial one.[10]

Underlying the vigor of Tabary's protest against the authorities, though, was a basic acceptance of their terms of reference. While acknowledging the pathogenic role of overwork and meager wages, his article railed at length against the unsanitary overcrowding that typified workshops and working-class housing. In fact, much of the dominant sociomedical etiology of tuberculosis—targeting exposure to the bacillus and cramped, unclean surroundings—stood unchallenged in Tabary's analysis. Only the blaming of workers for their own illness (through drink or other immoral behavior) was missing. Furthermore, of the three main weapons in Tabary's proposed fight against the disease—dispensaries, sanatoriums, and health insurance—the first two were fundamental (if largely unrealized) aspects of the official effort. Neither aimed at altering the social conditions by which tuberculosis spread throughout the working class. Tabary was well aware of this.

> Doubtless the creation of antituberculosis sanatoriums and dispensaries does not resolve the social question and does not change in the slightest the relations between capital and labor. It is just one reform among many others which directly interests the working classes.

Piecemeal, gradual reforms were essential, Tabary believed, to the long-term struggle for justice. "Even while having as our goal the transformation of society, our duty is to enact all possible democratic reforms." [11] His was a plea for step-by-step action, fighting the workers' fight on the authorities' battlefield.

Thiercelin shot back, still in the pages of the *Mouvement socialiste,* that such a fight was wrong-headed. *"The working class need not enter into a specific fight against tuberculosis,"* he repeated, and he found Tabary's arguments wholly unconvincing. [12] They proved only that "our doctor-legislators" were unwilling to face up to the failures of medicine and to its inability to solve social problems. All of the legislative proposals emanating from the medical community amounted to an elaborate attempt to hide the profession's total impotence against tuberculosis. Unable to come up with effective medication or a vaccine, doctors took refuge behind the age-old *cure hygiéno-diététique.* That the sanatorial regime of fresh air, rest, and abundant meals would temporarily "cure" symptoms of tuberculosis was self-evident, argued Thiercelin. Yet even if the money could be found to send workers to sanatoriums, their illness would resurface as soon as they were returned to their "natural" environment of overwork, malnutrition, and overcrowding. The vaunted cure hygiéno-diététique was, and always had been, a cure for the wealthy. [13]

Tabary and other observers often cited the example of Germany to support their call for the creation of sanatoriums, claiming that tuberculosis mortality there had declined markedly since the opening of numerous such institutions. Thiercelin rejected the example as irrelevant, because the sanatoriums were too new and had treated too few people—even the workers' facilities, subsidized by national insurance—to have affected the nation's mortality. More apropos, according to Thiercelin, was the experience of England: an industrial nation, with a poor climate and not a single sanatorium, it enjoyed the lowest death rates from tuberculosis of any major European country. The reason was simple and had nothing to do with medicine or medical care. "It is because the English worker, who benefits from the absence of military service, is especially privileged in that his workday is the shortest and his wages the highest." [14]

In dismantling the sanatorial myth and chiding Tabary's faith in such a futile institution, Thiercelin did not stop at the familiar arguments over therapeutic efficacy. Impulses more sinister than mere misguided medicine were at work, he seemed to contend. By posing as the advocates of the sanatorium, not only were doctors trying to "mask their complete failure" to find an antituberculosis serum but they were paving the way for the economically efficient quarantine of the sick. (Sanatorium treatment of workers would cost less, it was argued, than giving them equivalent medical care at home.) Thiercelin's ultimate judgment on sanatoriums in Germany is suggestive: "*Forced-rest homes, which bourgeois philanthropy offered to and imposed on workers, in order to imprison them in the event of tuberculosis.*"[15] Here, Thiercelin left the door open for a comprehensive analysis of the surveillance and containment impulse in the public health policies of the period, but for the most part, such an analysis was forthcoming neither from the socialists nor from the syndicalists.

Despite Thiercelin's polemical tone, his practical conclusions betrayed a remarkable degree of moderation. The first two of the four recommendations ending his article fit closely with the tenor of the entire piece: "that the working class not preoccupy itself with the war against various microbes" and that it keep in mind its "immediate goal," reduced hours and better wages. The last two, however, would have fit as well in Tabary's analysis (or in the medical establishment's journals) as in his own. They urged workers to pursue health and labor legislation to enhance their immediate "security" and "comfort."[16]

Among other things, Thiercelin suggested measures requiring crachoirs in the workplace and mandatory declaration of all contagious diseases. Sanitary spittoons had been a hallmark of the government's proposed defense measures since the first outlines of the War on Tuberculosis emerged. Many observers on the Left considered the matter an absurd displacement of concern from the vital issue of bodily resistance onto spitting a distraction at best.

An even more controversial issue, mandatory declaration had been the battle cry of hard-liners so fearful of contagion that they wished to force doctors to divulge publicly the names of all tuberculosis patients. The government could then disinfect the "contaminated" lodgings at regular intervals and after death. Even doctors fully committed to the dominant etiology of tuberculosis balked at mandatory declaration, which flagrantly violated doctor-patient confidentiality. It also raised the specter of unprecedented state surveillance of private citizens, which frightened libertarians as well as many socialists. Thiercelin grouped mandatory declaration with mandatory vaccination (for such diseases as smallpox) in his recommendations, apparently considering both to be medically necessary infringements on individual rights.[17] On the whole, it is striking how much both Thiercelin's and Tabary's socialist manifestos accept the dominant etiology; just as noteworthy is the way both blended a deep suspicion of the powers that be with a reliance on reform legislated from above.

The same puzzling mixture of radicalism and gradualism appeared in most articulations of the socialist current in the tuberculosis debate. Quite often, such texts would pay lip service to exploitation and over-work when discussing disease among workers, yet ignore such factors completely when making practical recommendations for fighting tuber-culosis. Tabary, for example, called the widespread distribution of spit-toons "uncontestably the most urgent measure" and also recommended outlawing marriage for "young people suspected of [having] tuberculo-sis."[18] Except for an occasional rhetorical nuance, the socialist current endorsed both the theory and practice of the mainstream antituberculo-sis campaign.

TUBERCULOSIS AS AN "OCCUPATIONAL DISEASE"

Some socialists were not content to criticize from within the mainstream model or simply to encourage philanthropy. Legislative officeholders in particular were at the forefront of a struggle during the first decade of the twentieth century to include tuberculosis in a category of "occupa-tional diseases" (maladies professionnelles) that would be subject to so-cial insurance benefits. The episode stands out as emblematic of the gradual drift toward reformism and electoralism in French socialism between 1880 and 1914. From the time the first socialist deputy was elected in 1881 and the first socialist group was formed within parlia-ment in 1886, there was pressure on the movement to increase and prove its strength through elections and legislative initiatives. Even one-time revolutionaries such as Jules Guesde and Edouard Vaillant evolved into reformists and parliamentarians, and the trend accelerated when conciliatory politicians such as Jean Jaurès assumed positions of influ-ence within the socialist movement.[19] On the specific issue of tuberculo-sis, this gradualist orientation can be seen in the socialists' tendency to accept the dominant etiology and to strive for piecemeal reforms in the area of public health.

The effort to classify tuberculosis as an occupational disease presents an interesting case study in the ideological appropriation of the disease by the Left as well as in socialist strategy. Because the project originated in a version of the alternative, syndicalist etiology and adopted the political tactics of the socialists, it provided an intermediate arena of potential overlap or intersection of the syndicalist and socialist currents. In the end, it proved to be fundamentally socialist and reformist—an illustration of the process by which radically oppositional ideas could be absorbed and diluted by the very system that they threatened. Representing tuberculosis as an occupational disease also paralleled the official War on Tuberculosis in directing attention to places of special concern. While mainstream physicians and public officials trained their sights on the cabaret and on the interior of working-class lodgings—dangerous or preoccupying spaces, in their view—the Left focused on the workplace, which it saw as the key locus of workers' oppression.

Edouard Vaillant, a socialist deputy, medical doctor, and veteran of the Paris Commune, introduced social insurance legislation in 1900 which was modeled after the German laws implemented by Bismarck in the 1880s. The bill came two years after the passage of France's landmark 1898 law on *accidents du travail,* which mandated employer compensation of workers injured on the job. Vaillant's *assurance sociale* would have provided benefits in cases of illness, accidents, invalidity, old age, and unemployment, among other "social risks." Moreover, tuberculosis was specifically targeted in the bill's preamble and supporting arguments.

> If one considers that tuberculosis kills 50 percent of all workers, by the fact of their work—*that is, their overwork*—by the insalubrity of their workshop, by their housing, by their too meager wages, . . . by their insufficient diet, one recognizes two consequences:
> 1. That tuberculosis is truly, for the working class, an occupational disease and that, like occupational diseases, it must, . . . because it is a result of the unhealthy and dangerous conditions of the occupation, be included in industrial accidents and confer rights to the same reparations.

Treating tuberculosis like industrial accidents was not only just, it was also the most effective means of curing the disease, by giving sick workers the opportunity (and the money) to escape temporarily the conditions that compromised their health in the first place.

> 2. [O]f all early-stage cases of tuberculosis, the worker's is particularly curable[;] removed from the occupation, the milieu, [and] the overwork by which he is perishing, [he] is reborn to good health, in a healthful climate and situation, as long as he is hygienically housed, clothed, and nourished.[20]

This excerpt from Vallant's proposed legislation represents a form of oppositional core narrative. In this case, instead of explaining the spread

of tuberculosis, the proto-story equates overwork with illness by telling
of the worker's recovery when removed from labor and poverty. Just as
in the mainstream core narratives, the subject is "he," the working-
class male, and women fade from consideration as victims of tuberculosis. By no means did narrative belong exclusively to the strategists in
the official War on Tuberculosis. To illustrate the causes of disease and
the morality of their position, the oppositional readings of tuberculosis
relied as much on core narratives as did the dominant etiology. It is
significant that in this bill, Vaillant did not restrict the designation of
"maladie professionnelle" to cases of tuberculosis that could have resulted from workplace exposure to certain specific particles or contaminants. For *all* workers, tuberculosis was an occupational disease.

Even more significant is the fact that in Vaillant's proposal, the
French parliament—and by extension, the nation's political leadership
as a whole—was confronted for the first time with the oppositional
etiology of tuberculosis. While the syndicalists might have quibbled
with a shade of meaning here or there and would certainly not have
accepted recourse to legislation as a means of action, Vaillant's bill (like
syndicalist agitation) proclaimed without ambiguity that through overwork, low wages, and their attendant ills, *wage labor caused tuberculosis*. Nevertheless, despite Vaillant's argument that to detect tuberculosis
early and nip it in the bud would cost less (as he claimed the German
experience had shown) than long-term care for terminally ill patients,
the social insurance bill failed to attract significant support in parliament.[21] Given the extreme reluctance of the legislature and the courts to
enforce even the weak industrial accidents law, the failure of Vaillant's
comprehensive plan was no surprise.

Yet the former Communard, by then one of the elder statesmen of
French socialism, did not give up. The following year, among many
proposed amendments to the 1898 law on accidents du travail, there
appeared one submitted by Vaillant. The amendment itself was simple
and straightforward. "Occupational diseases are included under industrial accidents and considered as such by this law. [¶] Tuberculosis in
workers and employees is held to be an occupational disease." Vaillant
made it clear that he did not expect the chamber to adopt his amendment as it stood, but he asked that his colleagues at least refer the question to the social welfare committee for examination. The extreme Left
of the chamber resounded with cries of "*Très bien! très bien!*" but some
deputies reacted with astonishment and consternation to the sweeping
proposal.[22]

Léon Mirman, the committee's *rapporteur* on the 1898 law amendments, cautioned that "the question is extremely delicate." Of course,
Mirman added, some diseases were obviously of occupational origin
and should be covered in the same fashion as accidents.

> The first difficulty . . . is to know which diseases should be considered occu-
> pational. There are certainly some which come to mind and which we could
> list, but I must admit I was somewhat astonished to see that in the additional
> clause proposed by M. Vaillant, tuberculosis was indicated as an occupa-
> tional disease.[23]

"It is above all a general disease," maintained Deputy Charles Ferry. "I
have always considered tuberculosis a general disease whose origins are
quite unclear," echoed Mirman. As proof of this uncertainty, Mirman
noted that he had seen posters in train stations, on boats, and on buses
urging passengers to avoid contagion by not spitting on the floor. (The
implication was that if tuberculosis was caused by spitting and contagion, it could not be caused by work and could not be considered an
occupational disease.) Vaillant countered that his proposal neither asserted nor denied the relevance of contagion. "I [only] declared," he
said, "that in workers predisposed by their working conditions, by their
insufficient wages, by the excessive length of the workday, by overwork,
etc., a general weakening ensued, and then tuberculosis." Because the
disease developed as the "inevitable result" of their occupations, it was
indisputably an occupational disease and an "accident du travail."[24]

Deputy Mirman remained unmoved, however. Pleading ignorance as
to whether or not tuberculosis was an occupational disease, he nevertheless left little doubt which answer the law would ultimately give.
"That its development is favored by certain hygienic conditions in
working-class housing or in factories, of this there is no doubt; but [as
for] whether it is an occupational disease or not, I did not believe so,
[but] I do not know [*je ne le croyais pas, et je n'en sais rien*]." Other
deputies pleaded with Vaillant to separate the two elements of his
amendment: the expansion of the 1898 law to occupational diseases
and the explicit recognition of tuberculosis as one of them. Separating
them (that is, acknowledging that the second part was unrealistic and
overly controversial) would facilitate the chances of eventually passing
an occupational diseases bill and would avoid alienating potential sup-
porters who might be frightened by extremist measures such as including tuberculosis. Vaillant resisted the pressure to dilute his amendment,
but it was eventually tabled in committee.[25]

Maladies professionnelles nevertheless continued to preoccupy socialist legislators intent on expanding the domain of the 1898 law. One
deputy in particular made occupational diseases a personal project and
pursued their legal recognition over two decades. Jules-Louis Breton, a
close colleague of Vaillant in politics and journalism since their younger
days together in the Cher, had become by 1903 a prominent spokesman
for the moderate socialists in parliament. In that year, Breton introduced another maladies professionnelles bill that also targeted tuberculosis as a common and deadly occupational disease. But this time the
universality of work-related tuberculosis was replaced by a much more
limited view of possible occupational causes of the disease. Once again,
the bill aimed at extending the protection of the industrial accidents law
to "diseases of occupational origin." However, tuberculosis enjoyed
quite a different status in this bill than in Vaillant's defiant proposal to
recognize it as broadly occupational in origin among the working class.

Breton affirmed the centrality of "pneumoconiosis" in the determination of occupational diseases. The word denotes a category of lung
disorders (at the time often indistinguishable from tuberculosis, now
seen as including asbestosis and silicosis) caused by the inhalation of
irritant particles. According to Breton's legislation, workers in jobs involving dust emissions or dusty surroundings ran a great risk of pneumoconiosis, which in turn "predisposed them by the alteration of their
lungs to contract tuberculosis." At issue in the text of the bill was not
whether occupational pneumoconiosis per se should be subject to compensation (Breton considered this a self-evident example of occupational disease) but whether the law should apply to *tuberculosis* of unknown origin in workers habitually exposed to dust or other harmful
particles. "In other words," the bill asked, "does the continual inhalation of these dusts predispose the worker to tuberculous infection to
such an extent that the employer owes in all fairness . . . the indemnity"
under the provisions of the 1898 law?[26]

Breton maintained that it did. Quoting a report by the extraparlia-
mentary Commission on Industrial Hygiene (appointed by the Ministry
of the Interior), he listed those industries in which workers were mas-
sively exposed to "animal," "vegetable," and "mineral" dusts.[27] The
role of workplace exposure in determining not only pneumoconiosis
but also tuberculosis was so well established in the view of the commission (and in Breton's mind) that it justified making tuberculosis an occupational disease under the law *for those industries.*[28]

While many deputies doubtless still considered this proposal too radical and a threat to business, it was certainly a major retreat from Vaillant's global inclusion of tuberculosis as a maladie professionnelle. Breton recognized full well that many cases of occupational tuberculosis would not be covered under his bill. Unfortunately, he explained, tailoring the bill to fit such cases would torpedo its chances of passage in the Chamber. This central stumbling block loomed large in the entire debate on maladies professionnelles. The necessity of compromise for the sake of getting legislation passed divided not only the antiparliamentary syndicalists from the socialists but also radicals from moderates within the socialist camp. Whereas Vaillant apparently preferred to stick to his principles and act as a gadfly by introducing bills that had not the slightest chance of passage, Breton toiled persistently at fashioning an occupational diseases bill that could become law. (When one finally did, after World War I, it bore his name, and he would come to be remembered as the father of maladies professionnelles.)

The risk of this strategy, of course, was watering down the legislation beyond the point of responsiveness to one's original constituency. Breton's willingness to compromise and tireless effort seem to have created a certain momentum for occupational disease legislation. Eventually, however, the substantial opposition to coverage of tuberculosis in any form wore him down. In 1907, the most recent incarnation of his bill (which, like the 1903 version, included tuberculosis in the "dusty" industries) faced off in committee against a drastically narrowed government-sponsored bill, which covered only lead and mercury poisoning. A government official testified before the social welfare committee that determining with certainty the occupational origin of a disease was problematic. "However," he said, "there are cases of diseases which we must resolutely exclude. We can say as much of tuberculosis, which has been admitted by M. Breton into the ranks of occupational diseases." Breton's response was a terse "There are special cases," to which the official answered, "One can generalize too easily." Shortly thereafter, the committee's minutes reported that "M. Breton agrees to exclude tuberculosis [because it] might cause the bill to fail." [29]

In the space of six years, then—a period that coincided with the height of public attention to the social aspects of tuberculosis—while parliament failed to pass any occupational disease legislation, proposals proceeded from Vaillant's universal coverage of tuberculosis to inclusion only of cases involving continual particle inhalation to no coverage of tuberculosis whatsoever. The center-Right composition of governmental coalitions and their extreme reluctance to challenge the prerogatives of private property and capital thwarted many efforts at social reform during the first half of the Third Republic. Faced with so many arguments against the feasibility of occupational disease legislation, it is perhaps unsurprising that socialists such as Vaillant and Breton could manage neither to keep tuberculosis in their proposals nor to pass any bill at all on the subject before World War I. Nevertheless, the story of their attempts—particularly the path traveled from Vaillant's resolute inclusion of all cases of tuberculosis to Breton's pragmatic abandonment of it altogether—illustrates a central feature of the socialist dilemma. Efforts to address the social causes of tuberculosis within the political arena were caught in the tension between the desire for radical change and a commitment to the system that made such change impossible.

REVOLUTIONARY SYNDICALISM AND THE DEVELOPMENT OF AN ALTERNATIVE ETIOLOGY OF TUBERCULOSIS

During the mid- to late 1890s, at roughly the same time that socialists were developing a critique of tuberculosis, the new ideology of revolutionary syndicalism began to address the disease in its propaganda. As the CGT and the *bourse du travail* movement (a network of local trade union organizations) articulated an intense opposition to electoral politics and a reliance on the working class alone in the struggle to remake society, workers' health assumed importance as an issue workers themselves needed to take charge of. Syndicalists rejected not only the socialists' electoralism and reformism in parliament but also the idea that any facet of the official War on Tuberculosis could help the working class.

What most distinguished the syndicalist perspective on tuberculosis from the others was its complete rejection of the medical establishment's strategy and terms of debate. In place of slum housing, exposure to the bacillus, and moral depravity, the syndicalists targeted overwork and low wages as the chief causes of the disease. They also rejected the casier sanitaire, legislation, sanatoriums, and private charity in favor of "direct action": intense propaganda and trade union organizing to press for economic demands, backed up by strikes and by the threat of the revolutionary general strike.

Given the syndicalists' attitude toward existing institutions and authorities, there were a limited number of avenues available to them through which to publicize their position on tuberculosis and other health issues. All organs of the medical establishment and the main-stream press were inaccessible to their subversive, revolutionary ideology. Their oppositional etiology of tuberculosis seems to have been spread largely in the following ways: word of mouth; occasional propaganda posters or pamphlets; union or bourse du travail activities and clinics; and two major publications, the CGT's *La Voix du peuple* and the more theoretically oriented anarchist journal *Les Temps nouveaux*.[30] The nature of these avenues of expression, combined with the elusive nature of the phenomenon itself, makes it impossible to measure either the diffusion or the reception of the syndicalist critique. However, the alternative etiology of tuberculosis can be assessed and understood contextually through an analysis of the key texts in its development. Although as a general rule, historians both of the French labor movement and of tuberculosis have ignored this aspect of syndicalist agitation, these texts reveal the development of a coherent, medically sophisticated, and relatively widespread understanding of the disease that aggressively took issue with mainstream medical knowledge.

One of the earliest signs that revolutionary syndicalism was developing its own explanation of working-class tuberculosis and consciously rejecting the dominant etiology appeared in a series of articles by Fernand Pelloutier published in various journals between 1894 and 1897.[31] Pelloutier, whom many historians consider to be the father of revolutionary syndicalism through his leadership of the bourse du travail movement, took a strong, unequivocal stand on tuberculosis. He ridiculed the bourgeois hygienists who ascribed high tuberculosis mortality to excessive population density and to working-class housing lacking sunlight and ventilation.

As noted above in chapter 4, Pelloutier contrasted two Parisian neighborhoods to prove his contention that poverty, not overcrowding, caused high death rates.

> The Temple quarter, one of the most unsanitary in central Paris, is occupied both by rich merchants who reside there and by a mass of workers who descend there every day from the quite healthful heights of Ménilmontant. So, where do more people die? In the Temple? No, in Ménilmontant. Isn't this because in the former, rest and wholesome diets triumph over unsanitary conditions, whereas in the latter, the purity of the air is powerless to neutralize the effects of extraordinary hardships?[32]

Rather than in overcrowding, Pelloutier saw the cause of tuberculosis (as well as of epidemic diseases) in "the weakening produced in the worker by a despicable diet and hard labor." Such diseases "would be extinguished at their source if poverty did not prepare soil favorable for their propagation." [33]

When Pelloutier first began the series of articles, which were later collected in *La Vie ouvrière en France,* it is likely that his was a voice crying out in the wilderness. By 1897, however, there were indications that some kindred political spirits were beginning to see tuberculosis and other health problems in the same light. In that year, the Groupe des étudiants socialistes révolutionnaires internationalistes de Paris (ESRI), an anarchist student group formed in 1891, published *Misère et mortalité,* the group's sixth in a series of educational pamphlets. The mere fact that disease and mortality warranted a spot in their periodical propaganda writings on contemporary political issues signified a new conception of the role of such questions in a revolutionary movement. Although it was unsigned, the pamphlet was probably written by Marc Pierrot, a doctor who had been active in the ESRI since medical school and who would later prove to be one of the leading syndicalist authorities on health matters in general and tuberculosis in particular. [34]

The pamphlet took pains to place individual diseases within a broad social and physiological context. To illustrate how this context affected the worker's body and health, the group used tuberculosis "as the archetype of these general diseases determined by social conditions." According to this analysis, the disease was most common where certain specific circumstances prevailed, and these circumstances fit exactly into a broad social profile.

> [Tuberculosis] strikes above all those who are *surmenés,* weakened by hardships and by overwork, living in a confined atmosphere, in unsanitary and overcrowded lodgings, in the middle of a dense population. It is therefore in the working class, where all of these conditions are realized, that it finds most of its victims.

Again, as in Pelloutier's argument, proof of the determinant role of social conditions in tuberculosis could be found in the statistical distribution of the disease in the arrondissements and *quartiers* of Paris. In the working-class districts, tuberculosis mortality reached levels nearly five times that of the fashionable eighth arrondissement. [35]

With the publication in 1897 of *Misère et mortalité,* an important step was taken in the elaboration of the new syndicalist etiology. For one thing, Pelloutier's dissenting voice found an echo in this anarchist manifesto against physiological exploitation. Moreover, as it was almost certainly written by a medical doctor (Pierrot), it presented a more fully theorized medical argument—at greater length and in more detail—than had Pelloutier's articles.

By 1904, both the ideology of revolutionary syndicalism and the issue of tuberculosis carried much more weight in France's public sphere. The syndicalist alternative to the dominant etiology had progressed significantly in terms of exposure and sophistication. Tuberculosis even showed signs of becoming part of the standard, familiar ammunition of labor propaganda. In spring 1904, for example, the local bourse du travail in Paris (at the time officially known as the Union des syndicats de la Seine) decided to publish a pamphlet on the causes of tuberculosis and its relevance to the workers' movement. Paul Delesalle, a veteran of ESRI and a leading figure in the CGT, initiated the proposal, and the executive committee of the Union des syndicats agreed that workers needed to know more about the disease they all too often experienced. The committee did not want a general work on tuberculosis but something that would shed light on "the determinant causes of this terrible illness among workers[:] . . . poverty, overwork, lack of substantial nourishment"; they wanted, "in a word, . . . a union propaganda brochure." A militant from the barbers' union, Raymond Dubéros, was chosen to write it.[36]

By the end of August, Dubéros had produced the pamphlet, and unions in the Paris region were working hard at getting it the widest possible audience. Dubéros had given the Union des syndicats the propaganda it had asked for; in fact, he managed in sixteen pages to turn a medical question into a trade union recruiting appeal. He based the appeal on a simple syllogism: "Tuberculosis is the sickness of poverty"; "to eliminate poverty is to eliminate tuberculosis"; "only [unions] are capable of effectively fighting tuberculosis, because only their action strives to eliminate poverty."[37] Not only was Dubéros's pamphlet the first of the syndicalist texts to be devoted exclusively to tuberculosis but it also crossed the indistinct line separating theoretical critique from pragmatic program. As a direct call to action, the union's brochure added a new dimension to the syndicalist etiology of tuberculosis.

Nearly simultaneously with Dubéros's pamphlet, there appeared in *Les Temps nouveaux* another document that marked a new stage in the syndicalist understanding of tuberculosis. Between July and December 1904, the newspaper published a series of nineteen articles by Dr. Marc Pierrot entitled "The War on Tuberculosis and the Sanatorium Question." Taken together, the articles represent no less than a complete medical textbook on tuberculosis—from an anarchosyndicalist perspective. Pierrot, who was a regular contributor to *Les Temps nouveaux* as well as an ESRI alumnus, took pains to explain germ theory, physiology and other medical concepts in a manner comprehensible and relevant to laymen. In place of inflammatory rhetoric or theoretical generalizations, Pierrot gave his readers an exhaustive exposition of the causes, prevention, and treatment of tuberculosis. He also gave household advice for avoiding the disease and for dealing with it rationally when it appeared. In sum, Pierrot attempted to combine an accessible medical treatise refuting the dominant antituberculosis strategy with a practical handbook on tuberculosis for working-class families.[38]

Pierrot's series of articles in *Les Temps nouveaux* and Dubéros's *La Tuberculose, mal de misère,* both of which appeared in 1904, presented the alternative etiology of tuberculosis in its mature form, fully articulated and taking its place within the political program of revolutionary syndicalism. It is significant that the oppositional view reached maturity at that time. The CGT's biennial congress in Bourges, at which it decided to focus its agitation on a single issue, the eight-hour day, took place in September 1904. The International Tuberculosis Congress in Paris, during which the disease was front-page news in all national newspapers, took place in October 1905. Dubéros's pamphlet was published and Pierrot's series in *Les Temps nouveaux* was well under way by the end of August 1904.

This chronology is important. Had these texts appeared slightly later, it might be plausible to dismiss the syndicalist antituberculosis propaganda on either of two grounds: that the movement attempted to refashion as many "workers' issues" as possible in terms of long workdays, having already put all of their eggs in that basket (at Bourges); or that syndicalists seized on tuberculosis as fodder for agitation once it became a familiar and highly visible issue in the public eye. In other words, syndicalist propaganda might have opportunistically seized on any issue, including tuberculosis, that was being discussed by mainstream newspapers or politicians or that suited its immediate strategic needs. Instead, it seems that ideological forces within revolutionary syndicalism itself led to the appropriation of tuberculosis as a major topic of propaganda. These forces were rooted in the movement's split from socialism and in its "holistic" tendencies, that is, its insistence (inspired by Pelloutier) on the importance of health, education, and general welfare in the overall economic struggle. A closer examination of the principal elements of the syndicalist critique illustrates the ways in which tuberculosis became a lightning rod and focal point of agitation.

EXPOSURE AND RESISTANCE TO INFECTION

The most salient medical feature of the syndicalist etiology was its emphasis on diminished resistance, rather than exposure, as the primary cause of tuberculosis. According to the ESRI group, the pathogenic effects of social conditions—including poor ventilation, malnutrition, overwork, and exposure to extremes of heat and cold—all had one thing in common: they "put the subject in a state of diminished resistance" (*la mise du sujet en état de moindre résistance*). The students' brochure also pointed out the various social factors that increased workers' chances of exposure to disease, including some common to the diminished resistance category. In fact, the "defective conditions" in which the working class lived and worked "put this class in a position remarkably favorable to receiving and developing various diseases." The various causes of exposure and susceptibility to illness "combine, add to each other, act parallel and concurrently." [39]

In the ESRI pamphlet, overwork, the greatest threat to workers' health, was presented as an inherent feature of capitalism. "The excessive length of the workday is a generalized economic phenomenon in the system of capitalist exploitation. . . . Overwork results in *surmenage,* which is characterized by general exhaustion." "General exhaustion" was not just a catchall category for that which could not be explained medically. Pierrot had begun to develop a medical explanation of exertion and fatigue.

> Physical exhaustion and nervous exhaustion lead to a general weakening and render the individual incapable of reacting against the invasion of any given disease. This weakening results from an accumulation in the body of excessive deposits, that is, from an actual poisoning. [40]

In other words, the by-products of muscular and nervous activity, which could no longer be absorbed by the body, built up in the bloodstream and slowly "poisoned" the worker by interfering with his defenses against infection. Pierrot would later refine this conception of *surmenage* and analyze it in depth as a biochemical process, but in *Misère et mortalité,* it made its appearance (however tentatively) in the early stages of a syndicalist reappraisal of disease. [41]

Dubéros even pointed to considerable evidence in mainstream medical literature to debunk the standard emphasis on exposure to the tubercle bacillus. Several studies, he argued, had shown that most (if not all) adults in France had been exposed to the bacillus; some of these studies pointed to bacilli found in saliva or tissue samples, others to autopsies commonly showing "healed" lesions from tuberculous infection in the lungs or other organs. With exposure or "contagion" so widespread, the crucial factor determining which bacilli caused illness and which remained harmless had to be the strength of the body's resistance. Tuberculosis preyed most often on workers, Dubéros explained, because their "organic losses" (through expenditure of energy) were not "compensated for" (by rest and proper nutrition). "Their organism is anemic; they do not have the means to recuperate the strength they use up every day in . . . their labor."[42]

ALCOHOLISM AND OTHER INCIDENTAL CAUSES

The syndicalist authors acknowledged that overwork and meager wages were not the only causes of tuberculosis. They insisted, however, that all of the other significant causes could be traced, directly or indirectly, to economic exploitation. As far as alcoholism was concerned, Dubéros simply turned the mainstream's moral etiology on its head. Alcoholic excesses could indeed contribute to tuberculosis by depressing the constitutional ability to fight off infection. But the *reasons* for consumption of alcohol—and therefore one of the causes of tuberculosis—differed, Dubéros maintained, between the working class and the class of "exploiters" and "parasites."

> As much as anyone, we deplore the ravages caused by alcoholism in the working class. But if members of the bourgeoisie drink alcohol in excess by habit or vice, they force workers, by the long and hard labor they impose on them, to do the same in order to obtain the temporary strength which will enable them just to hold out and accomplish their work.[43]

In the case of the overworked proletariat, drink was a desperate and understandable attempt at a fleeting illusion of strength regained; in the case of the idle bourgeoisie, there was no reason for it other than moral weakness. This theme was characteristic of syndicalist propaganda on working-class alcoholism; it ran through much of the movement's literature on tuberculosis as well, a corollary to the main axiom linking overwork to disease.

Pierrot also recognized that workplace issues such as wages and hours were not the only factors contributing to the prevalence of tuberculosis among workers. He devoted two installments in his series to the role of working-class housing and one each to alcoholism and child-rearing conditions. Yet each of these factors could ultimately be traced back to poverty; work and wages, too much of one and not enough of the other, conditioned all aspects of working-class life. For example, Pierrot saw alcohol consumption as an important cause of diminished resistance. Excessive and habitual drinking resulted in the "rapid usury [of the organism] with weakening and degeneration." If one investigated the origins and circumstances of alcoholism in France, he asserted, one would always find a social context that included either severe job-related fatigue, poor diets, or exposure to extremes of heat, cold, or humidity. In these contexts, alcohol reliably produced the necessary short-term *"coup de fouet"* needed to revive flagging spirits and energy. "In sum," Pierrot concluded, "it is the excess of labor that renders alcohol indispensable, so to speak, to the worker."[44]

Closely related to the question of alcoholism, according to the syndicalists, was that of nutrition. In *Misère et mortalité*, the ESRI bemoaned the deficiency of working-class diets in both quantity and quality. Low wages forced families to skimp constantly just to put something on the table.

> [The worker's] wages are not enough, in a large city, for him to afford the luxury of consuming all the substances necessary for his survival. He is often forced to play tricks with hunger, to eat soups with little nutritional value, to drink large quantities of coffee . . . , to eat bread scraped with a bit of butter, etc.

Moreover, many of the foods a poor family could afford contained harmful preservatives, fillers, and other adulterating substances. Cheap wines and spirits were made with highly toxic fortifying and coloring agents. Under such circumstances, malnutrition could even rival overwork as a determinant cause of tuberculosis.[45]

THE SANATORIUM AND BOURGEOIS PHILANTHROPY

Long hours, low wages, poor diet—all came with the territory of poverty, and the syndicalists saw them as inherent in the capitalist social order. What made the existing efforts to fight tuberculosis ineffectual, they argued, was that all were directed at the superficial manifestations of the disease and none aimed at the root cause—the social order itself.

In the first eight installments of his series in *Les Temps nouveaux*, Pierrot focused on the sanatorium as a weapon in the campaign against tuberculosis. Around the turn of the century, a wave of favorable publicity about Germany's experience with sanatoriums had generated a debate in France over the wisdom and feasibility of following the German example. According to many reports, the recent efforts of the German social insurance system to establish sanatoriums accessible to all sectors of society had already resulted in a significant decline in tuberculosis mortality. Although French republicans were loath to imitate the autocratic German regime, sanatoriums seemed an attractive option in an antituberculosis campaign that had been long on words and short on results.

Pierrot regarded the sanatorium as little more than a resort scam for the rich and a smokescreen for the working class. For one thing, there could never be enough sanatorium beds available for the vast number of Frenchmen afflicted with tuberculosis. Even if enough facilities could be built, there would never be enough money to support families whose breadwinners were idle in sanatoriums. Furthermore, even if a significant number of working-class people could be "treated" effectively in sanatoriums, they would be returned at the end of their treatment to the same overwork and poverty that caused their illness in the first place.[46]

The only effective treatment for tuberculosis, Pierrot argued, was prolonged rest, nourishment, and avoidance of all sources of debilitation, including overwork, malnutrition, and alcoholism. This treatment was a realistic possibility only for the wealthy, and there was no need for a sanatorium to administer it in any case. German statistics showing declining mortality from tuberculosis had been altered, Pierrot claimed, by doctors seeking to spare their patients the notoriety of mandatory declaration of the disease under the law. Figures showing favorable treatment results in sanatoriums were equally misleading, he maintained; any patient would show signs of improvement after several months of rest and fresh air—whether in a sanatorium or alone in a farmhouse. Once the patient left the sanatorium, there was little doubt in Pierrot's mind that the improvement would not last.[47]

In effect, Pierrot saw the sanatorium as nothing more than charitable window dressing; its appeal was limited to a bourgeoisie (and, to some extent, a government) eager to prove its benevolence and to show that it was doing *something* to fight France's number one killer. "Charity

... offers the 'compassionate elite' the opportunity to make itself known, to perform its social function, which is to dodge dangerous [social] demands by giving some scant alms, with the advantage of being able to glorify one's own good deeds."[48] Pierrot even tarred dispensaries (which could ostensibly reach more people and intervene at an earlier stage and at less cost than sanatoriums) with the same brush. Testing for the presence of bacilli or pulmonary lesions and dispensing advice along with occasional food vouchers and clean linen, they did nothing that practicing physicians and local bureaux de bienfaisance did not already do. As for early detection, dispensaries depended entirely on the patient's initiative to come in for a consultation—by which time the illness was usually quite advanced. And what good did early detection do, Pierrot asked, if the dispensary could not reduce the patient's work hours or support the patient's family? Many dispensaries, he concluded, were little more than fronts for unscrupulous doctors to enrich or make a name for themselves.[49]

Dubéros also ridiculed efforts to raise money for the construction of sanatoriums for the poor. What good would it do, he asked, for unions and other groups to help in these efforts, when even successful sanatorial treatment would be followed by a return to the same poverty that made the patient ill in the first place? To be effective, workers' action should combat the capitalist system that caused their poverty. "But by framing the issue in these terms, we know that we cannot count on philanthropy, nor on bourgeois charity, which will not follow us on this road because it is contrary to capitalist interests."[50] Disdain for bourgeois philanthropy was a staple of the syndicalist critique of tuberculosis. It was also the pivot on which Dubéros turned a medical argument about etiology into a CGT membership pitch. Since previous debates on how to combat tuberculosis had essentially focused on what type of institutions private charity could most effectively fund, and such a strategy was incapable of effecting real change, it followed that the fight had to come from a new source. According to Dubéros, that source had to be the workers themselves, represented by their trade unions and the CGT, because these were the only groups that targeted the real enemy, industrial capitalism.[51]

PRACTICAL STRATEGIES

It was sometimes more difficult for syndicalists to propose their own specific antituberculosis strategies than it was for them to criticize the official approach. The conclusion of the ESRI in 1897 typified the revolutionary syndicalist approach: since mortality and physical suffering among the poor stemmed from the existing social system, "let us put aside half-measures and partial reforms, which are nothing but deceptive stopgaps." The only real solution would be "international Communist revolution." [52]

However, the syndicalist credo of workers' self-reliance at least provided a principle on which to base a day-to-day strategy. Dubéros insisted that self-reliance applied as much to tuberculosis as to shop floor struggles or bread-and-butter issues. "Workers must rely only on themselves to improve their lot, and the only means they have for fighting effectively against poverty, against all ills and consequently against tuberculosis, is to join their respective trade union." [53]

The union's "mission" was, in fact, "to combat all the causes of tuberculosis": unemployment, low wages, long workdays, and unsanitary workplaces. Dubéros and other syndicalists saw no contradiction between seeking incremental gains in wages and hours while working to overthrow the system as a whole. The unions' "struggle against all the forces of oppression and exploitation" would necessarily enhance workers' well-being pending the realization of "the work of capitalist expropriation and social reorganization." Dubéros ended his pamphlet with an appeal to nonunionized workers and to unions not affiliated with the CGT. These workers and unions, he wrote, were unwitting accomplices in capital's assault on the health and welfare of the working class. [54]

Pierrot did not mention unions by name, but his message was similar. He ridiculed the superficial strategies of the mainstream doctors and functionaries.

> It must be pointed out that low wages ordinarily go hand in hand with prolonged workdays and intensive labor. . . . These are marvelous conditions for the blossoming of tuberculosis. What are we supposed to do about it? Avoid spitting on the ground? Create dispensaries? Elect better deputies? [55]

While such sarcasm was something of a departure from Pierrot's normally measured tone, his message was the same one syndicalists had always proclaimed: electing better deputies and adhering to the bourgeois agenda would get the working class nowhere. "Since workers have not yet obtained—because they have not taken it—the right to existence, they have only to wring as much as possible, by consent or by force, out of the propertied class . . . while waiting for something better."[56] In the case of tuberculosis, what workers had to wring out of employers were better wages, shorter workdays, and more hygienic workshops. To achieve these goals, Pierrot advocated "direct action," the syndicalist term denoting a rejection of electoral politics in favor of economic tactics such as the strike (sometimes supplemented by boycott and sabotage). "The tactic best adapted to the conditions" of industrial capitalism, direct action provided the opportunity for the proletariat to show its strength while building class consciousness in preparation for the "complete transformation of society."[57]

Pierrot concluded his nineteen-part series by comparing the bourgeoisie's reliance on fear—fear of tuberculosis, fear of the bacillus, and fear of people with tuberculosis—with his own prescription for fighting the disease. The enemy was not contagion, he insisted, it was capitalism.

> Tuberculosis is an illness of poverty. . . . It is the direct product of capitalist exploitation. . . . There is only one real way to combat tuberculosis, and that is to transform society, to abolish wage labor, to assure everyone of well-being through common ownership of the means of [production].

When capitalism disappeared, according to Pierrot, so would tuberculosis. When the principle of "from each according to his strength, to each according to his needs" became reality, the devastating disease would be "rarer than leprosy."[58]

THE SYNDICALISTS AND THE INTERNATIONAL TUBERCULOSIS CONGRESS OF 1905

When the world's most eminent doctors and an impressive number of France's political and philanthropic dignitaries gathered in Paris for the International Tuberculosis Congress in October 1905, many syndicalists watched closely to see what the establishment would do about the deadly scourge that affected the working class so severely. At least one observer claimed beforehand in the pages of *Les Temps nouveaux* that he knew exactly what was going to happen at the congress. Michel Petit (the pseudonym of Dr. Edouard Duchemin), an occasional contributor to the anarchist newspaper on medical issues, wrote a satirical article in May 1905 predicting the nature of the upcoming proceedings. The piece, entitled "A Fable for Grown-up Children," exuded sarcasm and contempt for the authorities.

"The fortunate ones of this world," Petit began his fable, "realized one day that it could be dangerous for them to allow diseases which

could one day strike them—and were already threatening the productive value of their employees—to propagate themselves among the
poor." Self-interest and "cowardice" made the bourgeoisie take notice
of tuberculosis, Petit continued, but what would they do about it? In
the past, blame had been laid squarely on the victims.

> Official science has stuck to the axiom "tuberculosis is a function of alcohol-
> ism," which they teach to schoolchildren, an easy formula to remember, and
> thanks to which it is natural to conclude that if a poor person falls ill it is
> his own fault, and one can only advise him to behave better![59]

Petit reasoned, however, that the congress would have to go beyond
such pat formulas. It would bring together in the glittering Grand Palais
France's most prominent business and civic leaders, along with their
wives and daughters (who would take advantage of the opportunity for
a shopping spree at the Parisian department stores), and would treat
them to lavish banquets and receptions—a festival of self-congratula-
tion for their generous humanitarian efforts. They would doubtless hear
a "harangue" from the president of the republic, reminding them of the
urgent task at hand: "safeguarding human lives" and "battling against
destructive forces."

> You know the slogans. That one is cliché number two. For example, it
> wouldn't do for him to pick the wrong box and take out cliché number
> one, which covers the necessity of arming oneself against the invader of the
> fatherland [and] the selflessness with which each citizen must sacrifice his
> life and especially that of his fellow man.

Petit surmised that the president's clichés would be followed by arcane
lectures on such topics as "saprophytic forms of the Koch bacillus" and
"tachycardia in pretuberculosis." Socialist collaborators in the governing coalition such as Alexandre Millerand would plead for reforms "to
better the lot of the needy," and the assembled throng would unanimously agree to do so—by forming another government commission or
even calling for a cabinet ministry of public health. "After that, they
will break out the champagne," Petit added caustically.[60]

  When the congress was over, Petit contributed a follow-up article to
Les Temps nouveaux, claiming that the first story "wasn't a fable" after
all. Not surprisingly, he reviewed the actual proceedings just as cyni-
cally as he had previewed them five months before.

> The ceremony took place, absurd, devoid of facts and useful ideas, full of
> demonstrations in which bluff competed with free advertising—in a word, a

carnival of vanities and appetites, in just the way our present society transfigures every action whose pretext is the betterment of humanity.

What few worthwhile presentations there were at the congress had been
"drowned in an uninterrupted series of pointless communications,
poured forth in incomprehensible jargon and mumbled at full speed"
(so as not to exceed the ten-minute time limit). Petit saw the congress
as a perfect illustration of the suppressive power structure within the
scientific community. The stranglehold of elite figures in universities,
publishing houses, and hospitals over the production of medical knowledge effectively silenced innovative thought by preventing its dissemina-
tion. Even congresses, he wrote, "which are designed—we tell the naive
ones—precisely to allow unknown and isolated [researchers] to deliver
their results to the public," fell prey to the stifling of new ideas, and the
tuberculosis congress had been no exception.[61]

Those who had attended the congress could have saved themselves a
great deal of time and money, Petit concluded, by replacing the entire
affair with a batch of posters proclaiming three propositions.

1. No longer will anybody have to work beyond the limits of his or her
strength;

2. Everyone will be able to eat his or her fill;

3. Persons living in unsanitary housing (that is, poorly ventilated, unex-
posed to sunlight, or too small) will have the right to move into any unoccu-
pied quarters.

With that, Petit announced, "tuberculosis will disappear from the human race."[62] While the congress gave him another chance to deride
some of the leading socialists who had joined in the mainstream fight
against tuberculosis, it also prompted Petit to present the syndicalist
etiology in a new light. Granted, the powers that be would never be
sympathetic to the social critique embodied in this oppositional medical
knowledge; but, he seemed to argue, even scientific research, past or
future, that might shed light on the true social causes of tuberculosis
would never be allowed to surface by the controlling elite in the medical
community.

Curiously, though, a hint of subversive knowledge did surface at the
congress. Dr. Albert Calmette, already an eminent figure in French medicine, had founded a dispensary in Lille in 1901 and published a report
on its operations in conjunction with the 1905 congress. Calmette hired
as medical director of his "preventorium" Désiré Verhæghe, a young

local physician, and apparently entrusted to him the section of the report dealing with the dispensary's medical statistics. Whether Calmette knew it or not, Verhæghe was also deeply involved in the labor movement. The result was a set of figures, along with some explanatory text, that deviated remarkably from the orthodox interpretation of tuberculosis—and appeared under Calmette's name.

For example, the report noted that 96 to 98 percent of the dispensary's patients showed signs of "physical surmenage" (the proportion varying slightly from year to year) and 67 to 76 percent suffered from malnutrition (*alimentation insuffisante*). In contrast, direct contagion was found to be responsible for tuberculosis in only 7 to 9 percent of patients, alcoholism in only 15 to 18 percent. The statistics and accompanying text read like a manifesto of the oppositional etiology, based on empirical evidence.[63] Surprisingly, although the report was discussed at the congress, it did not cause much of a stir. Some accounts of the proceedings mentioned the statistics (without comment), but the report as a whole served mainly to promote the cause of dispensaries in the War on Tuberculosis.

A week after the close of the congress, an article appeared in Lille's socialist newspaper decrying the bourgeoisie's impotence in the face of the tuberculosis problem. The article was signed simply "Max," but clues in its style and content reveal it to have been almost certainly the work of Verhæghe. Given his enviable position at Calmette's dispensary, it would have been unwise for him to write such a virulent piece under his real name. (It was not uncommon in some provincial cities for activists with syndicalist leanings to be published in local socialist newspapers, which were often more radical than their Parisian counterparts.)

After citing at length (his own) statistics from the Lille dispensary report, Verhæghe drew the conclusion that "the question of tuberculosis, as a disease of the urban working class, boils down to a question of wages and duration of work." He dismissed the congress's proclamations, philanthropic gestures, and the "half-measures" proposed by the authorities as a "safety valve against the potential explosions of anger from the exploited masses." "For us, socialists, truly effective action against tuberculosis . . . can only be that which . . . forces capitalism to limit its exploitation, pending . . . the complete transformation of society, [which will] free the working class from all exploitation." In a postscript to those "comrades" who had been asking him what to make of the flamboyant claims of some doctors at the congress that they had found a cure for tuberculosis, "Max" insisted that even if the Koch bacillus were to disappear from the earth, debilitated workers would still be vulnerable to other diseases that would take its place. "The surest remedy for tuberculosis, as for all human miseries," he wrote, "is revolution." [64]

After the heady days leading up to and following May Day, 1906, when the furor had subsided and organized labor had lost momentum in the struggle for the eight-hour day and other reforms, tuberculosis became a less prominent fixture of syndicalist propaganda. By 1909, the most active period of labor unrest theretofore seen in French history was over, and new issues such as the threat of war dominated public debate. Even in mainstream circles, tuberculosis had faded from the headlines. Nevertheless, the appearance of occasional pamphlets, articles, and trade union congress reports proved that the oppositional etiology of tuberculosis remained part of the revolutionary syndicalist program in the years immediately preceding the outbreak of World War I.

In the long run, certainly, left-wing agitation over tuberculosis was a failure. It never managed to change official policy to any significant degree, and reforms such as the eight-hour day were realized only later—granted from above rather than imposed from below, as the syndicalists had urged. The broader historical importance of this episode, however, is more difficult to gauge than are its immediate effects.

Labor historians today wonder why the workers' movement in nineteenth-century France never made working-class health a significant issue in its organizing activity and in its demands.[65] The answer is that it *did,* in a sustained and extremely vocal manner, but the voices have been lost in accounts of the theory of the general strike or the question of collaboration in bourgeois governments. If a cartoon representing tuberculosis could arouse (or even be expected to arouse) workers to strike for shorter workdays, then clearly some subversive ideas about the nature of disease had gained a certain amount of acceptance.

Similarly, the story of the Left challenging the authority and impartiality of the medical profession does not fit into the conventional history of medicine. Histories of tuberculosis and public health in France have been dominated by a model contrasting artistic romanticism with the gradual progress of dedicated men of science—supported by public consensus—toward ultimate victory over disease. The development of a militant oppositional understanding of tuberculosis at the turn of the century in France indicates that, on the contrary, the field of production and implementation of medical knowledge was hotly contested terrain.

The significance of this episode may even go beyond the existence of struggle behind the facade of scientific progress and consensus. In France and elsewhere, medicine and public health were critical domains in the "marginalizing" and "normalizing" functions of the dominant culture in its transition to modernity.[66] These sciences represented certain people and practices as pathological and others as normal, just as they diagnosed pathologies within the human body. Because the syndicalist movement challenged the basic tenets of mainstream medicine and public health through an alternative understanding of tuberculosis, it posed a qualitatively different threat to the institutional structures of modern capitalist society than did, for example, oppositional attacks limited to the domain of political economy. The syndicalist etiology of tuberculosis rejected both bacillophobia and the priority of surveillance and discipline in the fight against disease. Where mainstream medicine, philanthropy, and government proposed remoralizing the poor and monitoring dangerous public and private spaces, the extreme Left fought instead for the fortification of the individual worker's body. Viewed from this perspective, a scientific disagreement over the relative importance of exposure versus resistance to the tubercle bacillus becomes much more—truly a debate over the entire social and political order of modernity. The fact that the syndicalist challenge never fully realized its goals should obscure neither the reality nor the seriousness of the threat.

Moreover, the ever-increasing scientific sophistication of debates on disease control since the mid-nineteenth century should not be seen as foreclosing the possibilities of "alternative" interpretation. Far from narrowing the range of available answers, the proliferation of detailed epidemiological studies of the past century—regardless of their authors' or sponsors' intentions—has not shut off the dissenting perspectives that, for whatever reasons, make mainstream medicine uncomfortable. After all, the rise of germ theory did not *inevitably* result in the bacillophobia of the War on Tuberculosis; the syndicalists' focus on overwork and resistance to infection owed just as much to the science of germ theory as did the dominant etiology. That bacillophobia—and the oppositional etiology—did result says more about French society and politics than it does about bacteriology per se.

Conclusion

To end this history on the eve of the Great War is necessarily to tell an incomplete story. In the months before the war broke out in Europe, the martial metaphors of the French War on Tuberculosis—already in common usage—only gained in intensity. Newspaper headlines blared, "It is not enough to defend our borders / We must defend our race / It is threatened by tuberculosis, by slums, and by alcoholism." [1] Even the outbreak of hostilities in 1914 failed to slow the various legislative and philanthropic initiatives undertaken in peacetime. World War I did, however, mark a turning point in the overall orientation of French antituberculosis efforts. The nation's arsenal of dispensaries, sanatoriums, and related facilities—its *armement antituberculeux,* in the reformers' military terminology—was subject to increasingly anxious inventory and scrutiny.

Legislative campaigns during and after the war resulted in the passage of two laws aimed at rectifying France's perceived deficiencies in this regard. The 1916 Léon Bourgeois law (named after its chief sponsor in parliament, the chairman of the government's tuberculosis commission and former prime minister) provided for the widespread creation and administration of "dispensaries for social hygiene and protection against tuberculosis." While it stopped short of mandating such facilities in major cities, as some proponents had wished, the law created favorable terms and financing for partnerships of local authorities and philanthropies to open new dispensaries. The dispensaries would be the first line of defense in the fight against tuberculosis, serving as centers for triage and assistance and directing certain patients to hospitals and sanatoriums.[2] In 1919, the Honnorat law (named for its sponsor, Deputy André Honnorat) essentially did for sanatoriums what the earlier law did for dispensaries. It provided for their creation with the participation of local, departmental, and national governments, specifying the eligibility of patients for subsidized sanatorium treatment and the amounts to be contributed by the state for each patient.[3]

The Bourgeois and Honnorat laws signaled a shift in the French War on Tuberculosis from education, moralization, and information gathering to the implantation of specific antituberculosis facilities (principally dispensaries and sanatoriums) throughout the cities and countryside of France. Meanwhile, beginning in 1917, the Rockefeller Foundation sent experts from the United States on a six-year mission to France, with the goal of modernizing and rationalizing the French campaign against tuberculosis. The American hygienists instructed local authorities in, among other things, the proper management of dispensaries and the use of visiting nurses. Perhaps most important of all to the war-weary French, the "Rockefeller Mission" (as it was informally known) also brought substantial financial aid to the effort.[4]

Before these wartime and postwar initiatives, in the race to build new antituberculosis facilities, France had some catching up to do. The vigor and pace of institutional mobilization in other countries—in a climate of intense international rivalry—certainly contributed to the French sense of urgency. The most notable counterpoint was the German empire. Birthplace of the sanatorium and home of Bismarck's aggressive social insurance scheme inaugurated in the 1880s, Germany lacked the liberal tradition of reliance on private initiative and aversion to state control that dominated antituberculosis campaigns in France, Great Britain, and the United States. Yet even the latter two nations outpaced France in their institutional response to the disease. There were 26 antituberculosis dispensaries in France in 1902; two years later, Germany had the same number. However, by 1910, Germany's number had jumped to 321, and when the war broke out, it had skyrocketed to 1,145. There were only 52 dispensaries in France when the Rockefeller Mission began in 1917. England had 64 in 1911 and nearly 400 at war's end, while the United States already had approximately 450 dispensaries in 1915. Not until the end of the Rockefeller Mission in 1923 did France approach the figure of 500 dispensaries.[5] It is even more difficult to make international comparisons of sanatoriums given the many different types and varying numbers of beds. Nevertheless, there were more than 60 sanatoriums in Germany in 1900 to France's 6, and later figures suggest that until the interwar period, France was behind the other world powers in this regard as well.[6]

While France may have been slower than other countries to build antituberculosis facilities, it was hardly alone in allowing social anxieties and stereotypes to determine its response to the disease. What was unique to France was the particular shape of its anxieties and its response. Elsewhere, other preoccupations came to the fore when tuberculosis was perceived as a social problem or as a threat to the nation. In Great Britain, for example, there was a far greater focus on the problem of bovine tuberculosis; control of the milk and meat supply thus assumed greater urgency. The predominant British understanding of tuberculosis blamed the trinity of "bad food," "bad air," and "bad drink"—poor diet, unsanitary living and working conditions, and alcoholism—for the spread of the disease. British reformers placed special emphasis on personal responsibility in the fight against tuberculosis. They urged moderation, cleanliness, and a temperate lifestyle and denounced the "ignorance and folly" of those who brought illness on themselves. The ethos of individual responsibility in Britain left little room for heredity, which was downplayed as a cause of tuberculosis. In the aftermath of the Boer War, concern over endangered "national efficiency" led to an increased emphasis on protecting children in the antituberculosis campaign. Even though children suffered from the various forms of tuberculosis at much lower rates than did adults, it was considered vital in Britain to inculcate at an early age habits of temperance, responsibility, and vigorous outdoor living.[7]

The fight against tuberculosis in the United States was more decentralized than it was in France, and its appearance varied from city to city and state to state. In the years before World War I, there was comparatively little emphasis on the link between tuberculosis and "associated problems" such as slum housing and drinking; although American doctors and hygienists certainly denounced alcoholism, they seem to have done so less loudly and less insistently than did the French. Not surprisingly, the heterogeneity of the U.S. population resulted in a plethora of studies regarding differential racial and ethnic susceptibility to disease. The highest rates of tuberculosis were found in the Irish and Scandinavian immigrant communities as well as among Native Americans and blacks, while lower incidences were found among Jewish and Italian immigrants. Although some American proponents of eugenics argued for measures including laws restricting marriage for tuberculosis patients, the fact that the disease also struck "those of 'good stock' " gave pause to most eugenicists. Tuberculosis was not integrated into the rhetoric of degeneration in the United States to the extent that it was in France. Another striking difference is the amount of attention that was paid in mainstream American medical circles to the role of low wages in the epidemiology of tuberculosis.[8] Perhaps because the American authorities had less to fear than the French from an organized revolutionary labor movement, it was acceptable to articulate a connection between wages and health.

One aspect of the antituberculosis campaign in the United States before World War I startlingly parallels present-day responses to the disease. Public health officials around the country shared a preoccupation with the danger posed by "vicious" (that is, vice-prone) transient indigents suffering from tuberculosis. The institutionalization or confinement of these transients was considered imperative.[9] Today's widespread fear of homeless vagrants spreading tuberculosis echoes these concerns.

In Germany, efforts to curb the ravages of tuberculosis took place within a general framework that the historian Paul Weindling has called "the hygienization of private life." In the crusade to bring more "air, light, and space" into the everyday lives of all Germans, blame for tuberculosis was placed on crowded slums, the sharing of beds, and dirty linens as well as alcoholism. German physicians split into two opposing camps where the treatment of the disease was concerned: proponents of Robert Koch's tuberculin therapy (which was later found to have more diagnostic than therapeutic value), and advocates of rest, fresh air, nutrition, and exercise. Eugenicists in Germany, Weindling claims, "regarded the TB bacillus as 'the friend of the race' in that it eliminated the unfit," while other doctors sought to strike a balance between caring for the health of individuals, on the one hand, and "racial priorities," on the other.[10]

In all these countries, as in France, spitting figured prominently in the social etiology of tuberculosis.[11] Vigorous campaigns against spitting have been a nearly universal feature of battles against the disease for the past century. However, in none of these other countries do venereal disease, prostitution, or the cabaret appear to have been linked with tuberculosis as strongly as they were in France. Medicine in Europe and North America (as well as in the far-flung outposts of the colonial powers) at the turn of the century was certainly an international enterprise.

Knowledge was widely shared through specialized periodicals and congresses like the one in Paris in 1905. In the realm of medical textbooks, the causes of tuberculosis were well known. Nevertheless, it is still possible to speak of a uniquely "British" or "French" etiology of the disease. Just as French medical men concerned about degeneration and demographic decline spoke of the preservation of the "French race," the perspective of antituberculosis crusaders was decidedly national and their knowledge about tuberculosis was conditioned by national concerns.

Long-lasting and painful, clearly identifiable yet rarely disfiguring, tuberculosis was the most familiar face of death in nineteenth-century France. Because of its frequency and familiarity, and because of the sheer amount of suffering and death for which it was responsible, tuberculosis became a vessel into which could flow a variety of fears, grievances, and emotions. The interlocking worlds of medicine, government, and philanthropy presented a more or less unified front, emphasizing the threat posed by tuberculosis to national vitality and productivity. One story in particular suggests how deeply embedded tuberculosis was in the fear of national decline. It was reported that during a public health congress in Berlin around the turn of the century, Kaiser Wilhelm II took Paul Brouardel, the dean of French hygienists, aside in a lighthearted but candid moment. The kaiser was reported to have told Brouardel that if France could not stop the "forward march" of tuberculosis, Germany would be able to bring its rival to its knees without the slightest effort.[12] Whether the story was true or not, the fact that it was told and believed in France is quite significant. It played on the humiliation of 1870 and the loss of Alsace-Lorraine, and it gave added urgency to calls for national regeneration.

It was believed that regeneration could only be achieved through national unity and consensus. The leaders of the War on Tuberculosis regularly applauded what they saw as the dissolution of internal political division in the face of scientific truth and the common good. One philanthropist, speaking at a banquet in 1905, pointed with pride to the presence in the audience of elected officials from all political groupings: "Republicans, radicals, socialists; there are no longer any political nuances when it comes to uniting, . . . seeking out this foe, and fighting against it."[13] Another hygienist and adviser to industry urged the workers' movement to cooperate with management in health-related matters, setting aside "this class struggle which, in a democracy, does not correspond to reality." Between labor and capital, he insisted, there existed "mutual distrust and misunderstanding, rather than a real, absolute, and irreducible opposition of interests, and it is often up to science—which is the indisputable truth—to reconcile them." [14] Their positivist worldview infused the antituberculosis crusaders with the faith that material and ideological disputes could be neutralized by a transcendent truth. Science could become nothing less than the arbiter of all social conflicts.

Yet material interest and ideology never lay very far beneath the surface of the War on Tuberculosis. When organized labor heeded the hygienist's advice to join the struggle, it did not always find a sympathetic or cooperative reception. On the several occasions when aspects of the dissenting, left-wing explanation of tuberculosis were presented to a mainstream audience, reactions ranged from uneasy equivocation to outright rejection. In 1906, the government's permanent tuberculosis commission discussed for the only time in its history the possible role of surmenage—overwork and fatigue—in the etiology of the disease. At the time, the commission had one member representing working-class concerns: Auguste Manoury, secretary of a workers' health and safety association (the Association ouvrière de l'hygiène et de la sécurité des travailleurs). Manoury's interventions in the commission's deliberations were extremely rare, but the Senate was in the process of considering a bill that would make the *repos hebdomadaire*—one day off per week—every worker's legal right, and he felt the commission might have something to contribute to the debate. Manoury proposed a resolution that would have put the commission on record as supporting the repos hebdomadaire, "an effective aid in curbing the ravages of tuberculosis." [15]

Professor Brouardel, one of the commission's elder statesmen, immediately rose to oppose the resolution. "I have had the opportunity to study this question in depth, and I have unfortunately found that, on holidays, the extent to which workers frequent cabarets threatens to negate . . . the good effects of rest." Brouardel then retreated slightly from the implications of this hard-line position, saying, "I simply think we should not express a conclusion until after careful consideration." (Such a formula appears to have been, for this commission and for other governmental bodies, a fairly common way of advocating inaction.) Manoury countered that giving workers more leisure time on a regular basis would not necessarily lead them straight into the cabaret. "The six-day workweek will not, in my opinion, cause an increase in alcoholism; on the contrary, it is surmenage that leads workers to take refuge in alcohol, an illusory means of regaining lost strength." [16] This was as close as anyone ever came to endorsing the syndicalist etiology before the commission. Reducing the workweek would combat both tuberculosis and alcoholism, Manoury had said, because overwork diminished resistance to infection *and* contributed to excessive drinking.

Not all of the commission's members reacted to Manoury's resolution as decisively as had Brouardel. "That which weakens the organism's resistance," including surmenage, "is a cause of the spread of microbial diseases," one member admitted; another considered the role of overwork "undeniable." They were unsure only of the magnitude of the influence and questioned whether the commission would want to study the specific links further before arriving at a conclusion. Others concurred that overwork had a generally deleterious effect on health but objected that its effect on tuberculosis had not yet been "absolutely proven."[17] Nobody mentioned—even to refute—the report from Calmette's Lille dispensary, which had received considerable attention the previous year, in which Verhæghe had reported overwork as a factor in 96 to 98 percent of tuberculosis cases.[18]

Brouardel protested that he did not mean to cast aspersions on "the world of the working class, which is so worthy of our interest," but he added that more alcohol-related crimes were committed on holidays than on other days. "I declare that, as for me, I do not feel sufficiently enlightened and, as a result, I will abstain from any vote that we take." Coming from someone who was so highly regarded, the defensive and somewhat aggrieved tone of such statements could not be ignored. The commission's chairman, Léon Bourgeois, one of the few members who shared Brouardel's stature, intervened to find a middle ground. Bourgeois first objected that forcing workers to stay on the job was no way to fight alcoholism and that most would devote their extra free time to their families. He proposed that the commission put off for the future— but "as soon as possible"—a study of the specific relationship between overwork and tuberculosis. He also quickly substituted for Manoury's original text a new resolution, carefully worded in two clauses: it held that the repos hebdomadaire would diminish overwork and that any decrease in overwork would benefit workers' health. The Bourgeois resolution, with no mention of tuberculosis, passed unanimously; Manoury's text was never put to a vote.[19]

The oppositional etiology made the leaders of the mainstream War on Tuberculosis uncomfortable. Although it was only a mild version of the left-wing view, Manoury's resolution represented an affront to the illusion of consensus embraced by the medical and political mainstream. The underlying logic of industrial capitalism, the basis of France's political and economic life, was not among the predisposing causes of tuberculosis that could safely be discussed in medical or governmental circles. Surmenage could be addressed only through vague generalities, as in the Bourgeois resolution, but not in relation to tuberculosis or any other specific ailment. For the government's tuberculosis commission, the dilemma never recurred: shortly after the debate on the repos hebdomadaire, Manoury fell ill and disappeared from the group's minutes. He died in 1907, and the commission did not name another workers' representative to fill his position.[20]

The War on Tuberculosis appears to have had uneven but at times dramatic success in teaching the dominant etiology to the general public and in mobilizing local officials and charities on its behalf. Grass-roots protests and lawsuits in response to the threat of contagion from dispensaries and other treatment facilities suggest this much at least. However, there were certainly other voices speaking to the public about tuberculosis at the same time. The enduring popularity of Sarah Bernhardt and her consumptive roles, of the various adaptations of *La Dame aux camélias, Scènes de la vie de Bohème,* and *Les Misérables,* as well as of Thérèse of Lisieux, show that the redemptive-spiritual reading of tuberculosis resonated powerfully throughout French society at least until World War I. Moreover, it is clear that a medically sophisticated and unabashedly political opposition to the official campaign did exist and fought doggedly to counter mainstream antituberculosis propaganda with its own. It is impossible to determine with certainty how effective this effort was. Some sources report that the term *mal de misère,* or illness of poverty, was a popular synonym for tuberculosis.[21] If these (mostly polemical) reports are reliable, and the term was widely used or understood in this way, it would indicate either that left-wing propaganda concerning tuberculosis enjoyed some success or that many people empirically associated the disease with poverty based on the evidence of everyday life. Even though the left-wing opposition failed in its long-range battle to establish a new truth about tuberculosis, those battles illustrate the extent to which scientific knowledge is also social knowledge and fighting a deadly disease an inherently political enterprise.

The politics of overwork was not the only area in which tuberculosis came to be the object of controversy or uncertainty. The official response to tuberculosis in France consisted of an elaborate web of fear, anxiety, and positivist faith. Expressions (and moralizing narratives) of disgust and blame directed at the disease's victims took their place alongside preliminary steps toward surveillance and moralistic outreach, while an appreciable component of material intervention or assistance was notably lacking. Anxiety, surveillance, and outreach alike were directed in general at France's rapidly growing cities and, by extension, at the nation's population as a whole; in particular, they were targeted at the urban working class, now perceived not only as a political danger but also as a biological threat to bourgeois republican stability and prosperity. Meanwhile, throughout the nineteenth century, tuberculosis had an entirely different meaning as well. Judging from the popularity of Saint Thérèse of Lisieux and of various literary and theatrical works, the disease was understood by many not only as an *essential* affliction but also as a spiritually redemptive one. This reading of tuberculosis reinforced the sense that disease had a moral dimension, but it implicitly contested the authority of medical science to determine the true meaning of illness.

Even during a time when the amount of public and private resources devoted to fighting the disease was relatively small, the stakes were very high indeed. From various points of view, tuberculosis was seen as putting the survival of an individual, a family, a class, or the nation itself in jeopardy. As the nineteenth century drew to a close, all French citizens—doctors, politicians, trade union militants, actresses, nuns, and the mass of people intimately familiar with tuberculosis who left no record of their impressions—were struggling to address and assign meaning to an illness that, despite the discoveries of medicine, was still quite mysterious and threatening. They did so in ways that corresponded to their deepest hopes and fears, their self-image and their vision of society—just as we do today.

Notes

INTRODUCTION

1. Unnamed "spokesmen for the World Health Organization," quoted by William H. McNeill in his review of Frank Ryan, *The Forgotten Plague: How the Battle Against Tuberculosis Was Won—and Lost* (New York: Little, Brown, 1993), in *Washington Post Book World,* June 6, 1993, 1.

2. P. Sudre, G. ten Dam, and A. Kochi, "Tuberculosis: A Global Overview of the Situation Today," *Bulletin of the World Health Organization* 70 (1992): 149–159.

3. Michèle Biétry, "Tuberculose: Retour aux dispensaires," *Le Figaro,* October 7, 1993, 11.

4. See, for example, the five-part series "Tuberculosis: A Killer Returns" in the *New York Times,* October 11–15, 1992; Robert D. McFadden, "TB Kills 13th Inmate in New York Prison System," *New York Times,* November 17, 1991; Dennis Hevesi, "New York City Considering Quarantine of TB Patients," *New York Times,* February 22, 1992; and Geoffrey Cowley, "Tuberculosis: A Deadly Return," *Newsweek,* March 16, 1992, 52–57.

5. For example, Barbara Day, "Deadly TB strains could swell to AIDS proportions," *The Guardian* (New York), February 19, 1992; Cowley, "Tuberculosis: A Deadly Return," also emphasizes the role of poverty and "social deprivation" in the resurgence of tuberculosis, while also calling for surveillance-oriented public-health "control measures" as a first line of defense against the disease. See also the thoughtful historical review by Barron H. Lerner, "New York City's Tuberculosis Control Efforts: The Historical Limitations of the 'War on Consumption,' " *American Journal of Public Health* 83 (1993): 758–766.

6. There is already a vast and rapidly expanding literature on AIDS in cultural and historical perspective. See, among others, Susan Sontag, *AIDS and Its*

Metaphors (New York: Farrar, Straus and Giroux, 1989); Allan M. Brandt, *No Magic Bullet: A Social History of Venereal Disease in the United States since 1880*, expanded ed. (New York: Oxford University Press, 1987); and Elizabeth Fee and Daniel M. Fox, eds., *AIDS: The Burdens of History* (Berkeley, Los Angeles, and Oxford: University of California Press, 1988).

7. Even in the nineteenth century, anxiety over transmission of bovine tuberculosis to humans was less acute in France than it was, for example, in Great Britain or the United States. It has been estimated that in the days before widespread surveillance and regulation of milk and meat supplies, only 2 percent of all cases of pulmonary tuberculosis and 30 percent of nonpulmonary forms were attributable to bovine infection. This would amount to less than 10 percent of all cases of tuberculosis. Linda Bryder, *Below the Magic Mountain: A Social History of Tuberculosis in Twentieth-Century Britain* (Oxford: Clarendon Press, 1988), 3, 133.

8. For epidemiological developments since the mid-1980s, see Sudre et al., "Tuberculosis: A Global Overview of the Situation Today"; Asim K. Dutt, guest editor, "Update on Tuberculosis," *Seminars in Respiratory Infections* 4, no. 3 (September 1989); Peter F. Barnes et al., "Tuberculosis in Patients with Human Immunodeficiency Virus Infection," *New England Journal of Medicine* 324 (1991): 1644–1650; "Tuberculosis Outbreak Among HIV-Infected Persons," *JAMA* 266 (1991): 2058–2061; Stephen D. Ciesielski et al., "The Epidemiology of Tuberculosis Among North Carolina Migrant Farm Workers," *JAMA* 265 (1991): 1715–1719; Dixie E. Snider, Jr., et al., "Editorial: Tuberculosis and Migrant Farm Workers," *JAMA* 265 (1991): 1732.

9. See, for example, William W. Stead and Joseph H. Bates, "Epidemiology and Prevention of Tuberculosis," in Alfred P. Fishman, ed., *Pulmonary Diseases and Disorders*, 2d ed. (New York: McGraw-Hill, 1988), 3:1795; for other relatively accessible medical overviews of tuberculosis, see A. R. Rich, *The Pathogenesis of Tuberculosis*, 2d ed. (Springfield, Ill.: Charles C. Thomas, 1951); Paul T. Chapman, "Tuberculosis," in Franklin H. Top, Sr., and Paul F. Wehrle, eds., *Communicable and Infectious Diseases*, 7th ed. (St. Louis: C. V. Mosby, 1972), chap. 67; H. William Harris and John H. McClement, "Pulmonary Tuberculosis," in Paul D. Hoeprich, ed., *Infectious Diseases*, 3d ed. (Philadelphia: Harper and Row, 1983), 378–404; and National Tuberculosis and Respiratory Disease Association, *Introduction to Respiratory Diseases*, 4th ed. (n.p.: National Tuberculosis and Respiratory Disease Association, 1969), 31–45.

10. See, for example, Centers for Disease Control, "National Action Plan to Combat Multidrug-Resistant Tuberculosis," *Morbidity and Mortality Weekly Report*, June 19, 1992, 5; "D.C. Targets Homeless in TB Battle," *Washington Post*, January 11, 1993, A12; "Tuberculosis: A Killer Returns," *New York Times*, October 11, 1992, 44; Cowley, "Tuberculosis: A Deadly Return," 54.

11. Ian Sutherland, "Recent Studies in the Epidemiology of Tuberculosis," *Advances in Tuberculosis Research* 19 (1976): 1–63: "In those in whom progressive disease develops, it does so in the great majority within at most 1 or 2 years of infection" (44). S. H. Ferebee, "Controlled Chemoprophylaxis Trials in Tuberculosis: A General Review," *Advances in Tuberculosis Research* 17

(1970): 28–106; this latter article surveys the results of thirteen controlled studies (seven in the U.S., six in other countries) concerning the "risk of infection" and the "risk of disease" among stable populations studied over a period of years, as well as the role of preventive treatment with isoniazid in reducing the risk of disease for those infected. In these trials, the results of the placebo groups provide the figures for risk of disease in the general population. For another extremely detailed epidemiological study, see J. Frimodt-Møller, "A Community-Wide Tuberculosis Study in a South Indian Rural Population, 1950–1955," *Bulletin of the World Health Organization* 22 (1960): 61–170.

12. This is the view of, among others, René Dubos, the physician and historian/philosopher of medicine. See his *Mirage of Health: Utopias, Progress, and Biological Change* (New York: Harper, 1959), 63–64.

13. Arthur M. Dannenberg, Jr., and Joseph F. Tomashefski, Jr., "Pathogenesis of Pulmonary Tuberculosis," in *Introduction to Respiratory Diseases*, 1833–1837.

14. Thomas McKeown, *The Modern Rise of Population* (London: Edward Arnold, 1976); *The Role of Medicine: Dream, Mirage, or Nemesis?* (Princeton: Princeton University Press, 1979); and *The Origins of Human Disease* (London: Basil Blackwell, 1988).

15. Simon Szreter, "The Importance of Social Intervention in Britain's Mortality Decline, 1850–1914: A Re-interpretation of the Role of Public Health," *Social History of Medicine* 1 (1988): 1–37; Allan Mitchell, "An Inexact Science: The Statistics of Tuberculosis in Late Nineteenth-Century France," *Social History of Medicine* 3 (1990): 387–403; Leonard G. Wilson, "The Historical Decline of Tuberculosis in Europe and America: Its Causes and Significance," *Journal of the History of Medicine* 45 (1990): 366–396, and "The Rise and Fall of Tuberculosis in Minnesota: The Role of Infection," *Bulletin of the History of Medicine* 66 (1992): 16–52. For a partial response to this backlash, as far as nineteenth-century France is concerned, see David S. Barnes, "The Rise or Fall of Tuberculosis in Belle-Epoque France: A Reply to Allan Mitchell," *Social History of Medicine* 5 (1992): 279–290.

16. Mitchell, "An Inexact Science" and *The Divided Path: The German Influence on Social Reform in France after 1870* (Chapel Hill: University of North Carolina Press, 1991), 252–275; see also his "Obsessive Questions and Faint Answers: The French Response to Tuberculosis in the Belle Epoque," *Bulletin of the History of Medicine* 62 (1988): 215–235.

17. For a fuller statement of this argument, see Barnes, "The Rise or Fall of Tuberculosis in Belle-Epoque France."

18. Sources for tuberculosis mortality figures: *Recherches statistiques sur la ville de Paris et le département de la Seine*, 6 vols. (Paris: various publishers, 1821–1860), 1: 37, 6: 666, 671; Jacques Bertillon, "Etudes statistiques de géographie pathologique," *Annales d'hygiène publique*, 2d series, 17 (1862): 112, 114, 122; Bertillon, *De la fréquence des principales maladies à Paris pendant la période 1865–91* (Paris: Imprimerie administrative, 1894), 130–136; *Statistique sanitaire des villes de France* (Melun: Imprimerie administrative, yearly), 1887–1913.

19. McKeown, *The Role of Medicine*, 92–96.

20. Bertillon, *De la fréquence des principales maladies,* 130–136.

21. Maurice Lévy-Leboyer and François Bourguignon, *L'Économie française au XIXe siècle* (Paris: Economica, 1985), 19.

22. *Recherches statistiques,* 1: 37, 6: 666, 671; Bertillon, *De la fréquence des principales maladies,* 133.

23. Throughout the book, conforming to nineteenth-century usage, I use the somewhat awkward term "hygienist" to refer to public health experts or professionals. Some were medical doctors, and others were not, but they all concerned themselves primarily with the study and improvement of public health.

24. See, for example, Etienne Lanthois, *Théorie nouvelle de la phthisie pulmonaire,* 3d ed. (Paris: Adrien Egron, 1822), 236–237; P. C. A. Louis, "Note sur la fréquence relative de la phthisie chez les deux sexes," *Annales d'hygiène publique,* 1st series, 6 (1831): 49–57.

25. Alain Cottereau, "La Tuberculose, maladie urbaine ou maladie de l'usure au travail?" *Sociologie du travail* (1978): 192–224.

26. The most recent and melodramatic example of this approach is Frank Ryan, *The Forgotten Plague.* Others include, to varying degrees, Pierre Guillaume, *Du désespoir au salut: Les tuberculeux aux 19e et 20e siècles* (Paris: Aubier, 1986); Mark Caldwell, *The Last Crusade: The War on Consumption, 1862–1954* (New York: Atheneum, 1988); R. Y. Keers, *Pulmonary Tuberculosis: A Journey Down the Centuries* (London: Baillière Tindall, 1978); George Jasper Wherrett, *The Miracle of the Empty Beds: A History of Tuberculosis in Canada* (Toronto: University of Toronto Press, 1977); J. Arthur Myers, *Captain of All These Men of Death: Tuberculosis Historical Highlights* (St. Louis: Warren H. Green, 1977); Harley Williams, *Requiem for a Great Killer: The Story of Tuberculosis* (London: Health Horizon, 1973); and Charles Coury, *Grandeur et déclin d'une maladie: La tuberculose au cours des âges* (Suresnes: Lepetit, 1972). Three recent exceptions to some of these historiographical tendencies are Linda Bryder, *Below the Magic Mountain;* Dominique Dessertine and Olivier Faure, *Combattre la tuberculose* (Lyon: Presses universitaires de Lyon, 1988); and Michael Teller, *The Tuberculosis Movement: A Public Health Campaign in the Progressive Era* (New York: Greenwood Press, 1988).

27. Guillaume, *Du désespoir au salut;* Dessertine and Faure, *Combattre la tuberculose;* Isabelle Grellet and Caroline Kruse, *Histoires de la tuberculose: Les fièvres de l'âme, 1800–1940* (Paris: Ramsay, 1983); Bryder, *Below the Magic Mountain;* F. B. Smith, *The Retreat of Tuberculosis, 1850–1950* (London: Croom Helm, 1988); Barbara Bates, *Bargaining for Life: A Social History of Tuberculosis, 1876–1938* (Philadelphia: University of Pennsylvania Press, 1992); Caldwell, *The Last Crusade;* Teller, *The Tuberculosis Movement;* Ryan, *The Forgotten Plague.*

28. Guillaume, *Du désespoir au salut,* 8.

29. Grellet and Kruse, *Histoires de la tuberculose,* 15.

30. Joan Wallach Scott, *Gender and the Politics of History* (New York: Columbia University Press, 1988), 8.

31. Dominique Dessertine and Olivier Faure, "Malades et sanatoriums dans l'entre-deux-guerres," and Didier Nourrisson, "Tuberculose et alcoolisme, ou

du bon usage d'un aphorisme," in Jean-Pierre Bardet et al., eds., *Peurs et ter-reurs face à la contagion: Choléra, tuberculose, syphilis, XIXe-XXe siècles* (Paris: Fayard, 1988), 218–235 and 199–217, respectively.

32. William Coleman, *Death Is a Social Disease: Public Health and Political Economy in Early Industrial France* (Madison: University of Wisconsin Press, 1982); Richard J. Evans, *Death in Hamburg: Society and Politics in the Cholera Years, 1830–1910* (Oxford: Oxford University Press, 1987).

33. David Armstrong, *Political Anatomy of the Body: Medical Knowledge in Britain in the Twentieth Century* (Cambridge: Cambridge University Press, 1983), 7–11.

34. Brandt, *No Magic Bullet,* 5.

35. Otto Lorenz, *Catalogue général de la librairie française,* vols. 8–27 (Paris: various publishers, 1880–1920).

36. Joseph Grancher, "Sur la prophylaxie de la tuberculose," *Bulletin de l'Académie de Médecine,* 3d series, 39 (1898): 470, 478–479, 481. (Emphasis added.)

37. Commission de la tuberculose, *Moyens pratiques de combattre la prop-agation de la tuberculose* (Paris: Masson, 1900).

38. Commission permanente de préservation contre la tuberculose, *Recueil des travaux,* 4 vols. (Melun: Imprimerie administrative, 1903–1913).

39. Lionel Amodru, deputy, "Rapport fait au nom de la commission d'hy-giène publique sur les mesures à prendre pour arrêter les progrès de la tubercu-lose," *Journal officiel: Annexes de la Chambre des députés,* session of June 21, 1901, 782.

40. Ibid., 785–786.

41. Ibid., 787.

42. *Le Petit Havre,* October 3, 1905, 1.

43. On this period, see especially Dessertine and Faure, *Combattre la tuber-culose,* and Lion Murard and Patrick Zylberman, "L'autre guerre (1914–1918): La santé publique en France sous l'œil de l'Amérique," *Revue historique* 276 (1986): 367–398.

44. Susanna Barrows, *Distorting Mirrors: Visions of the Crowd in Late Nineteenth-Century France* (New Haven: Yale University Press, 1981), 2.

45. Robert A. Nye, *Crime, Madness, and Politics in Modern France: The Medical Concept of National Decline* (Princeton: Princeton University Press, 1984), xii–xiii. (Emphasis in original.)

46. Ibid., 139–140.

47. Louis Chevalier, *Laboring Classes and Dangerous Classes in Paris Dur-ing the First Half of the Nineteenth Century,* trans. Frank Jellinek (Princeton: Princeton University Press, 1981); Catherine J. Kudlick, "Disease, Public Health and Urban Social Relations: Perceptions of Cholera and the Paris Environment, 1830–1850" (Ph.D. dissertation, University of California, Berkeley, 1988); see also chap. 1, below.

48. See, for example, Nye, *Crime, Madness, and Politics,* 184–185.

49. Some of the best examples of this brand of history have come from Charles Rosenberg and his colleagues and students at the University of Pennsyl-vania. See, for example, Charles E. Rosenberg, *The Care of Strangers: The Rise*

of America's Hospital System (New York: Basic Books, 1987); Rosenberg, *Explaining Epidemics and Other Studies in the History of Medicine* (Cambridge: Cambridge University Press, 1992); Charles E. Rosenberg and Janet Golden, eds., *Framing Disease: Studies in Cultural History* (New Brunswick: Rutgers University Press, 1992). Another recent book has applied this patient-centered perspective to the history of tuberculosis in the United States: Bates, *Bargaining for Life.*

50. A recent collection of essays representing this approach is Andrew Wear, ed., *Medicine in Society: Historical Essays* (Cambridge: Cambridge University Press, 1992).

CHAPTER 1. SOCIAL ANXIETY, SOCIAL DISEASE, AND THE QUESTION OF CONTAGION

1. Chevalier, *Laboring Classes and Dangerous Classes,* 45.
2. See Kudlick, "Disease, Public Health and Urban Social Relations."
3. Jules Janin, review of Balzac, *Un Grand Homme de province à Paris* [1839], quoted in Chevalier, *Laboring Classes and Dangerous Classes,* 448 n. 3.
4. Jules Janin, *Un Hiver à Paris* [1845], quoted in Chevalier, *Laboring Classes and Dangerous Classes,* p. 67.
5. Lecouturier [1849], quoted in Chevalier, *Laboring Classes and Dangerous Classes,* 374.
6. R. T. H. Laënnec, *Traité de l'auscultation médiate et des maladies des poumons et du cœur,* 2d ed. [1826], facsimile reprint (Paris: Masson, 1927), 2 vols., 1: 647; Michel Peter, *De la tuberculisation en général,* agrégation thesis, Faculté de médecine, Paris, 1866 (Paris: Lahure, 1866).
7. Erwin H. Ackerknecht, *Medicine at the Paris Hospital, 1794–1848* (Baltimore: Johns Hopkins University Press, 1967), xi–xiv.
8. Ann F. La Berge, "The Early Nineteenth-Century French Public Health Movement: The Disciplinary Development and Institutionalization of *Hygiène Publique,*" *Bulletin of the History of Medicine* 58 (1984): 364; see also her *Mission and Method: The Early Nineteenth-Century French Public Health Movement* (Cambridge: Cambridge University Press, 1991).
9. Bernard-Pierre Lécuyer, "Démographie, statistique et hygiène publique sous la monarchie censitaire," *Annales de démographie historique* (1977): 215–245, 227; Coleman, *Death Is a Social Disease.*
10. William Coleman, *Yellow Fever in the North: The Methods of Early Epidemiology* (Madison: University of Wisconsin Press, 1987).
11. In fact, Laënnec had little in common with the "romantic" antiempirical system builders of his age. For a discussion of the problems involved in the use of the term "romantic medicine," see Ackerknecht, *Medicine at the Paris Hospital,* 76, 198, and George Rosen, "Romantic Medicine: A Problem in Historical Periodization," *Bulletin of the History of Medicine* 25 (1951): 149–158. On the "romantic" mystification of tuberculosis in fiction and the arts, see chap. 2, below.
12. Ackerknecht, *Medicine at the Paris Hospital,* 92, 111, 113, 160; Acker-

knecht, "Anticontagionism between 1821 and 1867," *Bulletin of the History of Medicine* 22 (1948): 562–593; see also his "Diathesis: The Word and the Concept in Medical History," *Bulletin of the History of Medicine* 56 (1982): 317–325.

13. Laënnec, *Traité de l'auscultation médiate,* 1: 650.

14. Ibid., 649.

15. Ibid., 650–651.

16. Peter, *De la tuberculisation en général,* 75–76.

17. Laënnec, *Traité de l'auscultation médiate,* 646–647.

18. Ibid., 645; Peter, *De la tuberculisation en général,* 54; Louis-Elie Beaufort, *Considérations sur les causes et le traitement prophylactique de la phthisie pulmonaire,* thesis, Faculté de médecine, Paris, 1819 (Paris: Didot Jeune, 1819), 9–14; G. Grandclément, *Considérations sur les causes principales de la phthisie,* thesis, Faculté de médecine, Paris, 1831 (Paris: Didot Jeune, 1831).

19. Peter, *De la tuberculisation en général,* 58–59; on the later leftist critique, see chap. 7, below.

20. Louis-René Villermé, *Tableau de l'état physique et moral des ouvriers employés dans les manufactures de coton, de laine et de soie,* 2 vols. (Paris: Jules Renouard, 1840), and "De la mortalité dans les divers quartiers de Paris," *Annales d'hygiène publique et de médecine légale* 3 (1830): 294–341.

21. Coleman, *Death Is a Social Disease,* 305. (Emphasis added.)

22. Lécuyer, "Les Maladies professionnelles dans les *Annales d'hygiène publique et de médecine légale,*" *Le Mouvement social,* no. 124 (1983): 50.

23. Coleman, *Death Is a Social Disease,* esp. 149–180; Lécuyer, "Demographie, statistique et hygiène publique sous la monarchie censitaire"; Coleman reviews the somewhat complicated publishing history of these Villermé articles at page 151 n. 1. In addition to these two secondary works, I have based my analysis primarily on the last of the three main Villermé articles, "De la mortalité dans les divers quartiers de Paris," *Annales d'hygiène publique et de médecine légale* 3 (1830): 294–341.

24. Villermé, "De la mortalité," 311–312.

25. Ibid., 312.

26. Coleman, *Death Is a Social Disease,* 85–92, 241–306.

27. Lécuyer, "Les Maladies professionnelles," 56.

28. See Coleman, *Yellow Fever in the North.*

29. Henri Lombard, "De l'influence des professions sur la phthisie pulmonaire," *Annales d'hygiène publique et de médecine légale* 11 (1834): 5–69.

30. Ibid., 26–27.

31. Ibid., 28.

32. Ibid., 28–38.

33. Ibid., 39.

34. Ibid., 41–50.

35. Ibid., 39–40.

36. Ibid., 40.

37. Louis-François Benoiston de Châteauneuf, "De l'influence de certaines professions sur le développement de la phthisie pulmonaire," *Annales d'hygiène publique et de médecine légale* 6 (1831): 5–48.

38. Ibid., 43–44.

39. Ibid., 18.

40. Cottereau, "La Tuberculose, maladie urbaine ou maladie de l'usure au travail?"

41. Benoiston de Châteauneuf, "De l'influence de certaines professions," 35.

42. Ibid.

43. Ibid.

44. Ibid., 36.

45. For a discussion of the role of such narratives, which became staples of the War on Tuberculosis around the turn of the century, see chaps. 3–5, below.

46. A landmark work of this era was Alexandre Parent-Duchâtelet's study, *La Prostitution à Paris au XIXe siècle* [1836], edited by Alain Corbin (Paris: Seuil, 1981).

47. Benoiston de Châteauneuf, "De l'influence de certaines professions," 37, 39.

48. Louis, "Note sur la fréquence relative de la phthisie chez les deux sexes," 49.

49. Ackerknecht, *Medicine at the Paris Hospital*, 9–10, 102–104; Coleman, *Death Is a Social Disease*, 132–135. Louis also wrote a book on tuberculosis: *Recherches anatomiques, pathologiques et thérapeutiques sur la phthisie* (Paris: J. B. Baillière, 1843).

50. Louis, "Note sur la fréquence relative de la phthisie chez les deux sexes," 49–50.

51. Ibid., 56.

52. Ibid., 56–57.

53. Ackerknecht, "Anticontagionism between 1821 and 1867."

54. See Bruno Latour, *Les Microbes* (Paris: A. M. Métailié, 1984), 35–38, and Jacques Léonard, *La Médecine entre les pouvoirs et les savoirs* (Paris: Aubier Montaigne, 1981), 243.

55. Peter, *De la tuberculisation en général;* on the contagion question, see 62–75.

56. Germ theory in its later, more developed form would argue that while the tubercle bacillus was most often introduced into the body through inhalation, the disease could subsequently take hold in any part of the body—though pulmonary localization was most common.

57. Jules Guérin, *Discours sur la tuberculose prononcé à l'Académie impériale de médecine dans sa séance du 2 juin 1868* (Paris: Gazette médicale, 1868), 24–27.

58. A. Coriveaud, "Pidoux" (obituary), *Journal de médecine de Bordeaux*, September 10, 1882, 60–61.

59. Hermann Pidoux, in "Discussion sur la tuberculose" (at Academy of Medicine, December 3 and 10, 1867), *Bulletin de l'Académie impériale de médecine* 32 (1866–67): 1254–1255, 1261.

60. Ibid., 1248; ibid., cited in Isidore Straus, *La Tuberculose et son bacille* (Paris: Rueff, 1895), 91.

61. Pidoux, in "Discussion sur la tuberculose," 1243. (Emphasis added.)

62. Ibid., 1253–1254.

63. Ibid., 1268–1269; Pidoux, *Introduction à une doctrine nouvelle de la phthisie pulmonaire* (Paris: Asselin, 1865), 7–8, and *Etudes générales et pratiques sur la phthisie* (Paris: Asselin, 1873), 521.

64. Ibid., 519–522, 533; Pidoux, in "Discussion sur la tuberculose," 1276.

65. Pidoux, *Etudes . . . sur la phthisie,* 517–518.

66. Ibid., 521–522, 528–529.

67. Ibid., 519–522, 533.

68. Pidoux, in "Discussion sur la tuberculose," 1298.

69. On efforts to combat contagion and on related "bacillophobia," see chap. 3, below.

CHAPTER 2. REDEMPTIVE SUFFERING AND THE PATRON SAINT OF TUBERCULOSIS

1. Arthur Gold and Robert Fizdale, *The Divine Sarah: A Life of Sarah Bernhardt* (New York: Alfred A. Knopf, 1991), 3–4, 33, 276.

2. Guy Gaucher, *Histoire d'une vie: Thérèse Martin* (Paris: Editions du Cerf, 1988), 227–228.

3. The most cogent discussion of narrative as a representational strategy is Hayden White's *The Content of the Form: Narrative Discourse and Historical Representation* (Baltimore: Johns Hopkins University Press, 1987), esp. 1–25. See also chap. 3, below.

4. This choice is somewhat narrow, and certainly open to criticism. These and other literary works are discussed in relation to tuberculosis in Guillaume, *Du désespoir au salut,* 81–105 ("Phtisie et sensibilité romantique"); in René and Jean Dubos, *The White Plague: Tuberculosis, Man, and Society,* 2d ed. (New Brunswick: Rutgers University Press, 1987), 44–66 ("Consumption and the Romantic Age"); and in Grellet and Kruse, *Histoires de la tuberculose.* This selection is not meant to convey a judgment of canonical status or of literary quality. Rather, I have tried to cover (chronologically) most of the nineteenth century and to call on familiar literary and artistic works that exemplify certain broad trends and themes in French culture and also address social issues (such as prostitution, class and gender relations, labor, and poverty). In addition, all of these works refer specifically to tuberculosis (rather than vaguely to some unspecified chronic illness, as do some of the works discussed by Grellet and Kruse), and two of them provided Sarah Bernhardt with some of her most famous stage moments; for reasons discussed below, I see Bernhardt as personifying in certain ways the nineteenth-century consumptive ideal.

5. See chap. 1, above.

6. See, for example, Guillaume, *Du désespoir au salut,* 81–105, and Grellet and Kruse, *Histoires de la tuberculose,* 133–142.

7. Alexandre Dumas *fils, La Dame aux camélias* [1848] (Paris: Calmann-Lévy, 1967).

8. Ibid., 86.

9. Ibid., 93, 101.

10. Ibid., 244.

11. Carlos M. Noël, *Les Idées sociales dans le théâtre de A. Dumas fils* (Paris: Albert Messein, 1912), 42–43, 47.

12. Roger J. B. Clark, introduction to Dumas *fils, La Dame aux camélias* (London: Oxford University Press, 1972), 44–45.

13. Henry Murger, *Scènes de la vie de bohème* [1851] (Paris: Gallimard, 1988).

14. In the opera version, *La Bohème* (1896), the character of Francine is folded into that of Mimi, and Mimi's death from tuberculosis is dramatized to such an extent that it plays a much more prominent part in the opera than does Francine's in the novel; as a result, later opera audiences perceive the death originally intended for Francine as more central to the drama than it is in Murger's text.

15. Murger, *Scènes de la vie de bohème*, 216–217.

16. See chap. 1, above.

17. Murger, *Scènes de la vie de bohème*, 281–282.

18. Ibid., 283–284, 287–289, 291.

19. Victor Hugo, *Les Misérables* [1862], trans. Lee Fahnestock and Norman MacAfee (New York: New American Library, 1987), 187.

20. Ibid., 182, 200–201, 257, 283–284, 294.

21. Jane P. Tompkins, "Sentimental Power: *Uncle Tom's Cabin* and the Politics of Literary History," in Elaine Showalter, ed., *The New Feminist Criticism: Essays on Women, Literature, and Theory* (New York: Pantheon, 1985), 81–104; quotation at 85.

22. Edmond and Jules de Goncourt, *Germinie Lacerteux* [1864] (Naples: Edizioni Scientifiche Italiane, 1982).

23. Ibid., 101–102.

24. Ibid., 142, 164.

25. Edmond and Jules de Goncourt, *Madame Gervaisais* [1869] (Paris: Gallimard, 1982), 93, 241.

26. Ibid., 209–210, 228.

27. Ibid., 241.

28. Elaine Aston, *Sarah Bernhardt: A French Actress on the English Stage* (Oxford: Berg, 1989), 122.

29. Edmond Rostand, *L'Aiglon* [1900] (Paris: Gallimard, 1986), 226.

30. Ibid., 90, 139.

31. Ibid., 231–236.

32. Ibid., 360–361.

33. Ibid., 360–361, 429 n. 109.

34. Among the best biographies of Thérèse are Gaucher, *Histoire d'une vie: Thérèse Martin*; Monica Furlong, *Thérèse of Lisieux* (New York: Pantheon, 1987); Jean-François Six, *Thérèse de Lisieux au Carmel* (Paris: Seuil, 1973); and René Laurentin, *Thérèse de Lisieux: Mythes et réalité* (Paris: Beauchesne, 1972).

35. Gérard Cholvy and Yves-Marie Hilaire, *Histoire religieuse de la France contemporaine, 1880–1930* (Toulouse: Privat, 1986), 142, 325–329; Furlong,

Thérèse of Lisieux, 124–128; Gaucher, *Histoire d'une vie,* 231–234.

36. See, for example, *Story of a Soul,* 157–159, 211; Furlong, *Thérèse of Lisieux,* 85–86.

37. *Story of a Soul,* 210–211.

38. Ibid., 210, 215, 265.

39. Furlong, *Thérèse of Lisieux,* 114–115.

40. John Clarke, ed., *St. Thérèse of Lisieux: Her Last Conversations* (Washington, D.C.: Institute of Carmelite Studies, 1977), 80, 98, 108.

41. Ibid., 217, 224. (Emphasis in original.)

42. Ibid., 224. This scene is rendered brilliantly in the film *Thérèse,* directed by Alain Cavalier (UGC Films, 1986).

43. Clarke, *St. Thérèse of Lisieux,* 229–230. (Ellipses in original.)

44. Ibid., 205, 230. (Ellipses in original.)

45. Joan Jacobs Brumberg, *Fasting Girls: The Emergence of Anorexia Nervosa as a Modern Disease* (Cambridge: Harvard University Press, 1988), 41–47.

46. Ibid., 61–100.

47. Ibid., 100.

48. Aston, *Sarah Bernhardt,* 48.

49. Susan Sontag, *Illness as Metaphor* (New York: Farrar, Straus and Giroux, 1978), 34–35; see also her *AIDS and Its Metaphors* (New York: Farrar, Straus and Giroux, 1989).

50. Claudine Herzlich and Janine Pierret, *Malades d'hier, malades d'aujourd'hui* (Paris: Payot, 1984), chap. 2, "De la phtisie à la tuberculose," 48–64.

51. Nicole Priollaud, "Avertissement," in Priollaud, ed., *La Femme au 19ᵉ siècle* (Paris: Levi/Messinger, 1983), 9. To a great extent, this was an international cultural phenomenon; in Anglo-Saxon cultures, as Sandra Gilbert and Susan Gubar have noted, society told women "that if they d[id] not behave like angels they must be monsters." In fact, they argue, the understanding of womanhood as inherently pathological so thoroughly penetrated society that, in addition to training girls in "docility, submissiveness, self-lessness . . . [and] renunciation . . . nineteenth-century culture seems to have actually admonished women to *be* ill." Sandra M. Gilbert and Susan Gubar, *The Madwoman in the Attic: The Woman Writer and the Nineteenth-Century Literary Imagination* (New Haven: Yale University Press, 1979), 53–54. (Emphasis in original.)

52. White, *The Content of the Form,* 1–25.

CHAPTER 3. *"GUERRE AU BACILLE!"*

1. See chap. 5, below.

2. I use this neologism to indicate not a single tenet or argument in discussions of the causes and prevention of tuberculosis but rather a general preoccupation with "seed" over "soil," with contagion over receptivity, and with the tracking down, isolation, and neutralization of the tubercle bacillus.

3. Louis Landouzy, "Comment et pourquoi on devient tuberculeux" (lecture series, Hôpital de la Charité, 1881), *Le Progrès médical* (1882): 685.

4. Ibid., 666–667.

5. Ibid., 667.

6. See, for example, the thematic issue of the journal *Literature and Medicine* (vol. 11, no. 1 [Spring 1992]) entitled "The Art of the Case History," and Kathryn Montgomery Hunter, *Doctors' Stories: The Narrative Structure of Medical Knowledge* (Princeton: Princeton University Press, 1991).

7. Hunter, *Doctors' Stories*, 152–153.

8. These categories break down roughly as follows:

> Annals typically list "events" without interpretation or conclusion: "Interval 1: The King died. Interval 2: Crops failed. Interval 3: the Queen died." A chronicle introduces selectivity and sequence, the germ of a story, but still lacks closure: "The King died, then the Queen died." Narrative implies causality or the operation of a moral principle: "The King died; then the Queen died of grief."

Ibid., 186 n. 5; Hayden White, "The Value of Narrativity in the Representation of Reality," *Critical Inquiry* 7 (1980): 5–27.

9. White, *The Content of the Form*, 1–25, quotation at 14.

10. Landouzy, "Comment et pourquoi on devient tuberculeux," 701–702.

11. Ibid., 701.

12. See chap. 1, above.

13. Landouzy, "Comment et pourquoi on devient tuberculeux," 702–703.

14. Jules Rochard, *Traité d'hygiène sociale* (Paris: Delahaye et Lecrosnier, 1888), 536–560.

15. See, for example, Latour, *Les Microbes*.

16. Michel Peter, *Leçons de clinique médicale,* vol. 3 (Paris: Asselin et Houzeau, 1893), 44–45, 57–58.

17. Ibid., 171.

18. See, for example, A. Mirabail, "Baiser et tuberculose," *La Médication martiale* (1904): 552–553.

19. Isidore Straus, *La Tuberculose et son bacille*, 466–468.

20. Charles Fauchon, *La Tuberculose, question sociale* (Paris: Asselin et Houzeau, 1903), 70; Albert Calmette, "La Lutte contre la tuberculose," *Revue philanthropique* 21 (1907): 570–571. (Emphasis in original.)

21. Edouard Fuster, "La Tuberculose, maladie sociale," *Revue d'hygiène et de police sanitaire* (1904): 27. (Emphasis in original.)

22. This phrase recurred quite frequently in antituberculosis literature; see, among others, Ernest Fernbach, *Deux conférences sur la tuberculose* (Paris: Fernand Nathan, n.d.): 10.

23. Allan Mitchell discusses spitting and the turn-of-the-century campaign against tuberculosis in "Obsessive Questions and Faint Answers: The French Response to Tuberculosis in the Belle Epoque," *Bulletin of the History of Medicine* 62 (1988): 215–235, esp. 223–225.

24. L.B., untitled article in *Hygiène ouvrière* (1912): 3–4.

25. Maurice Letulle, "La Lutte contre la tuberculose en France: Prophylaxie et traitement hygiénique dans les milieux ouvriers," *Bulletin mensuel de l'Alliance syndicale du commerce et de l'industrie* (January 1902): 11–14.

26. The space occupied by a sick worker in a factory or workshop was seen as particularly dangerous:

Ouvriers, qui travaillez dans des ateliers, vous connaissez tous la place maudite: vous savez que vous ne pouvez vous asseoir à cette place sans risquer de contracter la phtisie. Pourquoi: Parce qu'un de vos camarades, malade[,] y a travaillé, parce qu'il a éternué, toussé à cette place, parce qu'il a répandu ses crachats tout autour. Ces crachats se sont desséchés, se sont réduits en poussières; à chaque pas que vous faites vous soulevez ces poussières et vous respirez des bacilles tuberculeux par milliers.

Fernbach, *Deux conférences,* 7–8.

27. Roger Reveillaud, *La Tuberculose au point de vue social,* thesis, Faculté de médecine, Paris, 1908 (Paris: A. Maloine, 1908), 80.

28. Alain Corbin, *Le Miasme et la jonquille: L'odorat et l'imaginaire social, XVIIIe–XIXe siècles* (Paris: Flammarion, 1986); on attitudes toward crowding and filth in working-class housing, see chap. 4, below.

29. Norbert Elias, *The History of Manners,* trans. Edmund Jephcott (New York: Pantheon, 1978), 153–160.

30. Fuster, "La Tuberculose," 28.

31. Fauchon, *La Tuberculose,* 67–80.

32. See, for example, Samuel Bernheim and André Roblot, "Tuberculose et blanchisseries," *L'Hygiène familiale* (February 1906): 54–57.

33. Doctor Ox, "Livres et microbes," *Le Matin,* December 28, 1905.

34. Ibid.

35. Paul Cuq, "Le Baiser et ses dangers au point de vue de la tuberculose," *La Médication martiale* (1904): 481.

36. "Hygiène des bureaux de poste," *Revue médicale,* November 15, 1905, 912.

37. Fauchon, *La Tuberculose,* 62–64.

38. Fuster, "La Tuberculose," 28.

39. Reveillaud, *La Tuberculose au point de vue social,* 18–19.

40. "Recommandations publiées sur l'avis du Comité permanent de défense contre les épidémies et de la Société de préservation contre la tuberculose," *Bulletin municipal officiel,* Paris, September 23, 1905, 3293.

41. Reveillaud, *La Tuberculose au point de vue social,* 85; Fernbach, *Deux conférences,* 10.

42. Archives nationales [A.N.], C 7324, dossier 1496.

43. Archives Municipales de Nantes [A.M. Nantes], I^5, carton 20, dossier 1, and M^3, carton 4, dossier 5. See chap. 6, below, for similar dispensary-related controversies in Le Havre.

44. *La Ligue contre la tuberculose en Touraine contre M. le Comte de Lafont* (Tours: Paul Salmon, 1906), 8–12.

45. Ibid., 10, 20–22.

46. By this imprecise term, I mean the speeches, writings, and other works of the governmental officials, hygienists, professors, and doctors affiliated with the most prominent (usually Parisian) institutions prosecuting the War on Tuberculosis, including the Academy of Medicine, the Paris medical faculty, prestigious medical journals, and committees such as the Commission permanente de préservation contre la tuberculose.

47. Fuster, "La Tuberculose," 30.

48. Paul Brouardel, cited in Xavier Jousset, *Transmission de la tuberculose*

dans les rapports sociaux, thesis, Faculté de médecine, Paris, 1908 (Paris: Imprimerie de la Faculté de médecine, 1908), 7.

49. See, for example, his contribution to P. Budin et al., *Les Applications sociales de la solidarité* (Paris: Félix Alcan, 1904); the ramifications of solidarism on the War on Tuberculosis are discussed in chap. 4, below.

50. All cited in Doctor Ox, "Théorie et pratique," *Le Matin,* September 14, 1913.

51. Cited ibid.

52. Paul Cuq, "Le Baiser et ses dangers au point de vue de la tuberculose," *La Médication martiale* (1904): 479.

53. Ibid., 479–480.

54. Ibid., 480–481.

55. Mirabail, "Baiser et tuberculose," 552–553.

56. Ibid., 553.

57. Lucien Descaves, "Les Pestiférés," *Le Journal,* February 14, 1906.

58. Jousset, *Transmission de la tuberculose.* See chap. 7 on left-wing perspectives, below, for the full elaboration of class analysis as applied to tuberculosis at the time; the syndicalist and socialist "dissenters" were different in many respects from the likes of Cuq, Descaves, and Jousset, but they shared an emphasis on terrain and a deemphasis on contagion in the spread of tuberculosis.

59. Adolphe Leray, *Genèse de la tuberculose dans l'espèce humaine: Contagion ou auto-infection?* (Paris: Vigot Frères, 1906), 14–19.

60. Ibid., 18, 67–68.

61. Ibid., 32.

62. Ibid., 39.

63. Ibid., 74. (Paragraph separations omitted.)

64. Marcel Moine, *Recherches et considérations générales sur la mortalité à Paris depuis la Restauration* (Paris: Union des Caisses d'Assurances Sociales de la Région Parisienne, 1941), 25.

65. Georges Bourgeois, *Exode rural et tuberculose,* thesis, Faculté de médecine, Paris, 1904 (Paris: Félix Alcan, 1904), Table X.

66. Grellet and Kruse, *Histoires de la tuberculose,* 36–47, 95–107; Guillaume, *Du désespoir au salut,* 43–80. On the waxing and waning of symptoms with alternating periods of work and rest, see, for example, Marc Pierrot, "La Lutte contre la tuberculose et la question des sanatoriums," *Les Temps nouveaux,* nineteen installments between July 23–29 and December 10–16, 1904.

67. The best analysis of this aspect of "medicalization" in nineteenth-century France is Léonard, *La Médecine entre les pouvoirs et les savoirs;* see also Jack D. Ellis, *The Physician-Legislators of France: Medicine and Politics in the Early Third Republic, 1870–1914* (Cambridge: Cambridge University Press, 1990).

68. Grellet and Kruse, *Histoires de la tuberculose,* 36–47, 95–107; Guillaume, *Du désespoir au salut,* 43–80.

69. This imitation apparently began quite soon after the "preventorium" began operations in Lille. For example, it was evident in the announcement of the opening of a dispensary in Poitiers in February 1903. "Echos et nouvelles," *Revue internationale de la tuberculose* (February 1903): 150.

70. Albert Calmette, Désiré Verhæghe, and Th. Wœhrel, *Les Préventoriums, ou dispensaires de prophylaxie sociale antituberculeuse: Le Préventorium "Emile Roux" de Lille* (Lille: L. Danel, 1905), 5–6, 21.

71. Ibid., p. 22.

72. Calmette, "Nécessité du dispensaire," *L'Idéal du foyer,* May 1, 1903, 1.

73. Camille Savoire, discussion of Fuster's "La Tuberculose, maladie sociale," Société de médecine publique, meeting of December 23, 1903, *Revue d'hygiène et de police sanitaire* (1904): 158.

74. Alfred Fillassier, review of Ambroise Rendu, "Du rôle du dispensaire dans la lutte contre la tuberculose" [no further attribution given], in *L'Hygiène générale et appliquée* 3 (1908): 244–245.

75. Dr. Ernest Boureille, letter to the mayor of Le Havre, November 13, 1903, in Archives municipales du Havre [A.M.H.], Fonds contemporain [F.C.], M³2:6.

76. "Dispensaire du 6ᵉ canton de Nantes et de la commune de Chantenay crée pour la préservation et la guérison de la tuberculose," in A.M. Nantes, Q⁵12: 9, pp. 3–5, 8–14.

77. Since this question was never explicitly addressed, it is a murky area. But such phrases as "Si vous le voulez, vous supprimez les causes prédisposantes" and "Défiez-vous de la salive d'un tuberculeux" certainly imply that the intended reader would be avoiding tuberculosis for himself or herself. Ibid. See also, for the context in which the "catechisms" were given out, "Dispensaire de l'Œuvre Antituberculeuse de la Loire-Inférieure: Son fonctionnement depuis le 1ᵉʳ novembre 1904 au 30 avril 1905," A.M. Nantes, series Q⁵, carton 12.

78. Marius Devèze, "Proposition de loi tendant à la création de dispensaires antituberculeux dans les principaux centres," in A.N., C 7470: 1810, 7–8; Fuster, "La Tuberculose," 37.

79. Fuster, "La Tuberculose," 28.

80. Emile Vallin, "Compte-rendu des travaux des conseils d'hygiène," *Revue d'hygiène et de police sanitaire* 2 (1880): 780–782.

81. See, for example, Fauchon, *La Tuberculose,* 90–97.

82. Calmette, Verhæghe, and Wœhrel, *Les Préventoriums,* 3–4. (Emphasis in original.)

83. Dessertine and Faure, "Malades et sanatoriums dans l'entre-deux-guerres."

84. Fuster, "La Tuberculose," 28, 33.

85. Ibid., 32. (Emphasis in original.)

86. Jules Héricourt, "La Lutte contre la tuberculose," *La Revue,* October 1, 1905, 296–297.

87. Ibid.

88. Mireya Navarro, "Confinement for TB: Weighing Rights vs. Health, " *New York Times,* November 21, 1993. See also Michael Specter, "TB Carriers See Clash of Liberty and Health," *New York Times,* October 14, 1992; "Tuberculosis: A Deadly Return," *Newsweek,* March 16, 1992, 57.

89. Jules Héricourt, *Le Terrain dans les maladies* (Paris: E. Flammarion, 1927); Léonard, *La Médecine entre les pouvoirs et les savoirs.*

90. Michel Foucault, *Discipline and Punish: The Birth of the Prison,* trans. Alan Sheridan (New York: Pantheon, 1977), 304.

91. Ibid., 299.

92. Ibid., 297, 299, 302–303.

93. Recently, increased attention has been paid to the careful and effective orchestration of Pasteur's most famous experiments. See especially Bruno Latour, "Give Me a Laboratory and I Will Raise the World," in Karin D. Knorr-Cetina and Michael Mulkay, eds., *Science Observed: Perspectives on the Social Study of Science* (London: Sage, 1983), 141–170; see also Latour, *Les Microbes,* and Gerald Geison, "Pasteur, Roux and Rabies: Scientific versus Clinical Mentalities," *Journal of the History of Medicine and Allied Sciences* 45 (1990): 341–365.

94. Fauchon, *La Tuberculose,* 65–67, 81–82.

95. Paul Juillerat, "Le Choix d'un logement," *Annuaire de la tuberculose, 1907,* 166. (Emphasis added.)

96. See, for example, the numerous statistical tables in Bourgeois, *Exode rural et tuberculose.*

CHAPTER 4. INTERIORS

1. Cottereau, "La Tuberculose, maladie urbaine ou maladie de l'usure au travail?" One need not accept Cottereau's conclusions or adopt his political point of view to recognize this "ecological slippage" as a characteristic feature of the nineteenth-century science of public health.

2. Ann-Louise Shapiro, *Housing the Poor of Paris, 1850–1902* (Madison: University of Wisconsin Press, 1985), 82–83.

3. This description, which encompasses the following four block quotations, appeared in Robert Savary and Dr. Collet, "La Lutte contre la tuberculose en France," *Annales des sciences politiques* (1904): 490–491.

4. Ibid., 490; Georges Faugère, *La Défense individuelle contre la tuberculose* (Paris: Baillière, 1905): 15–16; Lucien Graux, "Les Causes sociales de la tuberculose," *Revue du XXe siècle* (January 1903): 18. See chap. 3, above, for a discussion of the hygienists' disgust.

5. Alain Corbin, *Le Miasme et la jonquille: L'odorat et l'imaginaire social, XVIIIe-XIXe siècles* (Paris: Flammarion, 1986); see esp. 263–270. The following comment applies particularly well to the War on Tuberculosis:

> Il faut toutefois prendre garde de ne pas exagérer la modernité des attitudes. . . . L'alliance entre le germe et la saleté—désormais identifiée à la crasse et à la poussière—fait toujours figure de dogme. . . . La puanteur n'est plus morbifique, mais elle présage la présence pathogène. Le peuple nauséabond a perdu son monopole infect, mais il demeure au plus haut point menaçant.

Ibid., 264–265.

6. Faugère, *La Défense individuelle:* 17; Graux, "Les Causes sociales de la tuberculose," 19. Actually, the earliest usages of the word *promiscuity* in English, dating from the mid-nineteenth century, closely resemble the French usage. One citation from 1868 in the *Oxford English Dictionary* refers to "men, women children huddled together in dirt, disorder, and promiscuity like that of

the lower animals." *The Compact Edition of the Oxford English Dictionary,* 2 vols. (Oxford: Oxford University Press, 1971), 2: 2322. Compare the current French definition of *promiscuité:* "Situation d'une personne placée dans un voisinage jugé désagréable ou choquant." *Petit Larousse illustré* (Paris: Larousse, 1983), 813.

7. On the commissions des logements insalubres, see, for example, Shapiro, *Housing the Poor of Paris,* 24–32.

8. Paul Juillerat, *Une Institution nécessaire: Le casier sanitaire des maisons* (Paris: Chaix, 1906), 30–33; arrêtés préfectoraux du 1 et 28 février 1893, in *Recueil des actes administratifs de la Préfecture du Département de la Seine,* 50ᵉ année (1893), Partie municipale (Paris: Imprimerie municipale, 1894), 69–70.

9. Juillerat, *Une Institution nécessaire.*

10. Juillerat, *Rapport à M. le Préfet sur les recherches effectuées au Bureau du casier sanitaire pendant l'année 1907* ... (Paris: Chaix, 1908), 7, 65; Juillerat, *Rapport à M. le Préfet sur les recherches effectuées au Bureau du casier sanitaire pendant l'année 1908* ... (Paris: Chaix, 1909), 109.

11. Paul Juillerat and Louis Bonnier, *Rapport à M. le Préfet sur les enquêtes effectuées en 1906 dans les maisons signalées comme foyers de tuberculose* (Paris: Chaix, 1907), 4.

12. Conseil municipal de Paris, *Rapport ... sur l'organisation du Bureau d'hygiène de la ville de Paris* (Paris: Imprimerie municipale, 1907), 284, 289–290, 303.

13. "Assainie" meant that the prescriptions of the casier sanitaire inspectors had been carried out. Approximately one-third of the prescribed remedies were actually prohibitions on the occupation of given units, in which cases keeping the units vacant—rather than any structural improvements—would constitute compliance and *assainissement.*

14. Juillerat, *Rapport à M. le Préfet sur les recherches effectuées au Bureau du casier sanitaire pendant l'année 1910* ... (Paris: Chaix, 1911), 6–8.

15. Ibid., 5; Juillerat, *Rapport à M. le Préfet ... 1908,* 5–7; Juillerat, *Rapport à M. le Préfet ... 1907,* 6.

16. Juillerat, *Rapport à M. le Préfet ... 1908,* 5.

17. Juillerat, *Rapport à M. le Préfet ... 1907,* 7, 63.

18. A.N., C 7470: 1798; Ellis, *The Physician-Legislators of France,* 188. On the problem of obligation versus voluntarism in French social welfare legislation in the Third Republic, see Mitchell, *The Divided Path.*

19. Victor-Henri Hutinel, "La Tuberculose, maladie sociale," *Gazette des hôpitaux* (1905): 1555.

20. Ibid., 1555–1556.

21. "E.L.," untitled article, *Revue socialiste* (July 1911): 24–32.

22. Ibid., 33–34.

23. For a more complete discussion of the extent to which socialists accepted the dominant etiology, see chap. 7, below.

24. Fernand Pelloutier and Maurice Pelloutier, *La Vie ouvrière en France* (Paris: Schleicher Frères, 1900), 256.

25. Juillerat, *Rapport à M. le Préfet ... 1908,* 115–117.

26. Ibid., 115–117, 119–121.

27. Alfred Fillassier, *Les Casiers sanitaires des villes et les œuvres d'assistance: Entente nécessaire,* Académie des sciences morales et politiques, séance du 28 octobre 1905 (Paris: Jules Rousset, 1906), 2.

28. Ibid., 4–8.

29. Conseil municipal de Paris, *Rapport . . . sur l'organisation du Bureau d'hygiène de la ville de Paris,* 305.

30. Juillerat, *Rapport à M. le Préfet . . . 1908,* 110. (Emphasis added.)

31. Louis Landouzy, *La Lutte contre la tuberculose* (Paris: L. Maretheux, 1902), 68–69.

32. The word *cabaret* is used here (following the usage of the time) to indicate any drinking establishment. See chap. 5, below.

33. For a discussion of core narratives, see chap. 3, above.

34. Jeanne Leroy-Allais, "Leçon de ménage et d'hygiène," *L'Idéal du foyer,* May 1, 1903, 122–124. (Emphasis in original.)

35. Ibid., 124.

36. Ibid. (Last ellipses in original.)

37. Ibid. (Ellipses in original.)

38. Ibid.

39. [Albert Calmette,] "Organisation et fonctionnement des Préventoriums," in Calmette, Verhæghe, and Wœhrel, *Les Préventoriums,* 20.

40. Ch. Leroux and W. Grunberg, "Enquête sur la descendance de 442 familles ouvrières tuberculeuses," *Revue de médecine* 32 (1912): 938.

41. Landouzy, *La Lutte contre la tuberculose,* 53–54. (Emphasis in original.)

42. Ibid., 54.

43. Ibid., 54–55.

44. Fuster, "La Tuberculose, maladie sociale," 40.

45. Madame le Dr. Edwards-Pilliet, "Conférence féministe de vulgarisation antituberculeuse: Du rôle de la femme dans la lutte antituberculeuse," *Revue internationale de la tuberculose* (June 1902): 415.

46. Ibid. (Emphasis added.)

47. Ibid., 415–416.

48. Bonnie Smith, *Ladies of the Leisure Class: The Bourgeoises of Northern France in the Nineteenth Century* (Princeton: Princeton University Press, 1981), 123–161, esp. 138.

49. The case of AIDS in the twentieth century is instructive on this point. To counter the widespread perception that only deviants of some sort get AIDS (a perception fostered by the commonly accepted social etiology of the disease), a vigorous educational campaign was launched whose message was "Anyone can get AIDS." Of course, even to the extent this constantly repeated message is consciously accepted among the population, it does not negate or even diminish the social stigma of the disease. A constant tension operates between the need to find scapegoats or to stigmatize and the need to fight complacency among nonstigmatized groups.

50. Graux, "Les Causes sociales de la tuberculose," 19.

51. Juillerat, "Le Choix d'un logement," *Annuaire de la tuberculose* (1907): 170–171.

52. Ibid., 173–175.

53. M. le Dr. Zuber, "Secret médical et tuberculose des domestiques," *La Revue médicale* (November 22, 1905): 929.

54. Ibid.

55. Ibid.

56. Ibid.

57. Ibid., 929–930.

58. A.N., C 7470: 1798.

CHAPTER 5. MORALITY AND MORTALITY

1. Louis Rénon, *Les Maladies populaires: Maladies vénériennes, alcoolisme, tuberculose* (Paris: Masson, 1905).

2. Around the turn of the century in France, the word *cabaret* did not specifically indicate a "café-concert" or "nightclub" type of establishment, as it does in English today. Equivalent to *débit de boissons,* it is used here (as it was then) to indicate any drinking establishment, including *marchands de vin, estaminets, brasseries, bistrots,* cafés, etc.

3. H. Triboulet, "Alcool—Tuberculose," *Congrès international de la tuberculose* (Paris, October 2–7, 1905), 3: 226. (Emphasis in original.)

4. Present-day medical textbooks generally regard alcoholism as a major "risk factor" predisposing to tuberculosis, based both on statistical correlations and the "considerable evidence that alcohol alters the defences of the body against infection and . . . assists the development of respiratory disease." The literature includes no such specific link between syphilis and tuberculosis. Among the several complications of syphilis listed in one textbook, tuberculosis is absent; in another, alcoholism is joined by "any chronic debilitating disease" among the risk factors for tuberculosis. William W. Stead and Asim K. Dutt, "Epidemiology and Host Factors," in David Schlossberg, ed., *Tuberculosis* (New York: Praeger, 1983), 12; Harold A. Lyons, "The Respiratory System and Specifics of Alcoholism," in E. Mansell Pattison and Edward Kaufman, eds., *Encyclopedic Handbook of Alcoholism* (New York: Gardner Press, 1982), 329; D. H. Marjot, "Mortality and Alcoholism," in P. Golding, ed., *Alcoholism: Analysis of a World-Wide Problem* (Lancaster: MTP Press, 1982), 247; Konrad Wicher and Victoria Wicher, "Syphilis," in Tsieh Sun, ed., *Sexually Related Infectious Diseases* (New York: Field, Rich, 1986), 23.

5. See Daniel Pick, *Faces of Degeneration: A European Disorder, c. 1848–1918* (Cambridge: Cambridge University Press, 1989).

6. Louis Chevalier, *La Formation de la population parisienne au XIXe siècle* (Paris: Presses Universitaires de France, 1950) and *Laboring Classes and Dangerous Classes.*

7. Theodore Zeldin, *France 1848–1945: Ambition and Love* (Oxford: Oxford University Press, 1979), 171–173; B. R. Mitchell, *European Historical Statistics, 1750–1975,* 2d rev. ed. (New York: Facts on File, 1981), 68–70; Bour-

geois, *Exode rural et tuberculose.*

8. For a discussion of "core narratives," see chap. 3, above.

9. Reveillaud, *La Tuberculose au point de vue social,* 64–65.

10. Fauchon, *La Tuberculose, question sociale,* 10–11.

11. Louis Renault, *La Tuberculose chez les Bretons,* cited in Bourgeois, *Exode rural et tuberculose,* 25–26.

12. Ibid., 26.

13. Hutinel, "La Tuberculose, maladie sociale," 1553.

14. Bourgeois, *Exode rural et tuberculose,* 78; Louis Cruveilhier, *Retour de la grande ville et tuberculose à la campagne* (Paris: Octave Doin, 1908), 5.

15. Bourgeois, *Exode rural et tuberculose,* 39. (Emphasis added.)

16. Ibid., 84–85.

17. Hutinel used a similar narrative to illustrate the migration–cabaret–tuberculosis cycle.

> Son alimentation est souvent insuffisante, son logis presque toujours étroit et mal ventilé; d'ailleurs il le déserte volontiers pour le cabaret où il glisse sur la pente de l'alcoolisme.... *L'alcoolisme* qui prend l'ouvrier au sortir du travail est en grande partie la conséquence [de] notre régime économique. Ne pouvant satisfaire son besoin de sociabilité, dans son intérieur dénué et misérable, l'ouvrier va au cabaret. «Là, pour quelques sous, il est le bienvenu et avec quelques verres à peine il peut s'évader un moment de la vie de souffrance et de privations dans laquelle demain le rejettera.» Or l'alcool est un poison phtisiogène.

Hutinel, "La Tuberculose, maladie sociale," 1553–1555.

18. For example, Cruveilhier explained that in his calculations, departments containing large cities were anomalous because they were loci of *immigration* more significantly than of *emigration* to Paris; wealthier regions such as Burgundy were anomalous because the stabling of animals was more widespread there, and those animals played a greater role in the spread of tuberculosis than did migration to Paris; and finally, coastal departments were anomalous because "there, tuberculosis is ordinarily a function of causes other than emigration." Cruveilhier, *Retour de la grande ville et tuberculose à la campagne,* 5.

19. Ibid., 7–8.

20. Ibid., 9.

21. "Il faut séparer les tuberculeux, rétrécir autant que faire se peut la sphère dans laquelle ils sont susceptibles de disséminer le germe morbide qu'ils portent et répandent. Il faut améliorer la police sanitaire des grandes cités." Bourgeois, *Exode rural et tuberculose,* 114.

22. See, for example, Bourgeois, *Exode rural et tuberculose,* 114.

23. M. Plicque, quoted in Bourgeois, *Exode rural et tuberculose,* 111–112.

24. Reconciling city and countryside via technological innovation surfaces in other policies and proposals as well, including efforts to recycle Paris sewage as countryside fertilizer. See Donald Reid, *Paris Sewers and Sewermen: Realities and Representations* (Cambridge: Harvard University Press, 1991), 53–70.

25. Graux, "Les Causes sociales de la tuberculose," 27.

26. Nourrisson, "Tuberculose et alcoolisme, ou du bon usage d'un aphorisme."

27. Cadet de Gassicourt, "Alcool," *Dictionnaire des sciences médicales* (Paris: C. L. F. Panckoucke, 1812), 1: 306; "Alcool," *Dictionnaire de médecine et de chirurgie pratiques* (Paris: Gabon, Méquignon-Marvis, J. B. Baillière, Crochard, 1829), 1: 468–469. See also "Alcool," *Dictionnaire de médecine,* 2d ed. (Paris: Béchet, 1833), 2: 140, 143–144.

28. Charles Roesch, "De l'abus des boissons spiritueuses," *Annales d'hygiène publique et de médecine légale* 20 (1838): 63–90.

29. Ibid., 304–311.

30. A. Fabre, "De l'alcoolisme pulmonaire," *Gazette des hôpitaux* 41 (1868): 493–494.

31. Ibid.

32. Ibid.

33. Ibid.

34. Louis Landouzy, "Comment et pourquoi on devient tuberculeux," 648, 684.

35. Joseph Grancher and Victor-Henri Hutinel, "Phthisie," *Dictionnaire encyclopédique des sciences médicales* (Paris: Masson, 1887), 24: 571.

36. Victor Hanot, "Phthisie," *Nouveau dictionnaire de médecine et de chirurgie pratiques* (Paris: J.B. Baillière, 1888), 27: 505–506.

37. Ibid., 506.

38. Constantin Thiron, "L'Alcoolisme, considéré comme une des grandes causes prédisposantes, par hérédité ou acquise individuellement, de la tuberculose," Congrès pour l'étude de la tuberculose chez l'homme et chez les animaux (Paris, 1898), *Comptes rendus et mémoires* (Paris: Masson, 1898), 737–749.

39. Ibid., 737–742.

40. Ibid., 748. (Emphasis in original.)

41. Ibid., 749.

42. L. Jacquet, "La Croisade contre la tuberculose et l'alcoolisme," *La Tribune médicale,* 2d series, 32 (1900): 701; E. de Lavarenne, "Alcoolisme et tuberculose," in Commission de la tuberculose, *Moyens pratiques de combattre la propagation de la tuberculose* (Paris: Masson, 1900), 299–302.

43. De Lavarenne, "Alcoolisme et tuberculose," 290.

44. Ibid., 295.

45. Rénon, *Les Maladies populaires,* 14.

46. Ibid., 296–297.

47. For the history of neo-Malthusianism in France, see Francis Ronsin, *La Grève des ventres: Propagande néo-Malthusienne et baisse de la natalite francaise, XIXe–XXe siècles* (Paris: Aubier Montaigne, 1980); Andre Armengaud, *Les Français et Malthus* (Paris: Presses universitaires de France, 1975); and A. Drouard, "Les Sources de l'eugénisme en France: Le néo-Malthusianisme (1896–1914)," *Population* 47 (1992): 435–460.

48. Isidore-Paul-Alphonse Ladevèze, *Comment les familles ouvrières parisiennes disparaissent par tuberculose,* thesis, Faculté de médecine, Paris, 1901 (Paris: Imprimerie de la Faculté de médecine, 1901), 44–47.

49. Ibid.

50. Ibid. The revolutionary syndicalists and other left-wing critics of the

dominant etiology attributed the gender differential to the pathogenic effects of overwork among men. See chap. 7, below.

51. Jacques Bertillon, "Alcool et phtisie," *Archives d'anthropologie criminelle* 25 (1910): 203–205.

52. Ibid., 208.

53. Ibid., 209.

54. Ibid.

55. Ibid., 202. Of course, research cited in Hanot's 1888 medical encyclopedia article reached precisely the opposite conclusion—that *cabaretiers* suffered very rarely from tuberculosis.

56. Robert Romme, *La Lutte sociale contre la tuberculose* (Paris: Masson, 1901), 32–36.

57. Louis Landouzy, *Le Rôle des facteurs sociaux dans l'étiologie de la tuberculose* (Paris: Masson, 1912), 21–22. (Emphasis added.)

58. Raoul Brunon, *La Tuberculose: Maladie évitable, maladie curable* (Paris: Steinheil, 1913), 167–168. (Emphasis added.)

59. Susanna Barrows, " 'Parliaments of the People': The Political Culture of Cafés in the Early Third Republic," in Susanna Barrows and Robin Room, eds., *Drinking: Behavior and Belief in Modern History* (Berkeley, Los Angeles, and London: University of California Press, 1991), 87–97; Didier Nourrisson, *Le Buveur du XIXᵉ siècle* (Paris: Albin Michel, 1990), 204–209.

60. Triboulet, "Alcool—Tuberculose," 220–221.

61. Ibid., 226. (Emphasis in original.)

62. Brunon, *La Tuberculose,* 197; Commission de la tuberculose, *Moyens pratiques,* 353–354 (emphasis added); Fuster, "La Tuberculose, maladie sociale," 42–43.

63. Nourrisson, *Le Buveur du XIXᵉ siècle,* 278–285.

64. Fauchon, *La Tuberculose, question sociale,* 48–50.

65. Dr. Lassabatie, "La Tuberculose et l'alcoolisme," *La Tribune médicale,* 2d series, 33 (1901): 369; *Compte rendu du Congrès contre l'alcoolisme et la tuberculose* (Toulouse: Edouard Privat, 1903), 48–49.

66. J. P. Maygrier, "Phthisie pulmonaire," *Dictionnaire des sciences médicales* (Paris: C. L. F. Panckoucke, 1820), 42: 28–33.

67. Ch. Vibert, "Syphilis," *Nouveau dictionnaire de médecine et de chirurgie pratiques* (Paris: J. B. Baillière, 1883), 34: 907, 912. This is not to say that such issues (particularly prostitution) were *absent* from prior discourse, only that they took on a new form and urgency amid the national anxieties of these later years.

68. Dr. Granier, "De la complication de la tuberculose par la syphilis," *Bulletin et mémoires de la Société de thérapeutique,* 2d series (1885): 142–143.

69. Ibid., 143.

70. Grancher and Hutinel, "Phthisie," 570–571; Hanot, "Phthisie," 502–503.

71. Louis Landouzy, "Associations morbides: Syphilis et tuberculose; terrains et graine," Congrès pour l'étude de la tuberculose chez l'homme et chez les animaux (Paris, 1891), *Comptes rendus et mémoires,* 185–186.

72. Ibid., 186.

73. Ibid., 187.

74. C. Potain, "Tuberculose et syphilis pulmonaires," *L'Union médicale,* 3d series (1894): 13–15.

75. René Jacquinet, *Contribution à l'étude de la tuberculose pulmonaire chez les syphilitiques,* thesis, Faculté de médecine, Paris, 1895; and "Tuberculose pulmonaire et syphilis," *La Presse médicale* (1895): 211–213.

76. Jacquinet, "Tuberculose pulmonaire et syphilis," 211.

77. Ibid.; Jacquinet, *Contribution à l'étude de la tuberculose pulmonaire chez les syphilitiques,* 89.

78. Jacquinet, *Contribution à l'étude de la tuberculose pulmonaire chez les syphilitiques,* 90.

79. For the best exposition of this issue, see Alain Corbin, "Le Péril vénérien au début du siècle," in Lion Murard and Patrick Zylberman, eds., *L'Haleine des faubourgs: Ville, habitat et santé au XIXᵉ siècle* (Fontenay-sous-Bois: Recherches, 1978).

80. Commission de la tuberculose, *Moyens pratiques,* 411–412. (Emphasis added.)

81. Ibid.

82. Ibid.

83. Commission permanente, *Recueil des travaux,* 3: 62 (session of November 21, 1908).

84. See, for example, Rénon, *Les Maladies populaires,* 12–13.

85. Ibid., 12.

86. Ibid., 112.

87. A. Forel (Chigny), "Alkohol und venerische Krankheiten," *VIII. Internationaler Congreß gegen den Alkoholismus,* Vienna, April 9–14, 1901 (Vienna: Verlag des Congresses, 1901), 11–12.

88. M. Barthélemy, "Influence de l'alcoolisme sur la syphilis," *Annales d'hygiène publique,* 3d series, 9 (1883): 66–68.

89. Ibid.

90. E. Tison, "Prophylaxie hygiénique de la tuberculose," Congrès pour l'étude de la tuberculose chez l'homme et chez les animaux (Paris, 1891), *Comptes rendus et mémoires,* 270–272.

91. Romme, *La Lutte sociale contre la tuberculose,* 21–22.

92. Rénon, "La Défense sociale contre la tuberculose," 200.

93. Ibid., 206–207. (Emphasis added.)

94. Rénon, *Les Maladies populaires,* 14.

95. *Compte rendu du Congrès contre l'alcoolisme et la tuberculose,* 16.

96. Susanna Barrows, "After the Commune: Alcoholism, Temperance, and Literature in the Early Third Republic," in John M. Merriman, ed., *Consciousness and Class Experience in Nineteenth-Century Europe* (New York: Holmes & Meier, 1979), 205; for an overview of the bourgeois view of the cabaret as a place of political subversion, among other things, see Jacqueline Lalouette, "Le Discours bourgeois sur les débits de boisson aux alentours de 1900," in *L'Haleine des faubourgs,* 315–347.

97. Nye, *Crime, Madness, and Politics in Modern France;* see also, among others, Gérard Jacquemet, "Médecine et 'maladies populaires' dans le Paris de la fin du XIXe siècle," in *L'Haleine des faubourgs,* 363–364.

98. On nineteenth-century meanings of heredity, see Nye, *Crime, Madness, and Politics in Modern France,* 119–131, and Carlos Lopez-Beltran, "Human Heredity, 1750–1870: The Construction of a Domain" (Ph.D. dissertation, King's College, London, 1992).

99. Corbin, "Le Péril vénérien," 282.

CHAPTER 6. LE HAVRE

1. Jean Legoy, *Le Peuple du Havre et son histoire, 1800–1914: La Vie politique et sociale* (Le Havre: Atelier d'Impression de la Ville du Havre, 1984), 308–311.

2. Jean Legoy, *Le Peuple du Havre et son histoire, 1800–1914: Le Cadre de vie* (Le Havre: Atelier d'Impression de la Ville du Havre, 1982), 181–314.

3. Ibid., 84.

4. Various advisory councils dealing with public health on the departmental and municipal levels had existed in France since the revolutionary and Napoleonic eras. See, for example, Dora B. Weiner, "Public Health under Napoleon: The Conseil de Salubrité de Paris, 1802–1815," *Clio Medica* 9 (1974): 271–284, and Ann Fowler La Berge, "The Paris Health Council, 1802–1848," *Bulletin of the History of Medicine* 49 (1975): 339–352. In contrast, Le Havre's Bureau d'hygiène was a department of the executive branch of municipal government, the first such health department in France.

5. Sanford Elwitt, *The Third Republic Defended: Bourgeois Reform in France, 1880–1914* (Baton Rouge: Louisiana State University Press, 1986); Legoy, *La Vie politique et sociale,* esp. 314–319.

6. Adolphe Lecadre, "Etude statistique, hygiénique et médicale relative au mouvement de la population du Havre en 1868," *Recueil des publications de la Société Impériale Havraise d'Etudes Diverses* (1868): 45–114, 91.

7. Ibid., 90.

8. Ibid., 91–92.

9. Lecadre, quoting his 1874 report, in "L'Année 1877 au Havre" (chap. 3, "Contribution à l'histoire de la phthisie pulmonaire"), *Recueil des publications de la Société Havraise d'Etudes Diverses* [S.H.E.D.] (1877): 70–73.

10. Ibid., 73. (Emphasis in original.)

11. Cottereau, "La Tuberculose, maladie urbaine ou maladie de l'usure au travail?"

12. Lecadre, "L'Année 1877 au Havre," 79.

13. Elwitt, *The Third Republic Defended,* 292; Legoy, *La Vie politique et sociale,* 319.

14. Jules Siegfried, *Les Cercles d'ouvriers,* lecture given in Le Havre, November 29, 1874 (Le Havre: Santallier, 1874), 4.

15. Ibid., 5–6.

16. Ibid., 5. (Emphasis in original.)

17. Quoted in Legoy, *La Vie politique et sociale,* 162.

18. Ibid., 318–319; Sanford Elwitt, *The Making of the Third Republic: Class and Politics in France, 1868–1884* (Baton Rouge: Louisiana State University Press, 1975), 210–213.

19. Siegfried, *Les Cercles d'ouvriers,* 14–15.

20. Ibid., 15.

21. Ibid.

22. Elwitt, *Making of the Third Republic,* 211, and *The Third Republic Defended,* 134–135; Legoy, *La Vie politique et sociale,* 162–163.

23. Legoy, *Le Cadre de vie,* 86–98.

24. Philippe Manneville, "La Lutte contre les logements insalubres au Havre (XIXe–XXe siècles)," *Actes du 110e Congrès national des sociétés savantes* (Montpellier, 1985), section d'histoire moderne et contemporaine, vol. 1 (Paris: C.T.H.S., 1985), 67–76.

25. Commission des logements insalubres, report of May 3, 1893, A.M.H. (F.C.), I^{5}13:11.

26. See, for example, Joan Scott, " 'L'Ouvrière! Mot impie, sordide . . .': Women Workers in the Discourse of French Political Economy, 1840–1860," in Scott, *Gender and the Politics of History,* 150.

27. Commission des logements insalubres, report of May 18, 1893, A.M.H. (F.C.), I^{5}13:11.

28. Ibid.

29. For a provocative interpretation of the disciplinary impulse behind the *cités ouvrières* and other communities of workers in the nineteenth century, see Lion Murard and Patrick Zylberman, *Le Petit Travailleur infatigable: Villes-usines, habitat et intimités au XIXe siècle* (Paris: *Recherches,* 1976). For a more empirical history of the problem of working-class housing in late-nineteenth-century Paris, see Shapiro, *Housing the Poor of Paris.*

30. Jules Siegfried, quoted in Legoy, "Les Débuts de l'habitat social au Havre: Utopies et réalités au XIXe siècle," *Recueil de l'Association des amis du vieux Havre* 47 (1988): 31–32.

31. A.M.H. (F.C.), Q^{4}7:1; Legoy, "Les Débuts de l'habitat social au Havre," 26–30.

32. Legoy, "Les Débuts de l'habitat social au Havre," 30–36; A.M.H. (F.C.), Q^{4}7:3, 6–7.

33. Legoy, "Les Débuts de l'habitat social au Havre," 36.

34. Ibid., 34.

35. "Rapport de M. Thillard sur les habitations économiques," *Recueil des publications de la S.H.E.D.* (1884): 63–65.

36. A. Mallet, "Société havraise des cités ouvrières: Assemblée générale annuelle du 23 avril 1885," unattributed newspaper clipping in A.M.H. (F.C.), Q^{4}7:3; H. Fénoux, in *Journal du Havre,* June 19, 1891 (A.M.H. [F.C.], Q^{4}7:5).

37. See, for example, the lively polemic in the pages of all Havrais newspapers during June and July of 1891, clippings of which are in A.M.H. (F.C.), Q^{4}7.

38. A. d'Euhaure, "Les Habitations ouvrières dites à bon marché," *Le Courrier du Havre,* August 15, 1893, 2.

39. Ibid.

40. A. Lécureur, "L'Hygiène des villes et les logements des travailleurs," *Le Havre* (newspaper), May 14, 1884.

41. Ibid.

42. Letter to the editor (anon.), *Petit Républicain,* June 11, 1891.

43. Ibid.

44. Ibid.

45. Legoy, *La Vie politique et sociale,* 235.

46. Joseph Gibert, speech to the Conseil municipal du Havre, quoted in Charles Vigné and Adrien Loir, *Trentenaire du Bureau d'hygiène du Havre* (Le Havre: O. Randolet, 1910): 14–15; "Création d'un Bureau d'hygiène municipal: Proposition faite par les docteurs Gibert, Fauvel et Lafaurie dans la séance du 11 février 1878," A.M.H. (F.C.), I⁵4:1; Legoy, *La Vie politique et sociale,* 317.

47. Le Havre city council minutes, meeting of March 5, 1879, reported in *Le Journal du Havre,* March 26, 1879, 2.

48. A.M.H. (F.C.), series I⁵; Vigné and Loir, *Trentenaire du Bureau d'hygiène du Havre,* 45–47.

49. A. Launay, "Bureau municipal d'hygiène: Rapport du directeur sur les opérations du 1ᵉʳ trimestre de l'année 1880," A.M.H. (F.C.), I⁵2:4, 14–15; and "Bureau municipal d'hygiène: Rapport du directeur sur les opérations de l'année 1884," A.M.H. (F.C.), I⁵2:4, 9.

50. See Didier Nourrisson, "Alcoolisme et anti-alcoolisme en France sous la troisième république: L'exemple de la Seine-Inférieure," doctoral dissertation, Université de Caen, 1986, 2 vols. (Paris: La Documentation Française, 1988).

51. Gibert, report on Le Havre in "Rapport des médecins des épidémies du département de la Seine-Inférieure en 1887," Archives départementales de la Seine-Maritime [A.D.S.M.], 5M:136, 98–101.

52. Commission consultative du Bureau d'hygiène, "Notes sur le Bureau municipal d'hygiène," A.M.H. (F.C.), I⁵4:3; Gibert, report on bureau operations for 1896, "Commission consultative du Bureau municipal d'hygiène: Compte-rendu de la séance du 30 janvier 1897," A.M.H. (F.C.), I⁵2:4, 3.

53. A.M.H. (F.C.), I⁵4:11, 13.

54. A.M.H. (F.C.), I⁵2:4, I⁵1:9. (Emphasis in original.)

55. Commission consultative du Bureau municipal d'hygiène, "Compte-rendu de la séance du 6 mars 1896," A.M.H. (F.C.), I⁵4:5, 1–2.

56. Medical topography traced its origins to the Hippocratic *Airs, Waters and Places*; the field enjoyed an early heyday of sorts in the late eighteenth century, with a proliferation of books, if not necessarily of spot maps per se. The shift toward mapping familiar, everyday diseases appears to have been a generalized international trend of the late nineteenth century; Le Havre was not necessarily unique in this respect, although it was clearly a pioneering city in France. George Rosen, *A History of Public Health* (New York: MD Publications, 1958), 176–180; G. Melvyn Howe, "The Mapping of Disease in History," in Edwin Clarke, ed., *Modern Methods in the History of Medicine* (London: Athlone Press, 1971), 335–357; James H. Cassedy, *American Medicine and Statistical Thinking, 1800–1860* (Cambridge: Harvard University Press, 1984), 8, 186, 217–219.

57. Louis Brindeau, preface to Bureau d'hygiène du Havre, *Relevé général de la statistique démographique et médicale, 1880–1889* (Le Havre, 1893).

58. Dr. A. Lausiès, "Mortalité par rue," in *Relevé général de la statistique démographique et médicale, 1880–1889.*

59. Ibid.

60. Gibert, "Phtisie pulmonaire," in *Relevé général de la statistique démographique et médicale, 1880–1889.*

61. Théodule Marais, preface to *Relevé général de la statistique démographique et médicale, 1890–1899* (Le Havre, 1903).

62. Henri Pottevin, "Statistique sanitaire de la ville du Havre pour une période de vingt ans, 1880–1899," in *Relevé général de la statistique démographique et médicale, 1890–1899.*

63. Ibid.

64. Adrien Loir, "Bureau municipal d'hygiène: Rapport sur l'année 1910," A.M.H. (F.C.), I^{5}2:4, 20–21.

65. Vincent-Pierre Comiti, "Histoire de la loi de la santé publique de 1902," *Revue française des affaires sociales* (April-June 1983): 81–88.

66. Ibid.

67. Georges Clémenceau, "Circulaire à MM. les préfets, relative à la nécessité d'appliquer intégralement la loi du 15 février 1902," *Revue philanthropique* 21 (1907): 536–537.

68. Henri Monod, "De l'exécution de la loi du 15 avril [*sic*] 1902," *Revue philanthropique* 25 (1909): 163–173; Ellis, *The Physician-Legislators of France*, 189.

69. A.M.H. (F.C.), I^{5}13:6–7.

70. A.M.H. (F.C.), I^{5}13:7.

71. Ibid.

72. A.M.H. (F.C.), I^{5}13:6.

73. A.M.H. (F.C.), I^{5}13:6–7.

74. A.M.H. (F.C.), I^{5}13:11.

75. Ibid.

76. A.M.H. (F.C.), M^{3}2:6.

77. Ibid.

78. Ibid.

79. Ibid.

80. Ibid.

81. Ibid.

82. Ibid.

83. Ibid. (Emphasis in original.)

84. Cottereau, "La Tuberculose, maladie urbaine ou maladie de l'usure au travail?", 192–224.

85. Michel Foucault, *The Birth of the Clinic: An Archaeology of Medical Perception,* trans. A. M. Sheridan Smith (New York: Vintage, 1973).

86. Armstrong, *Political Anatomy of the Body,* 7–11.

87. *Vérités* (the newspaper of the Union des syndicats du Havre), September 15–October 15, 1908, 4, and September 1, 1909, 4.

88. *Vérités,* September 15–October 15, 1908, 3, and February 1, 1911, 2; A.D.S.M., 4M: 528; A.N., F⁷: 13581, 13619.

CHAPTER 7. DISSENTING VOICES

1. *La Voix du peuple,* May 1, 1906, 3. (Ellipsis in original.)
2. See chap. 1, above, and Coleman, *Death Is a Social Disease.*
3. For example, Henri Napias, *Le Mal de misère* (Paris, 1876).
4. Several articles in the 1880 incarnation of Benoît Malon's *Revue socialiste* exemplify this tendency, including Louis Bertrand, "L'Influence de l'alimentation sur la mortalité," *Revue socialiste,* August 20, 1880, 481–492; and César de Pæpe, "De l'excès du travail et de l'insuffisance d'alimentation dans la classe ouvrière," *Revue socialiste,* June 5, 1880, 321–330.
5. Jules Thiercelin, "La Lutte contre la tuberculose," *Le Mouvement socialiste,* September 1, 1901, 291–292.
6. Ibid., 292–293.
7. Ibid., 293.
8. Ibid., 293–294.
9. Octave Tabary, "Le Parti socialiste et la lutte contre la tuberculose," *Le Mouvement socialiste,* October 15, 1901, 486–487.
10. Ibid.
11. Ibid., 483–484, 486.
12. Jules Thiercelin, "La Classe ouvrière et la tuberculose: Réponse au Docteur Tabary," *Le Mouvement socialiste,* October 15, 1901, 488. (Emphasis in original.)
13. Ibid., 488–491.
14. Ibid., 491–494.
15. Ibid., 493. (Emphasis in original.)
16. Ibid., 494–495.
17. Ibid.
18. Octave Tabary, *La Lutte contre la tuberculose dans la classe ouvrière* (Paris, 1900), 70–85.
19. F. F. Ridley, *Revolutionary Syndicalism in France: The Direct Action of Its Time* (Cambridge: Cambridge University Press, 1970), 45–55; R. D. Anderson, *France 1870–1914: Politics and Society* (London: Routledge & Kegan Paul, 1977), 125–136.
20. Text of bill in A.N., C 5623: dossier 386, 9. (Emphasis added.)
21. Ibid.
22. *Journal officiel: Chambre des députés, Débats parlementaires,* June 4, 1901 (session of June 3, 1901), 1223–1224.
23. Ibid.
24. Ibid., 1224.
25. Ibid., 1224–1225; A.N., C 5623: procès-verbaux de la Commission d'assurance et de prévoyance sociales.
26. Text of bill in A.N., C 7255: dossier 12, 95.
27. The industries included porcelain and ceramic manufacture; lime, plas-

ter, and cement work; stone and glass cutting; stone grinding; metal buffing and polishing (all of which involve "mineral" dusts); milling and baking; linen, hemp, and cotton carding and weaving ("vegetable" dusts); and the wool, silk, hide, feather, and mother-of-pearl industries ("animal" dusts). Ibid., 95–96.

28. Ibid. The report of the Commission d'hygiène industrielle is quoted at length in the bill's text, 243–245.

29. A.N., C 7343: dossier 245 (procès-verbaux de la Commission d'assurance et de prévoyance sociales).

30. The extent to which the syndicalist understanding of tuberculosis penetrated each of these means of communication is difficult to ascertain, with the exception of the two periodical publications. Word of mouth is the only one of those cited for which no hard evidence exists, but certain circumstantial evidence indicates that tuberculosis, its causes, and its prevention were discussed frequently among friends and co-workers. For example, numerous sources refer to the common nickname for tuberculosis among "the people": *le mal de misère,* "the illness of poverty." Beyond such basic formulas, it is impossible to know in exactly what terms workers—whether union activists or not—talked about the disease among themselves.

31. According to one of Pelloutier's biographers, Jacques Julliard, the contents of the posthumously published (1900) book, *La Vie ouvrière en France,* first appeared between 1894 and 1897 as articles in the journals *La Revue socialiste, La Société nouvelle,* and *L'Ouvrier des deux mondes.* I have not been able to determine exactly when the different parts of the book (including the parts dealing with tuberculosis) originally appeared. Fernand Pelloutier and Maurice Pelloutier, *La Vie ouvrière en France* (Paris: Schleicher Frères, 1900); Jacques Julliard, *Fernand Pelloutier et les origines du syndicalisme d'action directe* (Paris: Seuil, 1971), 273–276.

32. Pelloutier, *La Vie ouvrière en France,* 256.

33. Ibid.

34. On the history of this group and on Pierrot's leading role in particular, see Jean Maitron, "Le Groupe des Etudiants socialistes révolutionnaires internationalistes de Paris (1892–1902)," *Le Mouvement social,* no. 46 (1964): 3–26.

35. Groupe des Etudiants socialistes révolutionnaires internationalistes de Paris, *Misère et mortalité* (Paris: Imprimerie Jean Allemane, 1897), 5, 15.

36. Procès-verbaux du Comité général de l'Union des syndicats de la Seine (meeting of June 15, 1904), *Bulletin officiel de la Bourse du travail de Paris,* August 1, 1904, 2.

37. Raymond Dubéros, *La Tuberculose, mal de misère* (Paris: Union des Syndicats du Département de la Seine, n.d.[1904]), 12, 16; on publicity efforts after the pamphlet's publication, see, for example, *Bulletin officiel de la Bourse du travail de Paris,* September 1, 1904, 3.

38. Marc Pierrot, "La Lutte contre la tuberculose et la question des sanatoriums," *Les Temps nouveaux,* 19 installments between July 23–29 and December 10–16, 1904.

39. Groupe des ESRI, *Misère et mortalité,* 10–11.

40. Ibid., 8–10.

41. See Marc Pierrot, *Travail et surmenage* (Paris: *Les Temps nouveaux,* 1911).

42. Dubéros, *La Tuberculose, mal de misère,* 6–7.

43. Ibid., 7–8.

44. Pierrot, "La Lutte contre la tuberculose et la question des sanatoriums," October 22–28, 1904, 3–4.

45. Groupe des ESRI, *Misère et mortalité,* 8–10.

46. Pierrot, "La Lutte contre la tuberculose et la question des sanatoriums," September 3–9, 1904, 3–5, and September 10–16, 1904, 2.

47. Ibid.

48. Ibid., September 17–23, 1904, 3.

49. Ibid., September 24–30, 1904, 2–3.

50. Dubéros, *La Tuberculose, mal de misère,* 10.

51. Ibid., 10–11, 14–16.

52. Groupe des ESRI, *Misère et mortalité,* 32.

53. Dubéros, *La Tuberculose, mal de misère,* 10–11.

54. Ibid., 11–13.

55. Pierrot, "La Lutte contre la tuberculose et la question des sanatoriums," October 1–7, 1904, 4.

56. Ibid. (Ellipses in original.)

57. Ibid.

58. Ibid., December 24–30, 1904, 2–3.

59. Dr. E.D., "Le Congrès: Conte pour les grands enfants," *Les Temps nouveaux,* May 27, 1905, 2. Petit actually betrayed his own pseudonym to some extent by using his real initials in the byline of this piece. After the congress, when he wrote a follow-up article (see below) that referred to his authorship of this initial story, he signed it "Michel Petit," thereby inadvertently conceding that "Dr. E.D." and "Michel Petit" were one and the same. He is referred to as Michel Petit in the text because the bulk of his work throughout his career appeared under that name.

60. Ibid., 3.

61. Michel Petit, "Le Congrès de la tuberculose," *Les Temps nouveaux,* October 28, 1905, 1–2.

62. Ibid., 2.

63. Calmette, Verhæghe, and Woehrel, *Les Préventoriums,* 62–63. Verhæghe thereby cleverly defined *surmenage* as an average workday longer than eight hours, practically guaranteeing a result near 100 percent.

64. Max, "Contre la tuberculose," *Le Travailleur* (organe officiel de la Fédération du Nord, Parti socialiste, S.F.I.O.), October 19, 1905, 1.

65. This question was a prominent theme, for example, at the conference "Mouvement ouvrier et santé," Paris (Centre Malher), December 16–17, 1988.

66. Foucault hints at this role in *Discipline and Punish,* 297–305, and David Armstrong examines it in his *Political Anatomy of the Body.* See also the discussion of discipline and surveillance in chaps. 3 and 4, above.

CONCLUSION

1. *Le Matin,* May 22, 1913, 1.
2. Dessertine and Faure, *Combattre la tuberculose,* 36–41; Guillaume, *Du désespoir au salut,* 180–181.
3. Dessertine and Faure, *Combattre la tuberculose,* 36–43; Guillaume, *Du désespoir au salut,* 181–182.
4. Guillaume, *Du désespoir au salut,* 194–195; Grellet and Kruse, *Histoires de la tuberculose,* 173–174.
5. Louis Landouzy and Gilbert Sersiron, "Carte de l'armement antituberculeux," in Sersiron, *Moyens pratiques de placer un tuberculeux* (Paris: C. Naud, 1902); Paul Weindling, *Health, Race, and German Politics Between National Unification and Nazism, 1870–1945* (Cambridge: Cambridge University Press, 1989), 180; Bryder, *Below the Magic Mountain,* 34, 74; Guillaume, *Du désespoir au salut,* 195–196; Grellet and Kruse, *Histoires de la tuberculose,* 148.
6. Grellet and Kruse, *Histoires de la tuberculose,* 148, 173; Landouzy and Sersiron, "Carte de l'armement antituberculeux"; Dessertine and Faure, *Combattre la tuberculose,* 30; Bryder, *Below the Magic Mountain,* 23.
7. Bryder, *Below the Magic Mountain,* 17–22; Smith, *The Retreat of Tuberculosis,* 175–194.
8. Teller, *The Tuberculosis Movement,* 46–47, 57, 65–66, 97–98, 101–103.
9. Bates, *Bargaining for Life,* 257.
10. Weindling, *Health, Race, and German Politics,* 163–168, 180–181.
11. Bryder, *Below the Magic Mountain,* 18–19; Teller, *The Tuberculosis Movement,* 18, 55, 57, 60, 69–70, 104, 117; Weindling, *Health, Race, and German Politics,* 180.
12. A.N., C 7470: dossier 1810, 3.
13. M. Etienne, speech at the annual banquet of the Œuvre de la tuberculose humaine, April 8, 1905, in *Œuvre de la tuberculose humaine* (Paris: E. Arrault, n.d.), 3–4.
14. A. Imbert, "Congrès ouvriers et congrés scientifiques, " pamphlet reprinted from *Revue scientifique* (May 13, 1905), in A.N., F^{22}:526.
15. Commission permanente, *Recueil des travaux,* 2: 277–278.
16. Ibid., 278.
17. Ibid., 278–279.
18. Calmette, Verhæghe, and Woehrel, *Les Préventoriums,* 62–63.
19. Commission permanente, *Recueil des travaux,* 2: 279–280.
20. *L'Humanité,* May 9, 1907; *La Petite République,* September 9, 1907.
21. See, for example, Dubéros, *La Tuberculose, mal de misère.*

Selected Bibliography

ARCHIVAL SOURCES

Archives de l'Assistance publique de Paris: hospital death registers
Archives départementales de la Seine-Maritime (Rouen): series 5M (public health)
Archives municipales du Havre (Le Havre): Fonds contemporain, series I^5, M^3, Q^4 (low-income housing, public health)
Archives nationales, Paris: C 5623, C 7255, C 7324, C 7343, C 7470 (public health legislation)

PUBLISHED PRIMARY SOURCES

NEWSPAPERS AND OTHER PERIODICALS

Annales d'hygiène publique et de médecine légale
Bulletin de l'Académie de médecine
Le Courrier du Havre
Gazette des hôpitaux
L'Humanité
Le Journal (Paris)
Journal d'Hygiène
Le Journal du Havre
Le Matin
Le Mouvement socialiste
La Petite République (Paris)
Le Petit Havre
Le Petit Républicain (Le Havre)
La Presse médicale

Le Progrès médical
Recueil des publications de la Société havraise d'études diverses
Revue de médecine
Revue d'hygiène et de police sanitaire
Revue internationale de la tuberculose
La Revue médicale
Revue philanthropique
Revue scientifique
Revue socialiste
Statistique sanitaire des villes de France
Les Temps nouveaux
La Tribune médicale
L'Union médicale
La Voix du peuple

OTHER PUBLISHED PRIMARY SOURCES

Amodru, Lionel. "Rapport fait au nom de la commission d'hygiène publique
    sur les mesures à prendre pour arrêter les progrès de la tuberculose." *Journal
    officiel: Annexes de la Chambre des députés*, session of June 21, 1901, pp.
    782–793.
Benoiston de Châteauneuf, Louis-François. "De l'influence de certaines profes-
    sions sur le développement de la phthisie pulmonaire." *Annales d'hygiène
    publique et de médecine légale* 6 (1831): 5–48.
Bertillon, Jacques. "Etudes statistiques de géographie pathologique." *Annales
    d'hygiène publique*, 2d series, 17 (1862): 112–122.
———. *De la fréquence des principales maladies à Paris pendant la période
    1865–91*. Paris: Imprimerie administrative, 1894.
———. "Alcool et phtisie." *Archives d'anthropologie criminelle* 25 (1910):
    203–209.
Bourgeois, Georges. *Exode rural et tuberculose*. Thesis, Faculté de Médecine,
    Paris. Paris: Félix Alcan, 1904.
Brouardel, Paul. *Mortalité par tuberculose en France: Exposé de la question*.
    Melun: Imprimerie administrative, 1900.
Brunon, Raoul. *La Tuberculose: Maladie évitable, maladie curable*. Paris:
    Steinheil, 1913.
Bureau d'hygiène du Havre. *Relevé général de la statistique démographique et
    médicale, 1880–1889*. Le Havre, 1893.
———. *Relevé général de la statistique démographique et médicale, 1890–
    1899*. Le Havre, 1903.
Calmette, Albert, Désiré Verhæghe, and Th. Wœhrel. *Les Préventoriums ou
    dispensaires de prophylaxie sociale antituberculeuse: Le Préventorium
    "Emile Roux" de Lille*. Lille: L. Danel, 1905.
Commission de la tuberculose. *Moyens pratiques de combattre la propagation
    de la tuberculose*. Paris: Masson, 1900.
Commission permanente de préservation contre la tuberculose. *Recueil des tra-
    vaux*. 4 vols. Melun: Imprimerie administrative, 1903–1913.

Compte rendu du Congrès contre l'alcoolisme et la tuberculose. Toulouse: Edouard Privat, 1903.

Compte rendu du Congrès international de la tuberculose (Paris, 1905). Paris: Masson, 1906.

Congrès pour l'étude de la tuberculose chez l'homme et chez les animaux (Paris, 1891). *Comptes rendus et mémoires.* Paris: Masson, 1892.

Congrès pour l'étude de la tuberculose chez l'homme et chez les animaux (Paris, 1898). *Comptes rendus et mémoires.* Paris: Masson, 1898.

Conseil municipal de Paris. *Rapport . . . sur l'organisation du Bureau d'hygiène de la ville de Paris.* Paris: Imprimerie muicipale, 1907.

Dubéros, Raymond. *La Tuberculose, mal de misère.* Paris: Union des Syndicats du Département de la Seine, n.d. [1904].

Dumas, Alexandre *fils. La Dame aux camélias* [1848]. Paris: Calmann-Lévy, 1967.

Fauchon, Charles. *La Tuberculose, question sociale.* Paris: Asselin et Houzeau, 1903.

Fillassier, Alfred. *Les Casiers sanitaires des villes et les œuvres d'assistance: Entente nécessaire.* Paris: Jules Rousset, 1906.

Fuster, Edouard. "La Tuberculose, maladie sociale." *Revue d'hygiène* (1904): 25–45.

Goncourt, Edmond, and Jules de. *Germinie Lacerteux* [1864]. Naples: Edizioni Scientifiche Italiane, 1982.

———. *Madame Gervaisais* [1869]. Paris: Gallimard, 1982.

Grancher, Joseph. "Sur la prophylaxie de la tuberculose." *Bulletin de l'Académie de Médicine,* 3d series, 39 (1898): 470–529.

Graux, Lucien. "Les Causes sociales de la tuberculose." *Revue du XXᵉ siècle* (January 1903): 14–27.

Groupe des Etudiants socialistes révolutionnaires internationalistes de Paris. *Misère et Mortalité.* Paris: Imprimerie Jean Allemane, 1897.

Guéneau de Mussy, Noël. *Leçons cliniques sur les causes et sur le traitement de la tuberculisation pulmonaire.* Paris: A. Delahaye, 1860.

Héricourt, Jules. "La Lutte contre la tuberculose." *La Revue,* October 1, 1905, pp. 289–301.

Hugo, Victor. *Les Misérables* [1862]. Translated by Lee Fahnestock and Norman MacAfee. New York: New American Library, 1987.

Jousset, Xavier. *Transmission de la tuberculose dans les rapports sociaux.* Thesis, Faculté de Médicine, Paris. Paris: Imprimerie de la Faculté de Médecine, 1908.

Juillerat, Paul. *Rapport à M. le Préfet sur les recherches effectuées au Bureau du casier sanitaire pendant l'année 1907 . . . .* Paris: Chaix, 1908.

———. *Rapport à M. le Préfet sur les recherches effectuées au Bureau du casier sanitaire pendant l'année 1908 . . . .* Paris: Chaix, 1909.

———. *Rapport à M. le Préfet sur les recherches effectuées au Bureau du casier sanitaire pendant l'année 1910 . . . .* Paris: Chaix, 1911.

Juillerat, Paul, and Louis Bonnier. *Rapport à M. Le Préfet sur les enquêtes effectuées en 1906 dans les maisons signalées comme foyers de tuberculose.* Paris: Chaix, 1907.

Ladevèze, Isidore-Paul-Alphonse. *Comment les familles ouvrières parisiennes disparaissent par tuberculose.* Thesis, Faculté de médecine, Paris. Paris: Imprimerie de la Faculté de médecine, 1901.

Laënnec, R. T. H. *Traité de l'auscultation médiate et des maladies des poumons et du cœur.* 2d ed. [1826], facsimile reprint, 2 vols. Paris: Masson, 1927.

Landouzy, Louis. *La Lutte contre la tuberculose.* Paris: L. Maretheux, 1902.

———. *Le Rôle des facteurs sociaux dans l'étiologie de la tuberculose.* Paris: Masson, 1912.

Letulle, Maurice. "La Lutte contre la tuberculose en France: Prophylaxie et traitement hygiénique dans les milieux ouvriers." *Bulletin mensuel de l'Alliance syndicale du commerce et de l'industrie* (January 1902): 11–14.

La Ligue contre la tuberculose in Touraine contre M. le Comte de Lafont. Tours: Paul Salmon, 1906.

Lombard, Henri. "De l'influence des professions sur la phthisie pulmonaire." *Annales d'hygiène publique et de médecine légale* 11 (1834): 5–69.

Louis, P. C. A. "Note sur la fréquence relative de la phthisie chez les deux sexes." *Annales d'hygiène publique,* 1st series, 6 (1831): 49–57.

———. *Recherches anatomiques, pathologiques et thérapeutiques sur la phthisie.* 2d ed. Paris: Baillière, 1843.

Martin, Thérèse [St. Thérèse of Lisieux]. *Story of a Soul: The Autobiography of St. Thérèse of Lisieux* [1898]. Translated by John Clarke. Washington, D.C.: Institute of Carmelite Studies, 1976.

Max. "Contre la tuberculose." *Le Travailleur* (organe officiel de la Fédération du Nord, Parti socialiste, S.F.I.O.), October 19, 1905, p. 1.

Mirbeau, Octave. *Le Journal d'une femme de chambre* [1900]. Paris: Gallimard, 1984.

Murger, Henry. *Scènes de la vie de bohème* [1851]. Paris: Gallimard, 1988.

Napias, Henri. *Le Mal de misère.* Paris, 1876.

Pelloutier, Fernand and Maurice. *La Vie ouvrière en France.* Paris: Schleicher Frères, 1900.

Peter, Michel. *De la tuberculisation en général.* Agrégation thesis, Faculté de médecine, Paris. Paris: Lahure, 1866.

———. *Leçons de clinique médicale,* vol. 3. Paris: Asselin et Houzeau, 1893.

Pidoux, Hermann. *Introduction à une doctrine nouvelle de la phthisie pulmonaire.* Paris: Asselin, 1865.

———. *Etudes générales et pratiques sur la phthisie.* Paris: Asselin, 1873.

Pierrot, Marc. *Travail et surmenage.* Paris: Les Temps nouveaux, 1911.

Recherches statistiques sur la ville de Paris et le département de la Seine. 6 vols. Paris: various publishers, 1823–1960.

Rénon, Louis. *Les Maladies populaires: Maladies vénériennes, alcoolisme, tuberculose.* Paris: Masson: 1905.

Reveillaud, Roger. *La Tuberculose au point de vue social.* Thesis, Faculté de médecine, Paris. Paris: A. Maloine, 1908.

Rochard, Jules. *Traité d'hygiène sociale.* Paris: Delahaye et Lecrosnier, 1888.

Romme, Robert. *La Lutte sociale contre la tuberculose.* Paris: Masson, 1901.

Rostand, Edmond. *L'Aiglon* [1900]. Paris: Gallimard, 1986.

Savary, Robert, and Dr. Collet. "La Lutte contre la tuberculose en France." *Annales des sciences politiques* (1904): 19–30, 487–506.

Sée, Germain. *De la phtisie bacillaire des poumons.* Paris: Delahaye et Lecrosnier, 1884.

Siegfried, Jules. *Les Cercles d'ouvriers.* Lecture given in Le Havre, November 29, 1874. Le Havre: Santallier, 1874.

Straus, Isidore. *La Tuberculose et son bacille.* Paris: Rueff, 1895.

Tabary, Octave. *La Lutte contre la tuberculose dans la classe ouvrière.* Paris, 1900.

Villermé, Louis-René. "De la mortalité dans les divers quartiers de Paris." *Annales d'hygiène publique et de médecine légale* 3 (1830): 294–341.

SECONDARY SOURCES

Ackerknecht, Erwin. "Anticontagionism between 1821 and 1867." *Bulletin of the History of Medicine* 22 (1948): 562–593.

———. *Medicine at the Paris Hospital, 1794–1848.* Baltimore: Johns Hopkins University Press, 1967.

Armstrong, David S. *Political Anatomy of the Body: Medical Knowledge in Britain in the Twentieth Century.* Cambridge: Cambridge University Press, 1983.

Bardet, Jean-Pierre, et al., eds. *Peurs et terreurs face à la contagion.* Paris: Fayard, 1988.

Barnes, David S. "The Rise or Fall of Tuberculosis in Belle-Epoque France: A Reply to Allan Mitchell." *Social History of Medicine* 5 (1992): 279–290.

Barrows, Susanna. "After the Commune: Alcoholism, Temperance, and Literature in the Early Third Republic." In John M. Merriman, ed., *Consciousness and Class Experience in Nineteenth-Century Europe*, 205–218. New York: Holmes and Meier, 1979.

———. *Distorting Mirrors: Visions of the Crowd in Late Nineteenth-Century France.* New Haven: Yale University Press, 1981.

Barrows, Susanna, and Robin Room, eds. *Drinking: Behavior and Belief in Modern History.* Berkeley, Los Angeles, and London: University of California Press, 1991.

Bates, Barbara. *Bargaining for Life: A Social History of Tuberculosis, 1876–1938.* Philadelphia: University of Pennsylvania Press, 1992.

Bourdelais, Patrice, and Jean-Yves Raulot. *Une Peur bleue: Histoire du choléra en France, 1832–1854.* Paris: Payot, 1987.

Brandt, Allan M. *No Magic Bullet: A Social History of Venereal Disease in the United States since 1880.* Expanded ed. New York: Oxford University Press, 1987.

Brumberg, Joan Jacobs. *Fasting Girls: The Emergence of Anorexia Nervosa as a Modern Disease.* Cambridge: Harvard University Press, 1988.

Bryder, Linda. *Below the Magic Mountain: A Social History of Tuberculosis in Twentieth-Century Britain.* Oxford: Clarendon Press, 1988.

Castelain, Jean-Pierre. *Manières de vivre, manières de boire: Alcool et sociabilité sur le port.* Paris: Imago, 1989.

Chevalier, Louis. *La Formation de la population parisienne au XIXe siècle.* Paris: Presses Universitaires de France, 1950.

———. *Laboring Classes and Dangerous Classes in Paris during the First Half of the Nineteenth Century.* Translated by Frank Jellinek. Princeton: Princeton University Press, 1981.

Clark, T. J. *The Painting of Modern Life: Paris in the Art of Manet and His Followers.* New York: Knopf, 1984.

Clarke, John, ed. *St. Thérèse of Lisieux: Her Last Conversations.* Washington, D.C.: Institute of Carmelite Studies, 1977.

Coleman, William. *Death Is a Social Disease: Public Health and Political Economy in Early Industrial France.* Madison: University of Wisconsin Press, 1982.

———. *Yellow Fever in the North: The Methods of Early Epidemiology.* Madison: University of Wisconsin Press, 1987.

Corbin, Alain. *Le Miasme et la jonquille: L'odorat et l'imaginaire social, XVIIIe–XIXe siècles.* Paris: Flammarion, 1986.

———. *Le Temps, le désir et l'horreur: Essais sur le dix-neuvième siècle.* Paris: Aubier, 1991.

Cottereau, Alain. "La Tuberculose, maladie urbaine ou maladie du l'usure au travail?" *Sociologie du Travail* 20 (1978): 192–224.

Cowley, Geoffrey. "Tuberculosis: A Deadly Return." *Newsweek,* March 16, 1992, pp. 52–57.

Dessertine, Dominique, and Olivier Faure. *Combattre la tuberculose.* Lyon: Presses Universitaires de Lyon, 1988.

Dubos, René and Jean. *The White Plague: Tuberculosis, Man, and Society.* Rev. ed. Introductory essay by Barbara Gutmann Rosenkrantz. New Brunswick: Rutgers University Press, 1987.

Elias, Norbert. *The History of Manners.* Translated by Edmund Jephcott. New York: Pantheon, 1982.

Ellis, Jack D. *The Physician-Legislators of France: Medicine and Politics in the Early Third Republic, 1870–1914.* Cambridge: Cambridge University Press, 1990.

Elwitt, Sanford. *The Making of the Third Republic: Class and Politics in France, 1868–1884.* Baton Rouge: Louisiana State University Press, 1975.

———. *The Third Republic Defended: Bourgeois Reform in France, 1880–1914.* Baton Rouge: Louisiana State University Press, 1986.

Evans, Richard J. *Death in Hamburg: Society and Politics in the Cholera Years, 1830–1910.* Oxford: Oxford University Press, 1987.

Fee, Elizabeth, and Daniel M. Fox. eds. *AIDS: The Burdens of History.* Berkeley, Los Angeles, and London: University of California Press, 1988.

Fishman, Alfred P., ed. *Pulmonary Diseases and Disorders.* 2d ed. New York: McGraw-Hill, 1988.

Foucault, Michel. *The Birth of the Clinic: An Archaeology of Medical Perception.* Translated by A. M. Sheridan Smith. New York: Vintage, 1973.

———. *Discipline and Punish: The Birth of the Prison.* Translated by Alan Sheridan. New York: Pantheon, 1977.

Furlong, Monica. *Thérèse of Lisieux.* New York: Pantheon, 1987.

Gaucher, Guy. *Histoire d'une vie: Thérèse Martin*. Paris: Editions du Cerf, 1988.

Goldstein, Jan. *Console and Classify: The French Psychiatric Profession in the Nineteenth Century*. Cambridge: Cambridge University Press, 1987.

Grellet, Isabelle, and Caroline Kruse. *Histoires de la tuberculose: Les fièvres de l'âme, 1800–1940*. Paris: Ramsay, 1983.

Guillaume, Pierre. *Du désespoir au salut: Les tuberculeux aux 19ᵉ et 20ᵉ siècles*. Paris: Aubier, 1986.

Herzlich, Claudine, and Janine Pierret. *Malades d'hier, malades d'aujourd'hui*. Paris: Payot, 1984.

Kudlick, Catherine J. "Disease, Public Health and Urban Social Relations: Perceptions of Cholera and the Paris Environment, 1830–1850." Ph.D. dissertation, University of California, Berkeley, 1988.

La Berge, Ann F. *Mission and Method: The Early Nineteenth-Century French Public Health Movement*. Cambridge: Cambridge University Press, 1991.

Latour, Bruno. *Les Microbes*. Paris: A. M. Métailié, 1984.

Laurentin, René. *Thérèse de Lisieux: Mythes et réalité*. Paris: Beauchesne, 1972.

Lécuyer, Bernard-Pierre. "Demographie, statistique et hygiène publique sous la monarchie censitaire." *Annales de démographie historique* (1977): 215–245.

———. "Les Maladies professionnelles dans les *Annales d'hygiène publique et de médecine légale*," *Le Mouvement social*, no. 124 (1983): 45–69.

Legoy, Jean. *Le Peuple du Havre et son histoire, 1800–1914: La Vie politique et sociale*. Le Havre: Atelier d'Impression de la Ville du Havre, 1984.

———. *Le Peuple du Havre et son histoire, 1800–1914: Le Cadre de vie*. Le Havre: Atelier d'Impression de la Ville du Havre, 1982.

Léonard, Jacques. *La Médecine entres les pouvoirs et les savoirs*. Paris: Aubier Montaigne, 1981.

Mann, Thomas. *The Magic Mountain*. Translated by H. T. Lowe-Porter. New York: Vintage, 1969.

McKeown, Thomas. *The Modern Rise of Population*. London: Edward Arnold, 1976.

———. *The Role of Medicine: Dream, Mirage, or Nemesis?* Princeton: Princeton University Press, 1979.

———. *The Origins of Human Disease*. London: Basil Blackwell, 1988.

Merriman, John M. *The Red City: Limoges and the French Nineteenth Century*. New York: Oxford University Press, 1985.

———. *The Margins of City Life: Explorations on the French Urban Frontier, 1815–1851*. New York: Oxford University Press, 1991.

Mitchell, Allan. "Obsessive Questions and Faint Answers: The French Response to Tuberculosis in the Belle Epoque." *Bulletin of the History of Medicine* 62 (1988): 215–235.

———. "An Inexact Science: The Statistics of Tuberculosis in Late Nineteenth-Century France." *Social History of Medicine* 3 (1990): 387–403.

———. *The Divided Path: The German Influence on Social Reform in France after 1870*. Chapel Hill: University of North Carolina Press, 1991.

Murard, Lion, and Patrick Zylberman. *Le Petit travailleur infatigable: Villes-usines, habitat et intimités au XIXe siècle.* Paris: Recherches, 1976.

———. "Les Murs qui tuent." *Les cahiers médico-sociaux* 27 (1983): 285–294.

———. "L'Autre Guerre (1914–1918): La santé publique en France sous l'œil de l'Amérique." *Revue historique* 276 (1986): 367–398.

Murard, Lion, and Patrick Zylberman, eds. *L'Haleine des faubourgs: Ville, habitat et santé au XIXe siècle.* Fontenay-sous-Bois: Recherches, 1978.

Nourrisson, Didier. *Le Buveur du XIXe siècle.* Paris: Albin Michel, 1990.

Nye, Robert A. *Crime, Madness, and Politics in Modern France: The Medical Concept of National Decline.* Princeton: Princeton University Press, 1984.

Perrot, Michelle, ed. *A History of Private Life [vol. 4]: From the Fires of Revolution to the Great War.* Translated by Arthur Goldhammer. Cambridge: Harvard University Press, 1990.

Rabinbach, Anson. *The Human Motor: Energy, Fatigue, and the Origins of Modernity.* New York: Basic Books, 1990.

Reid, Donald. *Paris Sewers and Sewermen: Realities and Representations.* Cambridge: Harvard University Press, 1991.

Ridley, F. F. *Revolutionary Syndicalism in France: The Direct Action of Its Time.* Cambridge: Cambridge University Press, 1970.

Rosenberg, Charles E. *The Cholera Years: The United States in 1832, 1849 and 1866.* Chicago: University of Chicago Press, 1962.

———. *Explaining Epidemics and Other Studies in the History of Medicine.* Cambridge: Cambridge University Press, 1992.

Scott, James C. *Domination and the Arts of Resistance: Hidden Transcripts.* New Haven: Yale University Press, 1990.

Scott, Joan Wallach. *Gender and the Politics of History.* New York: Columbia University Press, 1988.

Shapiro, Ann-Louise. *Housing the Poor of Paris, 1850–1902.* Madison: University of Wisconsin Press, 1985.

Six, Jean-François. *Thérèse de Lisieux au Carmel.* Paris: Seuil, 1973.

Smith, F. B. *The Retreat of Tuberculosis, 1850–1950.* London: Croom Helm, 1988.

Sontag, Susan. *Illness as Metaphor.* New York: Farrar, Straus and Giroux, 1978.

———. *AIDS and Its Metaphors.* New York: Farrar, Straus and Giroux, 1989.

Szreter, Simon. "The Importance of Social Intervention in Britain's Mortality Decline, 1850–1914: A Re-interpretation of the Role of Public Health." *Social History of Medicine* 1 (1988): 1–37.

Teller, Michael. *The Tuberculosis Movement: A Public Health Campaign in the Progressive Era.* New York: Greenwood Press, 1988.

Traugott, Mark, ed. *The French Worker: Autobiographies from the Early Industrial Era.* Berkeley, Los Angeles, and London: University of California Press, 1993.

Weindling, Paul. *Health, Race, and German Politics Between National Unification and Nazism, 1870–1945.* Cambridge: Cambridge University Press, 1989.

White, Hayden. *Tropics of Discourse: Essays in Cultural Criticism*. Baltimore: Johns Hopkins University Press, 1978.

———. "The Value of Narrativity in the Representation of Reality." *Critical Inquiry* 7 (1980): 5–27.

———. *The Content of the Form: Narrative Discourse and Historical Representation*. Baltimore: Johns Hopkins University Press, 1987.

Wright, Peter, and Andrew Treacher, eds. *The Problem of Medical Knowledge: Examining the Social Construction of Medicine*. Edinburgh: Edinburgh University Press, 1982.

Index

Designer:	U.C. Press Staff
Compositor:	Maple-Vail Book Manufacturing Group
Text:	10/13 Sabon
Display:	Sabon
Printer:	Maple-Vail Book Manufacturing Group
Binder:	Maple-Vail Book Manufacturing Group